MALIGNANT TUMOURS
OF THE
MOUTH, JAWS
AND
SALIVARY GLANDS

MALIGNANT TUMOURS
OF THE
MOUTH, JAWS
AND
SALIVARY GLANDS

SECOND EDITION

JD Langdon

MB, BS, MDS, FDSRCS, FRCS

Professor and Head of Department
Department of Oral and Maxillofacial Surgery/Epithelial Cell Biology Unit
King's College School of Medicine and Dentistry, London and
Honorary Maxillofacial Surgeon
St George's Hospital, London and Royal Surrey and St Luke's NHS Trust, Guildford

JM Henk

MA, MB, BChir, FRCR

Consultant in Radiotherapy and Oncology
Department of Radiotherapy
Royal Marsden Hospital, London

Edward Arnold
A member of the Hodder Headline Group
LONDON   BOSTON   MELBOURNE   AUCKLAND

© 1995 Edward Arnold

First published in Great Britain as Malignant Tumours of the Oral
Cavity, 1985
Second edition published as Malignant Tumours of the Mouth, Jaws
and Salivary Glands, 1995

Distributed in the Americas by Little, Brown and Company
34 Beacon Street, Boston, MA 02108

British Library Cataloguing in Publication Data

Langdon, J. D.
  Malignant Tumours of the Mouth, Jaws and
  Salivary Glands
  I. Title   II. Henk, J. M.
  616.99

  ISBN 0-340-55794-X

Typeset in 10/11 pt Plantin by Rowland Phototypesetting Limited,
Bury St Edmunds, Suffolk.
Printed and bound in Great Britain for Edward Arnold, a division of
Hodder Headline PLC, 338 Euston Road, London NW1 3BH by
Butler & Tanner Ltd, Frome and London.

Preface

The cure rate of oral cancer has scarcely increased over the past 40 years despite real advances in surgery, especially in reconstructive techniques, anaesthesia, radiotherapeutic techniques and the era of cytotoxic therapy. Such developments as these have undoubtedly improved the quality of life of sufferers of this disease. As local control of the disease at the primary site and regional lymphatics has improved, our patients survive only to succumb to multiple primary tumours or to distant metastases. During the past twenty five years there has been extensive research and many publications but no clear consensus of opinion as to how mortality might be reduced. Debate continues on the relative merits of surgery and radiotherapy as primary treatment and in the management of lymph nodes in the neck. Despite initial enthusiasm, chemotherapy has proved to be of little value. Currently considerable research effort is being expended on the study of the fundamental growth control mechanisms with particular respect to the role of growth factors and oncogenes. It remains to be seen whether this research will ultimately lead to improved cure rates.

This book attempts to assess objectively the value of various types of treatment in current use for mouth cancer and malignant tumours of the jaws and salivary glands, while bearing in mind the necessity of fitting the treatment policy to the needs of the individual patient. In this context the necessity for joint consultation between clinicians from a variety of disciplines is stressed.

The basic principles underlying the use of surgery and radiotherapy, the treatment of the primary tumour and the management of the regional lymph nodes are each discussed in separate chapters. The authors' recommended policy for the disease according to site and stage is clearly stated, but it is stressed that this is only in the form of guidelines and may often need to be modified because of particular circumstances in an individual patient.

Aetiology, pathology, biology and diagnosis are discussed at some length as they are fundamental to an understanding of the underlying disease processes. During recent years there has been increased emphasis on the role of surgery in the management of these conditions and we include an overview of current surgical techniques. Cytotoxic chemotherapy and immunology are included but there is no evidence that any of the currently available agents can improve the outlook for patients with these tumours.

It is hoped that this book will be of value to all clinicians concerned in the management of malignant tumours of the mouth, jaws and salivary glands, and to postgraduate students in those disciplines concerned with this treatment.

JM Henk
JD Langdon

Contents

List of contributors

D Archer FDS, RCS, FRCS
Consultant Oral and Maxillofacial Surgeon, Head and Neck Unit, Royal Marsden Hospital, London

PF Bradley MD, BDS, FDS, FRCS
Professor of Oral and Maxillofacial Surgery, London Hospital Medical College and Honorary Consultant, Royal London Hospital, London

JW Eveson PhD, FDS, RCS, FDSRCPS, FRCPath
Reader and Consultant, Oral Medicine, Pathology and Microbiology, Centre for the Study of Oral Disease, Bristol Dental Hospital and School, Bristol

GH Forman MB, BS, BDS, MRCS, FDSRCS(Eng)
Consultant Oral and Maxillofacial Surgeon, King's College School of Medicine and Dentistry, London

JM Henk MA, MB, BChir, FRCR
Consultant in Radiotherapy and Oncology, Department of Radiotherapy, Royal Marsden Hospital, London

ME Gore PhD, MRCP
Consultant Cancer Physician, Department of Medicine, Royal Marsden Hospital, London

AF Jefferis MChir, FRCS
Consultant Ear, Nose and Throat Surgeon, Wexham Park Hospital, Wexham, Slough

AL Jones
Senior Registrar, Department of Medicine, Royal Marsden Hospital, London

JD Langdon MB, BS, MDS, FDSRCS, FRCS
Professor and Head of Department, Department of Oral and Maxillofacial Surgery/Epithelial Cell Biology Unit, King's College School of Medicine and Dentistry, London and Honorary Maxillofacial Surgeon, St George's Hospital, London and Royal Surrey and St Luke's NHS Trust, Guildford

M Partridge PhD, MPhil, BDS, FDSRCS
Senior Lecturer, Department of Oral and Maxillofacial Surgery/Epithelial Cell Biology Unit, King's College School of Medicine and Dentistry, London

C Scully PhD, MD, MDS, FDS, FFD, MRCPath
Professor of Oral Pathology, Department of Oral Medicine, Pathology and Microbiology, University of Bristol, Bristol Dental Hospital, Bristol

CJ Smith BDS, PhD, LDSRCS, FRCPath
Professor and Head of Department, Department of Oral Pathology, School of Clinical Dentistry, University of Sheffield and Honorary Consultant Oral Pathologist, Charles Clifford Dental Hospital, Sheffield Health Authority and Trent Region Health Authority, Sheffield

DS Soutar ChM, FRCS(Ed), FRCS(Glas), MB, ChB
Consultant Plastic Surgeon, West of Scotland Regional Plastic and Maxillofacial Surgery Unit, Canniesburn Hospital, Bearsden and Honorary Clinical Senior Lecturer, University of Glasgow, Glasgow

M Spittle MSc, FRC
Consultant Clinical Oncologist, Middlesex Hospital, London

I Taggart MB, ChB, FRCS(Glas)
Senior Registrar in Plastic Surgery, Frenchay Hospital, Bristol

RM Watson BDS, LDSRCS, MDS, FDSRCS(Eng)
Professor of Dental Prosthetics, King's College School of Medicine and Dentistry, London

1 Epidemiology and aetiology

CJ Smith

Introduction

Malignant disease in the head and neck region comprises a not inconsiderable proportion of the total burden falling upon the world's population. It has been estimated, for example, that in the early 1980s there would have been just over 250 000 new cases of cancers arising in the mouth and pharynx annually among men, representing approximately 8 per cent of all cancers in men.[1] Corresponding figures for women were about 120 000 new cases annually, comprising around 4 per cent of all malignancies in women.

When giving consideration to published information on the epidemiology and aetiology of malignant tumours in the oral region, it is particularly important to observe the methods used to collect original data, the anatomical sites included and the types of neoplasms involved. In this respect there are differences to be taken into account in relation to the sites covered by this Chapter – mouth, jaw and salivary glands – and whether information under consideration comes from hospital case records, pathological reports, cancer registries, case control studies, etc. Malignant tumours of the mouth are usually interpreted to be those affecting the mucosal lining of the oral cavity, but it is important always to identify whether those of the lip and oropharynx have also been included. A high proportion of oral malignant tumours are squamous carcinomas of the lining mucous membrane. Consequently any relation found to exist between registration or other epidemiological data for the broad category of oral malignant tumours and possible causative factors is usually interpreted as applying only to squamous carcinomas of the oral mucous membrane. It is important not to forget, however, that the minority of malignant tumours of the mouth that are not squamous cell carcinomas may include a wide variety of other tumours such as soft tissue sarcomas [amongst which there is a marked recent increase in Kaposi's sarcoma associated with human immunodeficiency virus (HIV) infection; see Chapter 18], malignant melanomas and various minor salivary gland neoplasms. As far as malignant tumours of the jaw are concerned, although they are much rarer than those of the mouth and there is correspondingly less information on their epidemiology and aetiology, the questions relating to accurate definition of site and type of tumour are equally valid.

Tumours affecting the major salivary glands are perhaps readily identifiable by site but there are problems in relation to the classification of some of the histological types as benign or malignant, which may vary from one report to another. At the level of cancer registration data there is an acknowledged difficulty with respect to pleomorphic salivary adenomas which, because of their tendency to recur, are included by some registries with malignant tumours.[2] Another factor is the extent to which tumours of the minor salivary glands may be considered alongside those of the major glands or whether they are included in the overall designation of oral cancers.

Epidemiology

Malignant tumours of the mouth

For a worldwide view of the distribution of oral cancer, one of the most useful recent publications is that showing data collected from registries in 36 different countries covering over 130 different population groups.[2] This compilation, produced under the auspices of the International Agency for Research on Cancer (IARC), represents the fifth volume in a series which shows increasing geographical coverage and by comparison with earlier volumes enables trends to be discerned in cancer incidence over the period 1960 to 1980.

The International Classification of Diseases (ICD) is used to provide a breakdown of anatomical sites affected by malignant tumours, and the overall category within which cancers of the mouth are found is that of 'buccal cavity and pharynx' (ICD 140–9). Many publications restrict themselves to this overall designation and some, probably inadvertently, mistakenly then interpret the data presented as being for 'oral cancer'. It is important, therefore, to realise that within the buccal cavity and pharynx there are marked differences in incidence of malignant tumours between the individual component sites from country to country (Table 1.1). In selecting only a few illustrative points from this Table, which it should be noted contains data only for men, there are obvious variations between the registries in that Hong Kong shows a preponderance of nasopharyngeal cancer, Newfoundland a high proportion of lip cancer, and even within the same registry (Connecticut) distinct population groups show different experiences of cancer incidence. As far as intra-oral cancer (ICD 141, 143–5) is concerned, the highest rate recorded in the world is that found in Bas-Rhin and it is of interest to see that in comparison with Bombay, with the second highest rate, there is a different relation between the figures for tongue (ICD 141) and other parts of the mouth (ICD 143–5). Table 1.1 contains data standardised to a world population, which is

a means whereby comparisons can be made between countries with populations of differing age structures.

Another way of expressing the occurrence of cancer in a population is to state the percentage of the total yield of cancers that is found to occur in a particular site. This is known as the relative frequency ratio and the data shown in Table 1.2 illustrate, for example, that 5.7 per cent of all newly registered cancers in men in Newfoundland around 1980 were cancers of the lip and 2.7 per cent of all newly registered cancers in women in Bombay were cancers of the tongue. Of course, what such figures do not necessarily convey is the variability in likelihood of detection, and consequently registration, of a cancer in a particular site. Cancer in the mouth is more likely to be noticed by the affected individual, and subsequently diagnosed by comparatively unsophisticated means, than is cancer of many internal organs. The availability of diagnostic procedures, accessibility to developed health services and cultural attitudes to disease will affect the extent to which cancer registries reflect the true incidence of malignant tumours. These are important points to bear in mind not only when studying statistics from cancer registries but also, perhaps even more so, when the source of data is records from a single hospital or limited group of hospitals, specialist centres or small population surveys.

In almost all parts of the world oral cancer is more common amongst men than women. To some extent this can be seen from Table 1.2, although

Table 1.1 Age-standardised* average annual incidence rates of malignant neoplasms per 100 000 men around 1980[2]

Site	Registry						
	Bas-Rhin (France)	Bombay (India)	Connecticut (USA) White	Connecticut (USA) Black	Hong Kong	Newfoundland (Canada)	Trent (UK)
Buccal cavity and pharynx (ICD 140–9)	49.1	34.3	14.5	28.7	38.6	21.3	5.5
Lip (ICD 140)	0.7	0.3	1.3	0.0	0.2	15.1	0.8
Tongue (ICD 141)	7.4	9.4	2.9	4.6	2.6	1.5	1.1
Salivary gland (ICD 142)	0.8	0.5	0.9	0.6	0.6	0.5	0.6
Mouth (ICD 143–5)	13.5	6.5	4.7	10.1	2.6	1.7	1.3
Oropharynx (ICD 146)	10.7	3.5	1.8	5.6	1.0	0.8	0.4
Nasopharynx (ICD 147)	1.1	0.8	0.6	1.5	30.0	0.8	0.4
Hypopharynx (ICD 148)	11.9	9.9	1.7	3.8	1.4	0.8	0.6
Pharynx, unspecified (ICD 149)	3.0	3.4	0.6	2.5	0.2	0.1	0.3

*Standardised to world population. ICD, International Classification of Diseases, 9th Revision.

Table 1.2 Relative frequencies of malignant neoplasms around 1980 (as a percentage of all malignant neoplasms)[2]

Registry	Lip (ICD 140)		Tongue (ICD 141)		Mouth (ICD 143–5)		Buccal cavity and pharynx (ICD 140–9)	
	Men	*Women*	*Men*	*Women*	*Men*	*Women*	*Men*	*Women*
Bombay (India)	0.2	0.1	6.5	2.7	4.6	4.0	23.9	10.8
Bas-Rhin (France)	0.2	0.0	2.2	0.4	4.1	0.4	14.7	1.7
Connecticut (USA)								
White	0.4	0.1	0.9	0.4	1.5	0.7	4.6	2.0
Black	0.0	0.0	1.2	0.4	2.6	1.0	7.6	3.2
Newfoundland (Canada)	5.7	0.2	0.6	0.1	0.7	0.3	8.1	1.3
Trent (UK)	0.5	0.1	0.4	0.3	0.3	0.3	2.1	1.4

Table 1.3 Age-standardised* average annual incidence rates for malignant disease of the lip, tongue and mouth per 100 000 population of men (SRM) and women (SRF) around 1980[2]

Region (country)	Lip (ICD 140)			Tongue (ICD 141)			Mouth (ICD 143–5)		
	SRM	*SRF*	*SRM/SRF*	*SRM*	*SRF*	*SRM/SRF*	*SRM*	*SRF*	*SRM/SRF*
Poona (India)	0.9	0.5	1.8	4.8	2.1	2.3	8.4	6.3	1.3
Isère (France)	2.2	0.2	11.0	4.2	0.4	10.1	5.6	0.6	9.3
Southern Ireland	11.6	1.2	9.7	1.4	0.1	14.0	1.2	0.4	3.0
Trent (UK)	0.8	0.1	8.0	1.1	0.6	1.8	1.3	0.6	2.2
Detroit (USA)									
Whites	1.3	0.2	6.5	3.0	1.3	2.3	4.2	1.7	2.5
Blacks	0.1	0.1	1.0	4.6	1.2	3.8	7.0	2.0	3.5
São Paolo (Brazil)	5.4	1.3	4.2	7.4	0.9	8.2	8.0	2.2	3.6
Alberta (Canada)	9.1	0.8	11.4	1.4	0.6	2.3	1.8	0.9	2.0

*Standardised to world population. ICD, International Classification of Diseases, 9th Revision.

Table 1.4 Average annual incidence rates* per 100 000 population for malignant disease of the tongue

Country (region)	Early 1960s[3]	Around 1980[2]
Germany (Hamburg)		
Men	0.8	1.3
Women	0.4	0.4
UK (Birmingham and the West Midlands)		
Men	1.9	0.9
Women	0.5	0.4

*Standardised to world population.

relative frequencies should strictly not be compared between the sexes because of the differential introduced by certain gender-specific sites (e.g. prostate, breast, cervix) in the overall cancer burden. The wide range of variation in gender ratio that can occur geographically and by anatomical site is shown in Table 1.3, where some of the more extreme examples are displayed. It should not be thought that such gender ratios remain static for they can vary quite substantially over time and may show different trends in what might seem to be rather similar populations (Table 1.4).

As with malignant tumours in many other sites, oral cancer is a disease that is more common with advancing age, usually demonstrating a sharply rising incidence rate after the age of 40 years or so (Fig. 1.1). Within this facet also it is instructive to observe trends that occur over time (Fig. 1.2), again emphasising the fact that the picture is constantly changing. In many populations there is evidence of a decline in incidence of oral cancer,[6] which is occurring particularly among the elderly, although there have been some recent reports from some countries suggesting that there may be a rising trend in incidence in younger men.[7–9] It is certainly the case that whatever collections of statistical data might show with respect to the most commonly affected age groups, clinicians need to maintain an

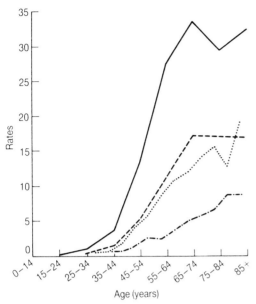

Fig. 1.1 Age-specific incidence rates per 100 000 persons for intra-oral cancer (International Classification of Diseases; ICD 141,143–5) in men and women in the USA (1983–87) and England and Wales (1986). Men, USA (———); women, USA (– – – –); men, England and Wales (......); women, England and Wales (·–·–·–·). Data derived from US Department of Health and Human Services Public Health Service (1992)[4] and Office of Population Censuses and Surveys (1991).[5]

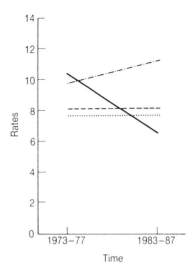

Fig. 1.2 Trends in incidence rates per 100 000 men at ages 55–64 years for lip and intra-oral cancer (International Classification of Diseases; ICD 140, 141, 143–5) in the USA between 1973 and 1977, and 1983 and 1987. Lip (———); tongue (·–·–·–); floor of mouth (......); other oral sites (– – – –). Data derived from US Department of Health and Human Services Public Health Service (1992).[4]

awareness of the fact that malignant tumours of the oral cavity may occur at any age.

The collection of comparative statistics for morbidity from malignant tumours is a relatively recent occurrence but data for mortality are available over a much longer period in many parts of the world. These mortality statistics tend to show similar variations and trends by gender, age and geographical region to those of morbidity statistics. Table 1.5 illustrates recent trends in mortality from malignant tumours of the buccal cavity and pharynx (ICD 140–9) for various European countries. As these data are crude rates and are not age-adjusted, apparent increases in rates may be accounted for, at least in part, by an increasing number of the elderly in the populations surveyed. The figures shown in Table 1.6, however, are age-adjusted and demonstrate that although the overall mortality rate (again for buccal cavity and pharynx in the USA) is declining, there are some states where the trend is in the reverse direction. Trends in mortality from cancer of the lip and tongue in England and Wales over the period 1868 to 1961[10] showed a steady

rise until around 1910 (except for a steady rate for tongue cancer in women), after which a gradual decline occurred.

Survival rates for patients with oral cancer have been reviewed by Binnie and Rankin,[11] whose analysis suggests there has been little or no change in 5 year relative survival rates for cancer of the lip, tongue and floor of mouth since 1950. Their review illustrated the point often made that localised lesions have a more favourable prognosis than more extensive ones and that survival rates tend to be better in women than in men. Some recently published data from the USA (Tables 1.7 and 1.8) reinforce these points.[4] The poorer prognosis for lip cancer amongst women is presumably because cancer of the lower lip, which is far more common in men, has a better prognosis than cancer of the upper lip. Otherwise, women have around 10 per cent better survival rates than men and they consistently present for diagnosis with their disease at a more localised stage.

Malignant tumours of the jaw

Registration data for malignant tumours of the jaw are incorporated into the categories for either bone

Table 1.5 Mortality rates per 100 000 population for malignant neoplasms of the buccal cavity and pharynx, 1965 to 1985 (crude rates not age-adjusted to a standardised population)

Country	1965		1975		1985*	
	Men	*Women*	*Men*	*Women*	*Men*	*Women*
Belgium	4.3	1.4	4.8	1.4	5.6	1.9
Denmark	3.1	1.4	2.6	1.6	4.4	2.1
France	12.8	1.4	18.4	2.0	19.6	2.1
Federal Republic of Germany	2.4	1.0	3.6	1.3	7.5	1.8
Greece	1.8	0.7	1.7	1.1	2.8	1.0
Republic of Ireland	5.9	2.8	5.3	2.8	5.3	2.8
Italy	6.7	1.3	7.9	1.5	9.3	1.9
Netherlands	2.4	1.0	2.5	1.0	3.0	1.4
Portugal	4.6	1.2	5.6	1.6	6.1	1.4
Spain	3.0	0.9	4.5	0.9	6.5	1.1
UK						
England and Wales	4.2	2.6	4.1	2.5	4.1	2.7
Scotland	4.8	1.9	4.4	2.0	4.6	3.6

*For Belgium 1984;
Sources: Various issues of *World Health Statistics Annual*. Geneva: WHO; 1965–1989.

Table 1.6 Age-adjusted mortality rates per 100 000 men for cancer of the buccal cavity and pharynx (ICD 140–9) for the USA and selected states[4]

Region	1973–77	1978–82	1983–87
Total USA	5.9	5.6	5.0
Alabama	4.7	4.8	5.0
California	5.7	5.6	4.7
Connecticut	7.1	7.1	5.6
District of Colombia	21.8	19.2	14.2
Florida	6.1	6.0	5.3
New York	6.8	6.5	5.7
South Carolina	5.5	5.6	6.8

Table 1.7 Five year relative survival rates (%) by site[4]

Site	Year of diagnosis		
	1974–76	*1977–80*	*1981–86*
Lip (ICD 140)			
Men	93.3	93.0	91.1
Women	80.7	89.4	83.7
Tongue (ICD 141)			
Men	36.8	36.9	42.8
Women	45.0	49.5	49.1
Floor of mouth (ICD 144)			
Men	53.3	46.9	49.8
Women	63.3	64.8	59.2
Other mouth (ICD 143, 145)			
Men	42.1	48.8	47.0
Women	58.5	58.4	63.3

neoplasms or neoplasms of sites within the oral cavity. Thus there is little information that can be obtained relating to the international distribution of jaw tumours. As Souhami[12] has pointed out, a significant proportion of malignant neoplasms in children and adolescents are primary bone tumours. Osteosarcomas are more common than chondrosarcomas or Ewing's sarcomas, and lower incidence rates for Ewing's sarcoma are found among Black and Chinese population groups than among Whites. It seems unlikely that the jaw bones would be significantly different from other bones in these respects. Malignant tumours of the odontogenic tissues are so rare that no meaningful statement can be made about their epidemiological characteristics and the same is true for metastatic

tumours located in the jaw bones. However, a malignant tumour arising predominantly in the jaws amongst African children was first described by Burkitt in 1958 and is now known as endemic Burkitt's lymphoma,[13,14] being characterised microscopically by a somewhat monotonous collection of lymphoblast-like cells amongst which are scattered sparse pale-staining macrophages. Following Burkitt's original description, the condition has since been described particularly in some other tropical countries.

Table 1.8   Stage distribution (%) and 5 year relative survival rates (%) by stage for oral sites, 1974 to 1986[4]

Site	Men					Women				
	Local	Regional	Distant	Unknown	Total	Local	Regional	Distant	Unknown	Total
Lip (ICD 140)										
Distribution	77	12	1	10	–	70	13	1	16	–
5 year survival	94	83	–	94	93	88	67	–	83	85
Tongue (ICD 141)										
Distribution	37	42	13	8	–	46	37	9	8	–
5 year survival	61	31	11	33	39	66	36	14	43	48
Floor of mouth (ICD 144)										
Distribution	36	51	6	7	–	42	47	4	8	–
5 year survival	70	41	14	37	50	77	54	20	46	62
Other mouth (ICD 143, 145)										
Distribution	31	45	11	12	–	37	44	8	11	–
5 year survival	64	44	17	42	47	80	52	31	46	60

Malignant tumours of the salivary glands

Cancer registration data for malignant tumours of the salivary glands show much less variation geographically and between the sexes than is found for cancer of the intra-oral sites. Rates standardised to a world population rarely exceed 1.0 per 100 000, with a suggestion that perhaps northern parts of Scotland, parts of South America and Australia may have slightly higher rates than elsewhere. Generally speaking, the relative frequency of cancer of the salivary glands is within the range 0.2 to 0.5 per cent and there is more often than not a slightly higher incidence in men than in women. Interpretation of statistics relating to malignant tumours of salivary glands is somewhat hazardous because coding conventions have changed over the years, there may not be consistency between registries and often the numbers involved are small. There is a slow rise in incidence with increasing age and trends over time show no distinctive pattern. Malignant tumours of salivary glands have been estimated to comprise about 8 per cent of all those in the buccal cavity and pharynx in the USA. The corresponding figure for the UK is around 11 per cent, with that for men 9 per cent and for women 14 per cent.

Previous reviews[15-18] of large series of neoplasms of minor salivary glands show that they represent 10 to 15 per cent of all salivary gland neoplasms, occur over a wide age range, affect both sexes approximately equally and may be more common in Black races. Malignant neoplasms are less common than benign ones, with the benign pleomorphic salivary adenoma being the most frequent of the histological types. Malignant and benign salivary gland neoplasms are more common in the palate than in other intra-oral sites and a higher proportion of minor salivary gland tumours is malignant compared with tumours of the major glands.

Mortality rates for malignant tumours of the salivary glands are slightly more favourable than for the buccal cavity and pharynx overall or for intra-oral sites individually.

Aetiology

There are many different types of malignant neoplasm that may arise in the head and neck region, for the majority of which there are hardly any clues as to what factor(s) might have contributed to their onset. The most common, however, squamous cell carcinoma, has been extensively studied and a strong association with potential aetiological agents has been identified by various types of investigation in a wide range of population groups. Other factors demonstrate a weaker link and still require more substantive proof that they are contributory.

Malignant tumours of the mouth

Discussion under this heading centres almost exclusively on squamous cell carcinomas arising from the lining epithelium, which form the greater part of the malignant neoplasms affecting the mouth. The extent to which agents identified as having an association with the development of oral cancer may be exerting a direct effect on the oral mucosa, or be making it more responsive to oncogenic viruses or to other carcinogens, is often not clear. Certainly it would seem that extrinsic and intrinsic influences may often combine in a way that magnifies their ability to produce malignant tumours, although the mechanisms responsible for such effects are, for the large part, not understood.

Sunlight

The increased incidence of lip cancer among those whose work is outdoors,[19,20] who are fair-skinned, who live in the country rather than the town, and particularly for all of these groups in areas where there is more sunlight,[21,22] has led to the conclusion that exposure to the sunlight is an important aetiological factor for cancer in the site. In this respect cancer of the lip is very much like cancer of the skin and the harmful component of sunlight is the ultraviolet light. As far as outdoor occupations are concerned, it is not possible to exclude entirely the potential influence of factors such as dust, spray, wind or unidentified carcinogens associated with a particular occupation. In parts of the world where there are White populations, it has long been recognised that lip cancer in men is much more common than in women and that the difference is largely accounted for by increased numbers of lower lip cancers. Whilst melanin pigmentation is known to exert a protective effect and can therefore account for the differential incidence between racial groups, the greater susceptibility of the lower lip in white males is more puzzling. Some have suggested it is because lipstick introduces a barrier effect,[23] others that it is due to men being more likely to follow an outdoor occupation.

Tobacco

There are many different varieties of tobacco and habits in which tobacco is used, most of them providing some evidence for a role for tobacco in oral cancer.[24-28] The most basic subdivision of tobacco habits is between those in which the tobacco is smoked and those in which unburned tobacco is maintained in contact with the oral mucosa and which can be conveniently collectively classified as tobacco chewing habits.

Tobacco smoking

There is a well established link between pipe smoking and cancer of the lip,[29-31] although there remains doubt about how much, if any, of a contribution is made by the heat produced or the materials from which the pipe stem is made. Similarly, it is possible that heat is a contributory factor in the increased prevalence of cancer of the palate observed amongst practitioners of the habit of reverse smoking.[32,33] In this habit, a cigarette or cigar is smoked with the burning end inside the mouth. There does not appear to be a similarly increased risk in those who show the signs of stomatitis nicotina on their palatal mucosa brought about by smoking a pipe in the more usual manner.

As far as cancer of other parts of the oral mucosa is concerned, smoking can be demonstrated to be a risk factor,[31,34,35] with cigar and pipe smoking being somewhat less of a risk than cigarettes. A study of more than 1.2 million people across 50 states of the USA followed over 4 years (1982–1986) has shown that men who smoked had an almost 30-fold increased risk of dying from oral cancer than non-smokers, whereas men who were former smokers had a nine-fold increased risk.[36] Women smokers had approaching a six-fold increased risk which was reduced to three-fold amongst former smokers. This study also concluded that 92 per cent of all deaths due to cancer of the buccal cavity and pharynx in men in the USA in 1989 were attributable to smoking (61 per cent for women). There are problems, of course, in the collection of sufficiently robust information to establish relations between particular types of smoking habit and specific intra-oral sites at risk. This is often because the anatomical sites may not be recorded and registered in sufficient detail, because a history of type and amount of tobacco use over past decades may not be entirely reliable, and because it is difficult to disassociate the effects of smoking and alcohol and both of these habits are commonly practised together. That complex inter-relations exist between aetiological factors for oral cancer is further borne out by the fact that in some countries where oral cancer has been declining over recent decades there had been, until recently in many instances, a long-term increasing trend in the consumption of cigarettes.[37,38]

Tobacco chewing

Evidence from many hospital-based studies and also from cancer registries has demonstrated the high incidence of intra-oral cancer in India and certain other parts of South-East Asia. An association between this occurrence and the widespread habit of betel quid chewing over a similar geographical region has been established[39,40] and there are numerous reports in the literature detailing various investigations into the possible role of each of the betel quid components.[41] Most contain tobacco in some form and most observers point to this as the significant carcinogenic agent; others, however, retain the view that possibly the slaked lime component is involved.

Tobacco is one of the many, often otherwise difficult to ascertain, ingredients of snuff and in some populations the method of using snuff is to place wads of it against the oral mucosa. The amount used, duration and site of application vary according to local custom or personal preference. This habit is often referred to as 'snuff dipping', and there is evidence both from some of the states in the south-eastern region of the USA[42,43] and from Sweden[44] that it is linked to the development of intra-oral cancer, particularly verrucous carcinoma, in these geographical regions. A more recent trend has been the manufacture and sale of sachets of tobacco, which have been promoted particularly among the young and often in association with a sporting context. In some countries the sale of such products has been banned on the grounds of potential harm based upon substantial evidence that links intra-oral tobacco use with a greater risk that oral cancer may develop.[45–49]

Alcohol

The consumption of alcohol on a regular and above-average basis is often associated with heavy tobacco usage and it is consequently difficult to ascertain the degree to which each might contribute to harmful effects.[31,50,51] Nevertheless, when the necessary correction factors can be applied, it leaves no doubt that alcohol has to be considered an important risk factor for oral cancer;[52–55] moreover, when the effects of alcohol and tobacco act together there is more than a simple summation of degrees of risk.[56] Although various attempts have been made to discover whether particular forms of alcoholic beverage represent more of a risk than others, there is no clear evidence pointing to any one type of drink;[56–58] nor has the potential role of contaminants or additives been eliminated. Much of the evidence implicating alcohol in the aetiology of oral cancer has come from the finding that the disease is more common amongst those who work in alcohol-related trades,[29,59,60] those who are or have

been alcoholics[51] or, conversely, that for those who are less likely to develop oral cancer it is because they shun alcohol.[50,61] As we have seen in some instances where tobacco consumption increases while oral cancer incidence rates fall, so similar trends can sometimes be observed as far as alcohol consumption is concerned.[62] In the interpretation of such data and drawing inferences from it, there are many caveats concerning latent period, form of alcohol consumption and its distribution in the population that have to be considered.

Infectious agents

Candida

This fungal organism is a frequent finding in so-called 'speckled' leukoplakia, which is associated with a greater tendency to show subsequent malignant change than other forms of leukoplakia.[63,64] Krogh et al.[65] have shown that candidal organisms recovered from oral precancerous lesions appear to have the potential to catalyse the production of a carcinogenic agent from its chemical precursors and that there is possibly a relation to the degree of histological change produced in the lesions by different strains. Other evidence in support of a potential role for candidal organisms in the development of oral cancer has been collated from experimental and clinical material.[66]

Treponema pallidum

Convincing evidence of a close association between syphilis and tongue cancer became apparent over 50 years ago[67] through comparison of registration data for both diseases in New York State. A later study[31] found that positive serological evidence of syphilitic infection, or a history of the disease, was twice as common in oral cancer patients than in an age- and gender-matched control group where account had also been taken of tobacco and alcohol habits. The anterior two-thirds of the dorsum of the tongue was particularly affected.

Since control of much of the damage produced by the late stages of syphilis has been possible through the use of antibiotics at an early stage in the infection, there has been little or no new evidence produced for its relation with oral cancer. This has led to the suggestion that perhaps it was not the syphilitic infection so much as the medicaments previously used to treat it (e.g. mercurials and arsenicals) that were acting as a causative agent for cancer of the dorsal surface of the tongue.

Human papillomaviruses

More than 60 types of human papillomaviruses (HPV) have now been recognised, many of which have been found in association with, or can be identified as being responsible for, various papillomatous or warty outgrowths involving epithelial surfaces. For cancer of the uterine cervix there appears to be an aetiological relationship with type 16 and possibly also type 18. As far as oral cancer is concerned, there is insufficient evidence of such a close association, although various HPV DNA and HPV antigens have been demonstrated in material from oral cancer.[68–72] Because normal mucosa and benign oral lesions may also be shown to exhibit evidence of the presence of HPV,[70] however, it is clear that the virus does not act alone as a causative agent for oral cancer.

Herpes simplex virus

Some patients with cancer of the head and neck region demonstrate raised serum antibody titres to antigenic components of herpes simplex virus (HSV) type 1.[73] Cigarette smoking is also associated with the presence of serum anti-HSV antibodies,[74,75] although there are higher mean antibody titres in cancer patients than in control subjects who smoke;[75] also, higher titres are found in individuals with large tumours compared with those who have small ones.[76] It is not possible at this stage to refute or confirm that HSV has a role in the aetiology of oral cancer, although if it does play a part there is every reason to suppose that it acts in conjunction with other factors.

Human immunodeficiency virus

There is one report[76] in which it appeared that oral cancer was more prevalent in a group of comparatively young men with acquired immune deficiency syndrome (AIDS) or earlier stages of HIV infection. These were not associated with lesions of hairy leukoplakia. The fact that subsequent studies and reports have yet to corroborate a link between HIV infection and oral cancer suggests that the original report may have identified a chance finding.

Patients with AIDS have an increased tendency to develop non-Hodgkin's lymphoma and Kaposi's sarcoma.[77] Both of these conditions may, of course, present orally but the frequency with which Kaposi's sarcoma affects the palatal mucosa is particularly noteworthy.

Nutritional deficiencies

Oral, pharyngeal and oesophageal cancers are more common in individuals with sideropenic dysphagia,[78,79] and this may be associated with the observation from both human and experimental studies that iron deficiency has an adverse effect upon the structure and function of the epithelium of the oral mucosa. It is possible that these effects render the epithelium more susceptible to the local action of carcinogenic substances, but as deficiencies of iron may also reduce the effectiveness of the immune system, there are other mechanisms that have to be considered for further study.

Low levels of serum vitamin A have been reported amongst patients with oral cancer,[80,81] although whether this could have been as a result of the malignancy rather than a contributory factor in causation is not known. Interest in the potential for vitamin A deficiency to be involved in oral cancer aetiology revolves around the importance of this vitamin in maintaining the structure and function of stratified squamous epithelia.

From the evidence of a single study[82] it appears that an adequate intake of fresh fruit may act as a protective factor against the development of oral and pharyngeal cancer.

Dental factors

It has been almost ritualistic for many years to cite dental sepsis and trauma as factors involved in the aetiology of oral cancer, although the evidence for such an association is extremely tenuous as it is largely based on individual cases rather than well controlled studies. There is, however, considerable difficulty in obtaining the evidence to establish, or hence to refute, whether dental factors have an influence on the development of oral cancer. Information about the dental status of individuals in the past, sufficient to make allowance for any latent period effect, is difficult to acquire, and at the time of diagnosis of an oral cancer any local traumatic factor is likely to be recognised and reported upon more readily than in a 'normal' individual. Subjects with oral cancer are likely to have teeth removed in association with its treatment, either for surgical reasons or because radiotherapy is given, and the fact that oral cancer patients may have fewer teeth than a suitable control group should not be taken necessarily to indicate an earlier state of poorer dental health. The evidence, such as it is, proves to be conflicting.[83–86]

Malignant tumours of the jaws

Aetiological factors for malignant bone tumours

appear to be growth, irradiation and Paget's disease. At the time of peak growth there is an increased incidence of long bone osteosarcomas, which is more marked in boys than girls. Evidence linking ionising radiation to malignant bone tumours is derived from two main sources: (1) following radiotherapy, usually for a previous malignant tumour; and (2) as a result of exposure to radioactive materials. With regard to the latter, Souhami[12] provides a fascinating historical account of the discovery that osteosarcomas developed in women employed to paint dials with luminous radioactive substances. In this example it is important to note that although the women readily developed osteoradionecrosis of the jaws, these bones were not especially affected by the sarcomas. However, carcinomas of the paranasal sinuses increased in frequency. The groups affected by radiation sarcomas of bone are spread broadly in the middle age range (median, 35–45 years).[87]

In a compilation of data from several series of cases, Souhami[12] has shown that the skull and jaws accounted for 13.5 per cent of all postradiation bone sarcomas.

Bone affected by Paget's disease is more susceptible to the development of osteosarcomatous changes, the tumours then being in older age groups and more frequent in men than in women. Around one-quarter of all bone sarcomas are found in bone affected by Paget's disease[12] and 5.5 per cent of osteogenic sarcomas have been found to be associated with Paget's disease.[88] It has been estimated from pooled data that around 3 per cent of Paget's sarcomas are found in the jaws, compared with 5 per cent of all osteosarcomas being located to the site.[12]

The prime aetiologic suspect for endemic Burkitt's lymphoma is the Epstein–Barr virus (EBV), which is able to immortalise B lymphocytes in culture, shows incorporation into tumour cell nuclear material and produces raised serum antibody titres in affected individuals.[13,14] Malaria infection, which acts to depress immune responses, together with EBV infection in infancy is believed to be the essential combination; in some way these produce the abnormal karyotype, comprising a chromosome 8, 14 translocation, that is found in a high proportion of affected individuals.[13,14]

Malignant tumours of salivary glands

There is little information in the literature on the aetiology of salivary gland neoplasms but Spitz

et al.[89] have found, in a case control study, that for malignant tumours the risk factors appear to include previous radiotherapy and, statistically established for women only, higher educational attainment, alcohol use and hairdye use. Malignant salivary gland neoplasms in women are more common amongst those individuals who also develop cancer of the breast.[90]

References

1 Parkin DM, Muir CS, Läärä E. *Global burden of cancer.* World Health Organization and International Agency for Research on Cancer Biennial Report 1986–87. Lyon: IARC, 1987: 11.
2 Muir C, Waterhouse J, Mack T *et al. Cancer incidence in five continents. Vol. V.* IARC Scientific Publications No. 88. Lyon: International Agency for Research on Cancer, 1987.
3 Doll R, Payne P, Waterhouse J. *Cancer incidence in five continents. A Technical Report.* International Union Against Cancer. Berlin: Springer-Verlag, 1966.
4 US Department of Health and Human Services Public Health Service. *Cancers of the oral cavity and pharynx: a statistics review monograph 1973–1987.* Atlanta, GA and Bethesda, MD: Centers for Disease Control and National Institutes of Health, 1992.
5 Office of Population Censuses and Surveys. *Cancer Statistics: Registrations. Cases of Diagnosed Cancer Registered in England and Wales, 1986.* London: HMSO, 1991.
6 Smith CJ. Oral cancer and precancer: background, epidemiology and aetiology. *British Dental Journal* 1989; **167:** 377–83.
7 Davis S, Severson RK. Increasing incidence of cancer of the tongue in the United States among young adults. *Lancet* 1987; **ii:** 910–11.
8 MacFarlane GM, Boyle P, Scully C. Rising mortality from cancer of the tongue in young Scottish males. *Lancet* 1987; **ii:** 912.
9 Møller H. Changing incidence of cancer of the tongue, oral cavity, and pharynx in Denmark. *Journal of Oral Pathology and Medicine* 1989; **18:** 224–9.
10 Binnie WH, Cawson RA, Hill GB, Soaper AE. *Oral cancer in England and Wales. A national study of morbidity, mortality, curability and related factors.* Office of Population Censuses and Surveys. Studies on Medical and Population Subjects, No. 23. London: HMSO, 1972.
11 Binnie WH, Rankin KV. Epidemiology of oral cancer. In: Wright BA, Wright JM, Binnie WH eds. *Oral Cancer: Clinical and Pathological Considerations.* Boca Raton, FL: CRC Press, 1988.
12 Souhami R. Incidence and aetiology of malignant primary bone tumours. In: Souhami R ed. *Bone*

Tumours. Bailliere's Clinical Oncology International Research and Practice 1987; **1**: 1–20.

13 Lenoir GM, O'Conor GT, Olweny CLM. *Burkitt's lymphoma: a human cancer model.* IARC Scientific Publications No. 6. Lyon: International Agency for Research on Cancer, 1985.

14 Isaacson PG. The non-Hodgkin's lymphomas. In: McGee JO'D, Isaacson PG, Wright NA eds. *Oxford Textbook of Pathology.* Oxford: Oxford Medical Publications, 1992: 1781–2.

15 Isacson G, Shear M. Intraoral salivary gland tumors: a retrospective study of 201 cases. *Journal of Oral Pathology* 1983; **12**: 57–62.

16 Eveson JW, Cawson RA. Tumours of the minor (oropharyngeal) salivary glands: a demographic study of 336 cases. *Journal of Oral Pathology* 1985; **14**: 500–9.

17 Chau MNY, Radden BG. Intraoral salivary gland neoplasms: a retrospective study of 98 cases. *Journal of Oral Pathology* 1986; **15**: 339–42.

18 van Heerden WFP, Raubenheimer EJ. Intraoral salivary gland neoplasms: a retrospective study of seventy cases in an African population. *Oral Surgery, Oral Medicine, Oral Pathology* 1991; **71**: 579–82.

19 OPCS. *Occupational mortality. The Registrar General's decennial supplement for England and Wales, 1970–72.* Series DS No. 1. London: HMSO, 1978.

20 Spitzer WO, Hill GB, Chambers LW, Helliwell BE, Murphy HB. The occupation of fishing as a risk factor in cancer of the lip. *New England Journal of Medicine* 1975; **293**: 419–24.

21 Dorn HF, Cutler SJ. *Morbidity from cancer in the United States.* Public Health Monograph No. 56. Washington DC: US Department of Health, Education and Welfare, 1958.

22 Lindqvist C, Teppo L. Epidemiological evaluation of sunlight as a risk factor of lip cancer. *British Journal of Cancer* 1978; **37**: 983–9.

23 Preston-Martin S, Henderson BE, Pike M. Descriptive epidemiology of cancers of the upper respiratory tract in Los Angeles. *Cancer* 1982; **49**: 2201–7.

24 US Public Health Service. *The health consequences of smoking. A report to the Surgeon General.* Public Health Service, DHHS (PHS) 821–50179. Washington DC: US Department of Health and Human Services, 1982.

25 International Agency for Research on Cancer. *Tobacco habits other than smoking: Betel quid and areca nut chewing; and some related nitrosamines. IARC monographs on the evaluation of the carcinogenic risk of chemicals to humans. Vol. 37.* Lyon: International Agency for Research on Cancer, 1985.

26 International Agency for Research on Cancer. *Tobacco smoking. IARC monographs on the evaluation of the carcinogenic risk of chemicals to humans. Vol. 38.* Lyon: International Agency for Research on Cancer, 1986.

27 Binnie WH. Risk factors and risk markers for oral cancer in low incidence areas of the world. In: Johnson NW ed. *Oral Cancer: Detection of Patients and Lesions at Risk.* Cambridge: Cambridge University Press, 1991: 64–87.

28 Daftary DK, Murti PR, Bhonsle RB, Gupta PC, Mehta FS, Pindborg JJ. Risk factors and risk markers for oral cancer in high incidence areas of the world. In: Johnson NW ed. *Oral Cancer: Detection of Patients and Lesions at Risk.* Cambridge: Cambridge University Press, 1991: 29–63.

29 Clemmesen JC. *Statistical Studies in the Aetiology of Malignant Neoplasms. Vol. 1. Reviews and Results.* Copenhagen: Munksgaard, 1965.

30 Levin ML, Goldstein H, Gerhardt PR. Cancer and tobacco smoking. *Journal of the American Medical Association* 1950; **143**: 336–8.

31 Wynder EL, Bross IJ, Feldman RM. A study of the etiological factors in cancer of the mouth. *Cancer* 1957; **10**: 1300–23.

32 Pindborg JJ, Mehta FS, Gupta PC, Daftary DK, Smith CJ. Reverse smoking in Andhra Pradesh, India. A study of palatal lesions among 10,169 villagers. *British Journal of Cancer* 1971; **25**: 10–20.

33 Reddy CRRM, Prahlad D, Ramulu C. Incidence of oral cancer with particular reference to hard palate cancer in 1 million population in the district of Visakhapatnam. *Indian Journal of Cancer* 1975; **12**: 72–6.

34 Wynder EL, Mushinski HM, Spirak JC. Tobacco and alcohol consumption in relation to the development of multiple primary cancers. *Cancer* 1977; **40**: 1872–8.

35 Kahn HA. The Dorn study of smoking and mortality among US veterans: report on eight and one-half years of observation. *Monographs/National Cancer Institute* 1966; **19**: 1–125.

36 Shopland DR, Pechacek TF, Cullen JW. Toward a tobacco-free society. *Seminars in Oncology* 1990; **17**: 402–12.

37 Smith CJ. Global epidemiology and aetiology of oral cancer. *International Dental Journal* 1973; **23**: 82–93.

38 Binnie WH, Rankin KV. Etiology. In: Wright BA, Wright JM, Binnie WH eds. *Oral Cancer: Clinical and Pathological Considerations.* Boca Raton, FL: CRC Press, 1988.

39 Hirayama T. An epidemiological study of oral and pharyngeal cancer in Central and South-East Asia. *Bulletin of the World Health Organization* 1966; **34**: 41–69.

40 Wahi PN. The epidemiology of oral and oropharyngeal cancer: a report of the study in Mainpuri District, Uttar Pradesh, India. *Bulletin of the World Health Organization* 1968; **38**: 495–521.

41 Gupta PC, Pindborg JJ, Mehta FS. Comparison of carcinogenicity of betel quid with and without tobacco: an epidemiological review. *Ecology of Disease* 1982; **21**: 3–9.

42 Vogler WR, Lloyd JW, Milmore BK. A retrospective study of etiological factors in cancer of the mouth, pharynx and larynx. *Cancer* 1962; **15**: 246–58.

43 Winn DM, Blot WJ, Shy CM, Pickle LW, Toledo A, Fraumeni JF. Snuff dipping and oral cancer among women in the southern United States. *New England Journal of Medicine* 1981; **304**: 745–9.

44 Sundström B, Mörnstad H, Axéll T. Oral carcinomas associated with snuff dipping: some clinical and histological characteristics of 23 tumours in Swedish males. *Journal of Oral Pathology* 1982; **11**: 245–51.

45 Editorial. Smokeless tobacco: a new oral health hazard. *British Dental Journal* 1986; **160**: 369–70.

46 Stephen KW. Health implications of smokeless tobacco: US National Institute of Health Consensus Development Conference. *British Dental Journal* 1986; **160**: 370–2.

47 US Public Health Service. *The health consequences of using smokeless tobacco. A report to the Surgeon General.* NIH Publication No. 86–2874. Bethesda, MD: US Department of Health and Human Services, 1986.

48 Winn D. Smokeless tobacco and cancer: the epidemiologic evidence. *CA: A Cancer Journal for Clinicians* 1988; **38**: 236–43.

49 Mattson ME, Winn DM. Smokeless tobacco: association with increased cancer risk. In: *National Cancer Institute Monograph No. 8. Smokeless tobacco use in the United States.* Bethesda, MD: National Cancer Institutes, 1989.

50 Lemon FR, Walden RT, Woods RW. Cancer of the lung and mouth in Seventh-Day Adventists. Preliminary report on a population study. *Cancer* 1964; **17**: 486–97.

51 Schmidt W, Popham RE. The role of drinking and smoking in mortality from cancer and other causes in male alcoholics. *Cancer* 1981; **47**: 1031–41.

52 Schwartz D, Lellouch J, Flamant R, Denoix PF. Alcool et cancer. Resultats d'une enquête rétrospective. *Revue Française d'Etudes Cliniques et Biologiques* 1961; **7**: 590–604.

53 Rothman KJ. The effect of alcohol consumption on risk of cancer of the head and neck. *Laryngoscope* 1978; **88** (suppl. 8): 51–5.

54 McCoy GD, Wynder EL. Etiological and preventive implications in alcohol carcinogenesis. *Cancer Research* 1979; **39**: 2844–50.

55 Brugère J, Guenel P, Leclerc A, Rodriguez J. Differential effects of tobacco and alcohol in cancer of the larynx, pharynx and mouth. *Cancer* 1986; **57**: 391–5.

56 Blot WJ, McLaughlin JK, Winn DM *et al.* Smoking and drinking in relation to oral and pharyngeal cancer. *Cancer Research* 1988; **48**: 3282–7.

57 Leclerc A, Brugère J, Luce D, Point D, Guenel P. Type of alcoholic beverage and cancer of the upper respiratory and digestive tract. *European Journal of Cancer* 1987; **23**: 529–34.

58 Kabat GC, Wynder EL. Type of alcoholic beverage and oral cancer. *International Journal of Cancer* 1989; **43**: 190–4.

59 Young M, Russell WT. *An investigation into the statistics of cancer in different trades and professions.* MRC Special Report No. 99. London: HMSO, 1926.

60 Herity B, Moriarty M, Bourke GJ, Daly L. A case-control study of head and neck cancer in the Republic of Ireland. *British Journal of Cancer* 1981; **43**: 177–82.

61 Lyon JL, Gardener JW, Klauber MR, Smart CR. Low cancer incidence and mortality in Utah. *Cancer* 1977; **39**: 2608–18.

62 Binnie WH. Epidemiology and etiology of oral cancer in Britain. *Proceedings of the Royal Society of Medicine* 1976; **69**: 737–40.

63 Cawson RA. Leukoplakia and oral cancer. *Proceedings of the Royal Society of Medicine* 1969; **62**: 610–15.

64 Pindborg JJ. Oral leukoplakia. *Australian Dental Journal* 1971; **16**: 83–93.

65 Krogh P, Hald B, Holmstrup P. Possible mycological etiology of oral mucosal cancer: catalytic potential of infecting *Candida albicans* and other yeasts in production of N-nitrosobenzylmethylamine. *Carcinogenesis* 1987; **8**: 1543–8.

66 Cawson RA, Binne WH. Candida leukoplakia and carcinoma: a possible relationship. In: Mackenzie IC, Dabelsteen E, Squier CA eds. *Oral Premalignancy.* Iowa City, IA: University of Iowa Press, 1980.

67 Levin ML, Kress LC, Goldstein H. Syphilis and cancer; reported syphilis prevalence among 7761 cancer patients. *New York State Journal of Medicine* 1942; **42**: 1737–45.

68 Syrjänen KJ, Pyrhonen S, Syrjänen SM, Lamberg MA. Immunohistochemical demonstration of human papilloma virus (HPV) antigens in oral squamous cell lesions. *British Journal of Oral Surgery* 1983; **21**: 147–53.

69 Löning T, Ikenberg H, Becker J, Gissman L, Hoepfer I, zur Hausen H. Analysis of oral papillomas, leukoplakias and invasive carcinomas for human papillomavirus type related DNA. *Journal of Investigative Dermatology* 1985; **88**: 417–20.

70 Scully C, Maitland NJ, Cox MF, Prime SS. Human papillomavirus DNA and oral mucosa. *Lancet* 1987; **i**: 336 (letter).

71 Gassenmeier A, Hornstein OP. Presence of human papillomavirus DNA in benign and precancerous oral leukoplakias and squamous cell carcinomas. *Dermatologica* 1988; **176**: 224–33.

72 Syrjänen SM, Syrjänen KJ, Happonen RP. Human papillomavirus (HPV) DNA sequences in oral precancerous lesions and squamous cell carcinoma demonstrated by *in situ* hybridization. *Journal of Oral Pathology* 1988; **17**: 273–8.

73 Silverman NA, Alexander JC, Hollinshead AC, Chretien PB. Correlation of tumor burden with *in vitro* lymphocyte reactivity and antibodies to herpes virus tumor-associated antigens in head and neck squamous carcinoma. *Cancer* 1976; **37**: 135–40.

74 Smith HG, Chretien PB, Henson DE, Silverman NA, Alexander JC. Viral-specific humoral immunity to herpes simplex-induced antigens in patients with

squamous carcinoma of the head and neck. *American Journal of Surgery* 1976; **132**: 541–8.

75 Shillitoe EJ, Greenspan D, Greenspan JS, Hansen LS, Silverman S. Neutralizing antibody to herpes simplex virus type 1 in patients with oral cancer. *Cancer* 1982; **49**: 2315–20.

76 Silverman S, Migliorati CA, Lozada-Nur F, Greenspan D, Conant MA. Oral findings in people with or at high risk for AIDS: a study of 375 homosexual males. *Journal of the American Dental Association* 1986; **112**: 187–92.

77 Biggar RJ. Cancer in acquired immunodeficiency syndrome: an epidemiological assessment. *Seminars in Oncology* 1990; **17**: 251–60.

78 Ahlbom HE. Simple achlorhydric anaemia, Plummer–Vinson syndrome, and carcinoma of mouth, pharynx and oesophagus in women. *British Medical Journal* 1936; **2**: 331–3.

79 Wynder EL, Hultberg S, Jaconsson F. Environmental factors in cancer of the upper alimentary tract. A Swedish study with special reference to Plummer–Vinson (Paterson–Kelly) syndrome. *Cancer* 1957; **10**: 470–87.

80 Wahi PN, Kehar U, Lahiri B. Factors influencing oral and oropharyngeal cancers in India. *British Journal of Cancer* 1965; **19**: 642–60.

81 Ibrahim K, Jafarey NA, Zuberi SJ. Plasma vitamin 'A' and carotene levels in squamous cell carcinoma of oral cavity and oro-pharynx. *Clinical Oncology* 1977; **3**: 203–7.

82 McLaughlin JK, Gridley G, Block G *et al*. Dietary factors in oral and pharyngeal cancer. *Journal of the National Cancer Institute* 1988; **80**: 1237–43.

83 Graham S, Dayal H, Rohrer T, Swanson M, Sultz H, Shedd D, Fischman S. Dentition, diet, tobacco and alcohol in the epidemiology of oral cancer. *Journal of the National Cancer Institute* 1977; **59**: 1611–18.

84 Trell E, Bjorlin G, Andréasson L, Korsgaard R, Mattiasson I. Carcinoma of the oral cavity in relation to aryl hydrocarbon hydroxylase inducibility, smoking and dental status. *International Journal of Oral Surgery* 1981; **10**: 93–9.

85 Zheng T, Boyle P, Hu H, Duan J, Jiang P, Ma D, Shui L, Niu S, Scully C, MacMahon B. Dentition, oral hygiene and risk of oral cancer: a case-control study in Beijing, People's Republic of China. *Cancer Causes and Control* 1990; **1**: 235–41.

86 Marshall JR, Graham S, Haughey BP, Shedd D, O'Shea R, Brasure J, Wilkinson GS, West D. Smoking, alcohol, dentition and diet in the epidemiology of oral cancer. *Oral Oncology, European Journal of Cancer* 1992; **28B**: 9–15.

87 Huvos AG, Woodard HQ, Cahan WG, Higinbotham NL, Stewart FW, Butler A, Bretsky SS. Postradiation osteogenic sarcoma of bone and soft tissues: a clinicopathologic study of 66 patients. *Cancer* 1985; **55**: 1244–55.

88 Huvos AG, Butler A, Bretsky SS. Osteogenic sarcoma associated with Paget's disease of bone: a clinicopathologic study of 65 patients. *Cancer* 1983; **52**: 1489–95.

89 Spitz MR, Fueger JJ, Goepfert H, Newell GR. Salivary gland cancer: a case-control investigation of risk factors. *Archives of Otolaryngology – Head and Neck Surgery* 1990; **116**: 1163–6.

90 Berg JW, Hutter RVP, Foote FW. The unique association between salivary gland cancer and breast cancer. *Journal of the American Medical Association* 1968; **204**: 113–16.

2 Biology of cancer

M Partridge

Cancers arise as a result of alterations of cellular growth control processes together with changes in the interactions between cells and their surroundings, giving rise to invasion and metastasis. The control of cell growth is a consequence of signals which positively or negatively regulate cell proliferation. Tumour development arises from the accumulation of genetic events that affect these processes. These events include the activation of cellular oncogenes and inactivation of tumour suppressor genes by mutation or deletions. The isolation of these genes, together with the characterisation of the proteins that they encode, has led to remarkable developments in our understanding of the molecular basis of cancer.

Cellular oncogenes

The clue that certain genes are involved in the pathogenesis of cancer came from the study of experimentally induced tumours. Many RNA tumour viruses (retroviruses) cause cancer in animals. These viruses have very few genes but additional sequences of DNA associated with the development of cancer have been found. These viral genes were termed v-*onc*, an abbreviation for viral oncogenes,[1] and given three-letter code names derived from the type of animal or tumours from which they were first isolated. For example, the v-*src* gene was so called as it causes *sarc*oma in chickens, v-*ras* causes sarcomas in *ra*ts.

It soon became apparent that these genes are not viral genes at all but are present in normal mammalian cells.[1] The normal cellular sequences are termed cellular oncogenes or c-*onc*. These genes are better termed proto-oncogenes as they play an important role in cell growth and differentiation. They have oncogenic potential only when they are

altered, perhaps as a result of a mutation following exposure to a chemical carcinogen, or as a consequence of gene amplification resulting in extra copies of a gene. The retroviruses that cause cancers in animals carry the altered forms of these cellular oncogenes which were acquired during the course of infection of a human cell (Fig. 2.1).

Oncogenes can be classified into two broad groups by the location of their protein products.

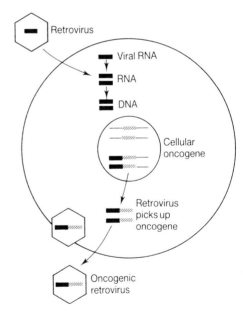

Fig. 2.1 The relation between viral and cellular oncogenes. When a retrovirus infects a human cell its RNA genome is converted into DNA using an enzyme called reverse transcriptase. DNA becomes integrated into the host cell genome. Integration may occur at the site of an activated oncogene. When the virus replicates and buds from the cell it may pick up the adjacent cellular oncogene and become an oncogenic retrovirus.

Some oncogenes function at the cell membrane or within the cytoplasm; a second group play a role in events occurring within the nucleus. Altered expression of a single oncogene is generally insufficient to induce full transformation and in most cases activation of both nuclear and cytoplasmic oncogenes contributes to the tumourigenic process.[2]

Functions of oncogene-encoded proteins

The exact biochemical functions of the proto-oncogene products have been only partially defined but available evidence suggests that they play a vital role in transducing the signal for cell division across the cell membrane to the nucleus (Fig. 2.2). Some oncogenes encode growth factors, the molecules that initiate the signals for cell division. For example, the oncogene of the simian sarcoma virus v-*sis*, which was the first oncogene to be identified,[3] is derived from the cellular gene encoding the β-chain of platelet-derived growth factor (PDGF; Fig. 2.2). Increased amounts of PDGF are produced and secreted by some tumours and may stimulate tumour cell division via an autocrine or paracrine growth control loop, since this growth factor can exert its action by binding to receptors on the same or adjacent cell. PDGF may also simulate the development of tumour vascularisation since it stimulates the formation of new blood vessels.

Another group of oncogenes encode cell surface receptors for growth factors that are associated with cytoplasmic signalling mechanisms (Fig. 2.2). The *erb* B oncogene encodes the intracellular domain of the epidermal growth factor (EGF) receptor and *fms* the receptor for colony stimulating factor.[1] Both oncogenes encode protein kinases which phosphorylate tyrosine residues in their target proteins.[4,5] Alterations in the structure and activity of these enzymes changes the pattern of signals influencing cell growth.

A third group of oncogenes act to couple extracellular signals to cytoplasmic signalling mechanisms often termed 'second messengers'. These include adenylate cyclase, phospholipase C and phosphoinositol; they help to transfer the signal for cell division from the cell membrane to the nucleus. The *ras* genes code for p21, a protein of 21 kD, located on the inner plasma membrane of the cell, which functions as a G protein, binding guanosine triphosphate (GTP) in its active state.[6] Mutations in the *ras* gene probably cause the protein to remain active. The *src* gene product encodes a protein tyrosine kinase which phosphorylates another component of one of the second messenger systems.[7]

A final group of oncogenes encode proteins involved in the control of gene transcription and the duplication of DNA. Several oncogenes function as transcription factors, which are the molecular switches controlling gene expression. The *fos* and *jun* oncogenes form a heterodimer (a molecule having two different polypeptide chains) which makes up a portion of the transcription factor AP-1.[8] These factors (proteins influencing synthesis of messenger RNA) bind to specific DNA sequences, termed AP-1 sites, and enhance transcription of adjacent genes. The *myc* gene is another example of a nuclear oncogene and codes for a 62 kD protein, p62, which plays a role in DNA duplication and cell division.

Evidence for involvement of oncogenes in oral cancer

Activated oncogenes were initially identified in head and neck cancers by transfection studies (experimental techniques allowing foreign DNA to cross the cell membrane and integrate into the genome).[9] DNA was isolated from oral squamous cell carcinoma, mixed with insoluble calcium phosphate and layered onto cells in tissue culture. The foreign DNA is taken up and integrated into the genome (a collective term for all the genetic ma-

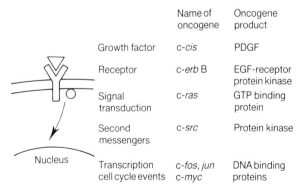

	Name of oncogene	Oncogene product
Growth factor	c-*cis*	PDGF
Receptor	c-*erb* B	EGF-receptor protein kinase
Signal transduction	c-*ras*	GTP binding protein
Second messengers	c-*src*	Protein kinase
Nucleus		
Transcription cell cycle events	c-*fos, jun* c-*myc*	DNA binding proteins

Fig. 2.2 Signal transduction mechanisms involving oncogene products. PDGF, platelet-derived growth factor; EGF, epidermal growth factor; GTP, guanosine triphosphate.

terial within a cell) of the cultured cells. When a fragment of DNA containing an oncogene is expressed by these cells transformation results, with loss of contact inhibition, unrestricted growth and piling up of cells. Cells from these transformed foci can produce tumours in experimental animals. DNA obtained from these tumours can be analysed to isolate and characterise the activated oncogene in each case.

The most frequently activated oncogenes in human cancers are the *ras* and *myc* oncogenes.[10,11] The possible role of these oncogenes in the pathogenesis of oral squamous cell carcinoma has also been studied. Amplification of the *ras* gene has been detected in oral squamous cell carcinoma in some studies[12] but is not a consistent finding. The incidence of mutations in the *ras* gene in oral tumours is low, being only 2–4 per cent of all cases reported in the developed world.[13] However, mutations in the *ras* gene occur with high frequency in patients with oral squamous cell carcinoma from the Indian subcontinent,[14] suggesting that the difference in the incidence of *ras* mutations may be related to betel chewing in the Indian population.

Amplification of the *myc* oncogene has been reported in 17 per cent of oral tumours[12] and elevated levels of *myc* protein can be detected in aggressive disease,[15] suggesting that expression of this oncogene may play a role in the altered growth control of late stage oral cancer. However, studies have shown that tumour cells show an increased rate of proliferation when compared with normal cells,[16] so in some tumours increased levels of the *myc* oncogene product may be merely the result of the increased growth rate of the tumour rather than altered expression of these genes.

Genes located on the long arm of chromosome 11, termed *hst* and *int 2*, may also be involved in the pathogenesis of oral tumours. These genes encode proteins similar to acidic and basic fibroblast growth factors which have diverse biological effects including a role in angiogenesis. Co-amplification of *hst* and *int 2* correlates with distant metastasis in breast and oesophageal squamous cell carcinoma,[17] and provides a prognostic marker for oesophageal carcinoma. Amplification of *int 2* has also been detected in head and neck squamous cell carcinoma[18] and may be important in the pathogenesis of oral cancers. The bcl (breakpoint cluster locus) is another region on this chromosome that is involved in a reciprocal translocation with the immunoglobulin locus on chromosome 14 in B cell lymphomas. It is assumed that another oncogene which lies close to the bcl locus is activated as a result of this translocation. Thirty five per cent of head and neck squamous cell carcinomas show amplification of this locus, implying that genes in this region are likely to be important in the development of oral cancers.[19]

Anti-oncogenes or tumour suppressor genes

The second group of genes implicated in the pathogenesis of cancer are the tumour suppressor genes, encoding proteins that have the ability to suppress cell division. During tumour development these genes often become mutated or deleted and lose their normal function of negatively regulating cell growth. These genes may thus play a crucial role in the development of neoplasia.

Alterations in a tumour suppressor gene manifest in a 'recessive' manner such that a single normal copy of a tumour suppressor gene is sufficient to limit proliferation and prevent tumour development. If both copies of the gene are altered as a result of deletion or mutation, the growth suppressive function is lost and uncontrolled growth or tumour formation results. The best characterised tumour suppressor gene is the retinoblastoma gene, which is found on chromosome 13.[20] In cases of retinoblastoma an affected individual carries a defective allele at one locus and a tumour may develop following loss of the remaining normal allele from the other chromosome.

Allelic loss of tumour suppressor genes also plays a role in the development of sporadic tumours. Identical chromosomal deletions have been reported in several tumour types, including colorectal cancers which show deletions of regions of chromosomes 5, 17 and 18, and breast tumours which may have deletions of chromosomes 17 and 18. Deletions of a region of chromosome 13 are frequently seen in small cell lung carcinomas, breast tumours, bladder tumours and osteosarcomas.[21] Other chromosomal deletions appear to be cell type specific; for example, deletion of chromosome 1 occurs in melanoma, deletions of 3 in small cell lung cancer and deletions of 22 in acoustic neuroma.[22] The p53, Rb (retinoblastoma) and DCC (deleted in colorectal carcinoma) genes (see below) have been identified as the deleted genes on chromosomes 17, 13 and 18, respectively.[20,23,24] Since these deletions appear to be common to many tumour types these findings suggest that these genes may play a central role in controlling growth in many tissues and act as negative regulators of cellular proliferation allowing the cell to respond to growth inhibitory signals.

The retinoblastoma tumour suppressor gene

The retinoblastoma, Rb, gene encodes a protein of 105–110 kD. Several forms of Rb occur as this protein has multiple phosphorylation sites. The underphosphorylated form is thought to mediate its growth regulatory properties. The Rb protein can bind to sequences present in oncogenic DNA viruses including the adenovirus E1A protein, SV40T and human papilloma viruses.[25–27] These associations are thought to mimic the role of a normal cellular protein that is critical for growth regulation. Several other proteins have been shown to form complex interactions with the Rb product. These include binding of Rb to the E2F transcription factor[28] which limits the ability of E2F to function as a transcription factor. Rb also binds to the *myc* oncogene product,[29] members of the cyclin family of molecules[30] and two other proteins termed RBP-1 and RBP-2.[31] The significance of the latter interactions is not yet clear but probably plays a crucial role in determining whether or not cells enter the S phase of the cell cycle. Taken together these associations suggest that Rb limits cellular proliferation by binding to several nuclear proteins involved in proliferation and that the viral oncoproteins transform cells by releasing these proteins from inactive complexes.

Rb may not only function as a tumour suppressor gene since Meling *et al.*[32] have demonstrated amplification of the Rb gene in colorectal carcinoma. Amplification is a phenomenon usually associated with the oncogenes and suggests that Rb may also have an oncogene-like action in some tumour types.

The p53 tumour suppressor gene

p53 (so termed as it is a protein with a molecular weight of 53 kD) is a nuclear phosphoprotein discovered as it forms a complex with SV40T antigen which is required to initiate replication of this virus in transformed cells.[33] All known mutants of p53 fail to bind T antigen. This suggests that p53 binds with a cellular homologue of T antigen which is responsible for initiating replication and entry into S phase. p53 may also function as a nuclear transcription function.[34]

Alterations in the p53 gene are also very common in human cancers and have been found in tumours of the lung, colon and breast.[35–37]

p53 is present in minute concentrations in normal cells and is difficult to detect by standard laboratory techniques such as immunohistochemistry. Mutation stabilises p53 and extends the life of the protein which means that any p53 protein detected by immunohistochemistry is very probably in the mutant configuration.[38] Studies using an antibody which recognises the mutant form of p53,[39] termed Ab240,[40] show that mutant p53 protein can be detected in 80 per cent of oral squamous cell carcinomas. High levels of expression of p53 were reported in tumours obtained from patients who were heavy smokers and drinkers, suggesting that alterations in the p53 gene may be one of the sites of genetic damage in this group of patients.[41]

A number of studies have helped to determine the molecular basis for loss of function of normal p53 and overexpression of the mutant protein in malignant tissues and cells. The p53 gene lies on chromosome 17. When colon, breast or lung tumours are examined 75–85 per cent show alteration of both p53 alleles, one through gene deletion, the other through point mutation.[35–37] A point mutation in this gene together with loss of the normal gene may lead to accumulation of mutant p53 within the cell. Mutations in the p53 gene convert it from a tumour suppressor gene to a dominant oncogene that can act with other oncogenes to transform cells.[42] Thus a mutation of one p53 allele together with loss of the other allele would remove the normal regulatory function of p53 and at the same time transform p53 into a dominantly acting oncogene.

Mutations in the p53 gene are generally clustered in four highly conserved regions involving exons 5–10 (coding regions within a gene) although intronic (non-coding) mutations have also been reported.[43] A single base pair mutation, which is consistent with mutations produced by aflatoxin, has been reported for hepatocellular carcinoma.[44] Other studies suggest that not all mutations have the same functional effects on p53;[45] thus it is important to analyse the precise spectrum of mutations found in each tumour type.

The presence of mutations occurring at two different sites in cell lines derived from head and neck tumours has been demonstrated by Gusterson *et al.*[46] In a different study involving analysis of lung cancers 15 of 25 mutations were found to be G to T transversions, a pattern that could be produced by benzo{a}pyrene, a carcinogen in cigarette smoke.[35] Determination of the frequency of allelic loss at chromosome 17 and direct sequencing of the p53 gene obtained from oral tumours should be performed to demonstrate whether mutation and deletions of the p53 gene occur in oral tumours.

Co-operation between tumour suppressor genes may also occur. Studies have shown that mutation of the p53 gene may occur together with abnormalities of the Rb gene,[47] suggesting that coincident inactivation of more than one tumour suppressor gene may be required for tumour development in some cases.

Several other tumour suppressor genes have been characterised including the DCC gene which encodes a protein with similarities to cell adhesion molecules. Loss of DCC function may result in loss of contact inhibition or impairment of membrane transduction. The DCC gene is also the deleted gene on chromosome 18 reported in breast cancer.[48] The MCC gene (mutated in colorectal carcinoma) is important in the pathogenesis of 25 per cent of lung tumours as well as colorectal cancer.[49]

For some types of cancer the nature of these genetic events involved in tumour development and the order in which they are most likely to occur has been determined. For example, a model has been proposed for colorectal carcinoma in which alteration of a gene on chromosome 5 (MCC) leads to abnormal proliferation of cells. Subsequent loss of methylation of DNA is then associated with the development of a benign adenoma. Mutation in the *ras* gene increases the rate of cell proliferation, and further events involving loss of the DCC gene on chromosome 18 and p53 gene from chromosome 17 may result in the transition of the lesion to a carcinoma.[50]

Chromosomes 1 and 3 may also carry tumour suppressor genes. Deletions of chromosome 1 occur in breast and bladder tumours and have been reported in cell lines derived from head and neck tumours.[51] Deletion of chromosome 3 occurs in squamous cell carcinoma of the lung[52] and in head and neck squamous cell carcinoma cell lines.[53] Many patients with lung or oral tumours are heavy smokers and the common genetic events found in these tumours may reflect exposure to similar carcinogens.

Determination of the genetic events that play a role in the pathogenesis of oral cancer will ultimately provide a classification system for these tumours according to the type of activated oncogenes or deleted tumour suppressor genes they contain. This may provide a more powerful prognostic indicator of tumour behaviour than the histological data currently available. Early detection of malignant change in areas of leukoplakia or erythroplakia may also be improved through knowledge of the molecular pathogenesis of the development of this disease. Evaluation of the genetic alterations may also define new targets for therapy.

Growth factors

Many oncogenes encode growth factors or growth factor receptors (Fig. 2.2). These molecules play a crucial role in stimulating cell proliferation, so evidence of production of growth factors or changes in expression of growth factor receptors has been sought for a number of tumour types.

Transforming growth factor-α (TGFα) is a small polypeptide, related to EGF, which stimulates cell growth by binding to the EGF receptor. TGFα was originally characterised as a factor secreted by fibroblasts infected with a retrovirus that could transform normal cells.[54] The identification of these transforming growth factors led to the proposal of an autocrine hypothesis of growth control with transformed cells able to respond to self-produced growth factors.[55]

TGFα is also synthesised and secreted by normal epithelial cells.[56,57] The physiological roles of TGFα are unclear, but it can prolong the life of cultured epidermal cells suggesting a role in epidermal homeostasis;[58] experiments with transgenic mice suggest that it plays a role in determining epidermal thickness during development and differentiation.[59]

Several studies suggest that aberrant expression of TGFα is associated with the development of oral cancer. TGFα is synthesised and secreted by cell lines derived from head and neck tumours including oral squamous cell carcinoma.[57] Infiltrating eosinophils associated with these tumours have been shown to be an important source of TGFα.[60]

A number of studies have examined the pattern of expression of the receptor for TGFα in oral squamous cell carcinoma by immunohistochemistry, using antibodies which recognise the EGF receptor.[57,61,62] Oral squamous cell carcinomas express the EGF receptor at the cell membrane, but the level of expression is variable with some tumours showing high levels of receptor whereas others express only low levels. In well differentiated squamous cell carcinomas a gradation of staining intensity is observed, with the keratinising elements losing their EGF receptors. This suggests that the levels of receptor on a given cell may reflect its state of differentiation within the tumour population. An example of this pattern of EGF receptor expression is shown in Fig. 2.3. A semiquantitative assessment of the level of receptor present for each tumour can be made by assigning a score value based on the level of receptor expression and the proportion of tumour cells in the specimen.[57] When levels of TGFα detected in each tumour are compared with the level of EGF receptors a highly significant inverse correlation is found; the highest levels of TGFα are seen in the tumours with the lowest levels of EGF receptor. This suggests that binding of TGFα to the EGF receptor may stimulate proliferation of the tumour. However, this example of an autocrine growth control loop takes no account of other multiple growth factor interactions which affect cell growth and is clearly just one facet of a complex growth regulatory mechanism.

Many growth inhibitory molecules have also been characterised. These include transforming growth factor-β (TGFβ), which is a member of a complex family of structurally related growth and differentiation factors. TGFβ can be present in transformed cells which produce TGFα and has been identified in a wide range of malignant cell lines.[63] Most cells secrete TGFβ in a latent form which cannot bind to cell surface receptors[64] and the activation of latent TGFβ is a key regulatory event. *In vitro*, acidification or protease digestion appears to activate latent TGFβ.

TGFβ has a growth inhibitory effect on normal epithelial cells and can be detected in oral squamous cell carcinoma.[57] It has been postulated that TGFβ plays an important role in the regulation of normal epithelial cell growth with lack of response leading to altered growth in carcinomas.[57,65] A number of squamous cell carcinoma cell lines, including those derived from head and neck tumours, fail to respond to the growth inhibitory effects of TGFβ. The reasons for this are unclear but it may be that TGFβ is present in a latent form which cannot bind to its receptor, the receptor may be absent, or there may be alterations in the postreceptor signalling pathways which fail to deliver a growth inhibitory signal to the nucleus.[66] These studies have led to a proposed model for the role of TGFα and β in the growth control of normal and malignant cells, with an increase in stimulatory or a decrease in growth inhibitory signals playing a role in neoplastic transformation (Fig. 2.4).

Recognition of growth factors and receptors that influence the proliferation of tumour cells provides attractive targets for new forms of therapy. Preliminary studies designed to downregulate growth

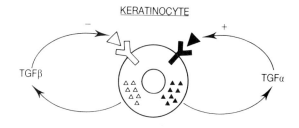

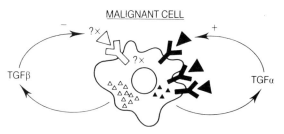

Fig. 2.4 Potential stimulatory/inhibitory growth regulation of epithelial cells. In normal cells transforming growth factor-α (TGFα) provides a stimulatory signal whereas TGFβ is growth inhibitory. Altered growth in tumour cells may result from increased production of TGFα and/or loss of a negative growth inhibitory signal. This may arise due to failure to activate latent TGFβ, loss of TGFβ receptors or changes in postreceptor signalling mechanisms.

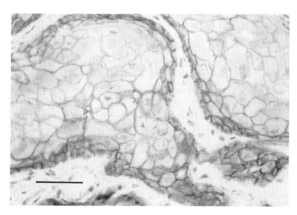

Fig. 2.3 Immunohistochemical detection of the epidermal growth factor receptor on oral squamous cell carcinoma. Scale bar, 50 microns.

stimulatory signals include attempts to use agents which block TGFα binding to its receptor, inhibit EGF receptor dimerisation or inhibit protein tyrosine kinase activity. Tumour specific growth factors would provide a more attractive target for new forms of therapy. However at the present time no growth factor has been identified which is synthesised by malignant but not by normal cells.

Monoclonal antibodies raised against growth factor receptors have been radiolabelled with ^{131}I and used to detect metastasis for some tumour types. Extensive studies are now being carried out to determine whether drugs, toxins or radiolabelled nuclides can be coupled to these monoclonal antibodies and so used to destroy tumours.

Tumour invasion and metastasis

The mechanisms responsible for the induction of metastatic potential in tumour cells have yet to be fully elucidated. It is generally considered that not all cells within a given tumour population have the ability to metastasise, and that the ability to form a new tumour colony reflects the general phenomenon of tumour heterogeneity. To produce a metastatic colony cells must be able to leave the primary tumour, penetrate the basement membrane, invade the local tissues, escape host immune killing, enter the lymphatic circulation or the blood, extravasate at a distant site and proliferate to form a new tumour. Invasion of tissues involves changes in cell adhesion and locomotion. A number of agents increase locomotion and affect cell positioning, including tumour autocrine mobility factors and scatter factors.[67]

Tumour cells also secrete, or induce host cells to secrete, increased levels of protease enzymes which result in localised lysis of matrix allowing the cell to migrate through tissue barriers.[68] Migration only occurs where the accumulation of enzyme exceeds the level of natural protease inhibitors present.

A cascade of proteases are thought to be important in dissolution of matrix components; these include metalloproteinases, serine proteinases and heparanases. The metalloproteinases, secreted as inactive zymogens which require activation, are subdivided into groups depending on the type of substrates which they attack preferentially. The three groups comprise the interstitial collagenases which degrade type 1 collagen, type 1V collagenase which selectively cleaves type 1V collagen, and the stromeolysins which are a group of related proteins

that degrade a variety of matrix components including proteoglycans, laminin and fibronectin.

Natural inhibitor proteins, produced by the host or tumour cells, block the action of latent or active metalloproteinases. These are termed TIMP-1 and TIMP-2 (tissue inhibitors of metalloproteinases).[69] TIMP-2 binds to both the latent and activated forms of type 1V collagenase whereas TIMP-1 acts as a general inhibitor of metalloproteinases. These inhibitory proteins are natural inhibitors of tumour invasion; studies have confirmed an inverse correlation between levels of TIMP detected in tumours and the invasive potential of the tumour cells.[70] Levels of TIMP are increased as a result of exposure to TGFβ1[71] although whether the active form of TGFβ is present in oral squamous cell carcinoma has yet to be determined. Other factors that influence the levels of proteinases and their inhibitors in squamous cell carcinoma have yet to be elucidated but may show a relation to tumour morphology or behaviour.

Immunological changes and immunotherapy

A mononuclear cell infiltrate is often present beneath dysplastic oral epithelium and has been reported to be a good prognostic marker.[72] This infiltrate is heterogeneous but composed largely of T lymphocytes and probably represents a cell mediated immune response to the tumour. Immunoglobulins are also deposited around oral squamous cell carcinomas. However in the majority of cases tumours are ultimately able to avoid both immune surveillance and the inflammatory responses mounted by the host.

A number of immunological abnormalities have been reported in patients with head and neck squamous cell carcinoma which result in depression of the cell mediated immune reponse.[73] These abnormalities include a reduction in the number of T lymphocytes[74] and impairment of lymphocyte function.[75] Circulating immune complexes are also found in patients with oral squamous cell carcinoma and may be one of the factors contributing to the depressed cell mediated immune response.[76] Leukotrienes and prostaglandins may also influence the immune system in patients suffering from oral squamous cell carcinoma.[77]

In the last decade new biological treatments for cancer have been proposed based on stimulating the natural immune responses against this disease.

Rosenberg[78] was the first to establish biological therapies based on the administration of interleukin 2 (IL-2) or giving IL-2 in combination with lymphokine activated killer (LAK) cells. LAK cells are non-MHC (major histocompatability complex) restricted killing cells capable of lysing tumour but not normal cells. LAK cells are obtained from a venous blood sample and stimulated with IL-2 in the laboratory. The mechanism of action of this immunotherapy does not depend only on the activation of LAK cells; IL-2 also stimulates other populations of lymphocytes expressing IL-2 receptors, including cytotoxic lymphocytes already reacting to the tumour.

Clinical trials based on this form of therapy have been conducted and significant antitumour responses were observed in patients with advanced melanoma, renal cell carcinoma, colon cancer and non-Hodgkin's lymphoma. Ten per cent of patients with advanced melanoma or renal cell carcinoma went into complete remission.[79] However, the beneficial response to therapy with IL-2 has to be considered in relation to the high incidence of toxic side effects.

Subsequently techniques were developed for isolating tumour infiltrating lymphocytes (TIL). These lymphocytes are obtained from single cell suspensions of tumour biopsy material and are capable of recognising unique antigens present on tumour cells. When first isolated from the tumour these cells are not cytotoxic but expansion and activation of these cells in response to IL-2 generates several forms of cytotoxicity. These include MHC restricted cytotoxic cells that are reactive to the tumour, non-MHC restricted cytotoxicity (LAK) cells and natural killer (NK) activity. This therapy is potentially more tumour specific as the lymphocytes are reactive to the tumour. Current techniques for generating TIL depend on the use of low doses of IL-2, which generates cells with more specific cytotoxic activity than high levels of IL-2. Clinical trials to evaluate this form of therapy are currently in progress.

Gene therapy of cancer

Techniques that allow the expression of foreign genes in mammalian cells have created new possibilities for the therapy of cancer. TIL have been modified by introducing the gene encoding tumour necrosis factor into these cells. The rationale for this experiment is that tumour necrosis factor can cause necrosis and regression of tumours.[80] In theory TIL can travel directly to the tumour and secrete high local concentrations of tumour necrosis factor. This therapy is being used in a study to treat cases of advanced melanoma and if clinical benefit is shown then additional genes such as those which code for IL-2, IL-6 or γ-interferon may be introduced into TIL or into the tumour cells themselves.

In the last decade increased understanding of the molecular mechanisms responsible for tumour development together with some success in the application of biological therapies offers hope that new strategies for the treatment of malignant disease can be developed, aimed at the alterations in growth control that contribute to the pathogenesis of this disease.

References

1 Bishop JM, Varmus H. Functions and origins of retroviral transforming genes. In: Weiss RA, Teich N, Varmus H, Coffin J eds. *RNA Tumour Viruses*. New York: Cold Spring Harbor Laboratory, 1982: 988–1108.

2 Land H, Parada LF, Weinberg RA. Tumorigenic conversion of primary embryo fibroblasts requires at least two cooperating oncogenes. *Nature* 1983; **304**: 596–602.

3 Waterfield MD, Scrace GT, Whittle N *et al*. Platelet-derived growth factor is structurally related to the putative transforming protein p28 of simian sarcoma virus. *Nature* 1983; **304**: 35–9.

4 Downward J, Yarden Y, Mayes E *et al*. Close similarity of epidermal growth factor receptor and v-*erb* B oncogene protein sequences. *Nature* 1984; **307**: 521–9.

5 Sherr CH, Rettenmeir CW, Sacca R, Roussel MF, Look AT, Stanley ER. The c-*fms* proto-oncogene product is related to the receptor for the mononuclear phagocytic growth factor CSF-1. *Cell* 1985; **43**: 665–76.

6 Barbacid M. *Ras* genes. *Annual Review of Biochemistry* 1987; **56**: 779–827.

7 Sugimoto Y, Whitman M, Cantley LC, Erikson R. Evidence that the Rous sarcoma transforming gene product phosphorylates phosphatidylinositol and diacylglycerol. *Proceedings of the National Academy of Sciences USA* 1984; **81**: 2117–21.

8 Bohmann D, Bos TJ, Admon A, Nishimura T, Vogt PK, Tijan R. Human proto-oncogene c-*jun* encodes a DNA binding protein with structural and functional properties of transcription factor AP-1. *Science* 1987; **238**: 1386–92.

9 Friedman WH, Rosenblum BN, Loewenstein P, Thornton H, Katsantonis G, Green M. Oncogenes:

their presence and significance in squamous cell cancer of the head and neck. *Laryngoscope* 1985; **95**: 313–16.

10 Bos JL, Fearon ER, Hamilton SR *et al.* Prevalence of *ras* gene mutation in human colorectal cancers. *Nature* 1987; **327**: 293–7.

11 Alitalo K, Schwab M. Oncogene activation in tumour cells. *Advances in Cancer Research* 1986; **47**: 235–81.

12 Saranath D, Panchal RG, Nair N *et al.* Oncogene activation in squamous cell carcinoma of the oral cavity. *Japanese Journal of Cancer Research* 1989; **80**: 430–7.

13 Rumsby G, Carter RL, Gusterson BA. Low incidence of *ras* oncogene activation in human squamous cell carcinomas. *British Journal of Cancer* 1990; **61**: 365–8.

14 Saranath D, Chang SE, Bhoite LT *et al.* High frequency mutations in codons 12 and 61 of H-*ras* oncogene in chewing tobacco-related human oral carcinoma in India. *British Journal of Cancer* 1991; **63**: 573–8.

15 Field JK, Spandidos DA, Stell PM, Vaughan ED, Evan GI, Moore JP. Elevated expression of the c-*myc* oncoprotein correlates with poor prognosis in head and neck squamous cell carcinoma. *Oncogene* 1989; **4**: 1463–8.

16 Wong DTW. Histone gene (H3) expression in chemically transformed oral keratinocytes. *Experimental and Molecular Pathology* 1988; **49**: 206–14.

17 Kitagawa Y, Ueda M, Ando M, Shinozawa Y, Shimizu N, Abe O. Significance of int 2/hst-1 coamplification as a prognostic factor in patients with oesophageal carcinoma. *Cancer Research* 1991; **51**: 1504–8.

18 Zhou D, Casey G, Cline M. Amplification of human int-2 in breast cancers and squamous carcinomas. *Oncogene* 1988; **2**: 279–83.

19 Berenson JR, Yang J, Mickel RA. Frequent amplification of the *bcl*-1 locus in head and neck squamous cell carcinomas. *Oncogene* 1989; **4**: 1111–16.

20 Friend S, Horowitz JM, Gerber MR *et al.* Deletions of a DNA sequence in retinoblastomas and mesenchymal tumours: organisation of the sequence and its encoded protein. *Proceedings of the National Academy of Sciences USA* 1987; **84**: 9063–95.

21 Horowitz JM, Park SH, Bogenmann E *et al.* Frequent inactivation of the retinoblastoma anti-oncogene is restricted to a subset of human tumours. *Proceedings of the National Academy of Sciences USA* 1990; **87**: 2775–9.

22 Weinberg R. The retinoblastoma gene and cell growth control. *Trends in Biological Sciences* 1990; **15**: 199–202.

23 Baker SJ, Fearon ER, Nigro JM *et al.* Chromosome 17 deletions and p53 gene mutations in colorectal carcinomas. *Science* 1989; **244**: 217–21.

24 Fearnon E, Cho KR, Nigro JM *et al.* Identification of a chromosome 18q gene that is altered in colorectal carcinoma. *Science* 1990; **247**: 49–56.

25 Scheffner M, Werness BA, Huibregtse JM, Levine AJ, Howley PM. The E6 oncoprotein encoded by human papillomavirus types 16 and 18 promotes the degradation of p53. *Cell* 1990; **63**: 1129–36.

26 Whyte P, Williamson NM, Harlow E. Cellular targets for transformation by the adenovirus E1A proteins. *Cell* 1989; **56**: 67–75.

27 DeCaprio JA, Ludlow JW, Figge J *et al.* SV40 large tumor antigen forms a specific complex with the product of the retinoblastoma susceptibility gene. *Cell* 1988; **54**: 275–83.

28 Bagchi S, Weinmann R, Raychauhuri P. The retinoblastoma protein copurifies with E2F-1, an E1A-regulated inhibitor of the transcription factor E2F. *Cell* 1991; **65**: 1063–72.

29 Rustgi AK, Dyson N, Bernards R. Amino-terminal domains of c-*myc* and N-*myc* proteins mediate binding of the retinoblastoma gene product. *Nature* 1991; **352**: 541–4.

30 Bandara L, LaThangue N. Adenovirus E1a prevents the retinoblastoma gene product from complexing with a cellular transcription factor. *Nature* 1991; **351**: 494–7.

31 Defeo-Jones D, Huang PS, Jones RE *et al.* Cloning of cDNAs for cellular proteins that bind to the retinoblastoma gene product. *Nature* 1991; **352**: 251–4.

32 Meling GI, Lothe RA, Borresen A-L *et al.* Genetic alterations within the retinoblastoma locus in colorectal carcinomas. Relation to ploidy pattern studied by flow cytometric analysis. *British Journal of Cancer* 1991; **64**: 475–80.

33 Lane DP, Crawford LV. T-antigen is bound to host protein in SV 40 transformed cells. *Nature* 1979; **278**: 261–3.

34 Field S, Jang SK. Presence of a potent transcription activating sequence in the p53 protein. *Science* 1990; **249**: 1046–9.

35 Iggo R, Gatter K, Bartek J, Lane D, Harris A. Increased expression of mutant forms of p53 oncogene in primary lung cancer. *Lancet* 1990; **335**: 675–9.

36 Bartek J, Bartkova J, Vojtesek B *et al.* Patterns of expression of the p53 tumour suppressor in human breast tissues and tumours *in situ* and *in vitro*. *International Journal of Cancer* 1990; **46**: 839–44.

37 Rodrigues N, Rowan A, Smith MEF, Kerr IB, Bodmer WF, Gannon JV, Lane DP. p53 mutations in colorectal cancer. *Proceedings of the National Academy of Sciences USA* 1990; **87**: 7555–9.

38 Lane DP, Benchimol S. p53: oncogene or anti-oncogene? *Genes and Development* 1990; **4**: 1–8.

39 Bartek J, Iggo R, Lane DP. Genetic and immuno-chemical analysis of mutant p53 in human breast cancer cell lines. *Oncogene* 1990; **5**: 893–9.

40 Gannon JV, Greaves R, Iggo R, Lane DP. Activating mutations in p53 produce a common conformational effect. A monoclonal antibody specific for the mutant

form. *European Molecular Biology Organisation Journal* 1990; **9**: 1595–602.

41 Langdon JD, Partridge M. Expression of the tumour suppressor gene p53 in oral cancer. *British Journal of Oral and Maxillofacial Surgery* 1992; **30**: 214.

42 Hinds P, Finlay C, Levine AJ. Mutation is required to activate the p53 gene for co-operation with the *ras* oncogene and transformation. *Journal of Virology* 1989; **63**: 739–46.

43 Takahasi T, d'Amico D, Chiba I, Buchhagen DL, Minna JD. Identification of intronic point mutations as an alternative mechanism for p53 inactivation in lung cancer. *Journal of Clinical Investigation* 1990; **86**: 363–9.

44 Hsu IC, Metcalf RA, Sun T, Welsh JA, Wang NJ, Harris CC. Mutational hot spots in the p53 gene in human hepatocellular carcinomas. *Nature* 1991; **350**: 427–9.

45 Halevy O, Michalovitz D, Oren M. Different tumour-derived p53 mutants exhibit distinct biological activities. *Science* 1990; **250**: 113–16.

46 Gusterson BA, Anbazhagan R, Warren W *et al.* Expression of p53 in premalignant and malignant squamous epithelium. *Oncogene* 1991; **6**: 1785–9.

47 Stratton MR, Moss S, Warren W *et al.* Mutation of the p53 gene in human soft tissue sarcomas: association with abnormalities of the RB1 gene. *Oncogene* 1990; **5**: 1297–301.

48 Devilee P, van Vliet M, Kuipers-Dijkshoorn N, Pearson PL, Cornelisse CJ. Somatic changes on chromosome 18 in breast carcinomas: is the DCC gene involved? *Oncogene* 1991; **6**: 311–15.

49 Ashton-Rickardt PG, Wyllie AH, Bird CC *et al.* MCC, a candidate familial polyposis gene in 5q.21, shows frequent allele loss in colorectal and lung cancer. *Oncogene* 1991; **6**: 1881–6.

50 Fearnon EF, Vogelstein B. A genetic model for colorectal tumorigenesis. *Cell* 1990; **61**: 759–67.

51 Hauser-Urfer IH, Stauffer J. Comparative chromosome analysis of nine squamous cell carcinoma lines from tumours of the head and neck. *Cytogenetics and Cell Genetics* 1985; **39**: 35–9.

52 Sozzi G, Miozzo M, Tagliabue E *et al.* Cytogenetic abnormalities and overexpression of receptors for growth factors in normal bronchial epitheli and tumour samples of lung cancer patients. *Cancer Research* 1991; **51**: 400–4.

53 Heo DS, Snyderman C, Gollin SM *et al.* Biology, cytogenetics and sensitivity to immunological effector cells of new head and neck squamous cell carcinoma lines. *Cancer Research* 1989; **49**: 5167–75.

54 DeLarco JE, Todaro GJ. Growth factors from murine sarcoma virus transformed cells. *Proceedings of the National Academy of Sciences USA* 1987; **75**: 4001–5.

55 Sporn MB, Todaro GJ. Autocrine secretion and malignant transformation of cells. *New England Journal of Medicine* 1980; **303**: 878–900.

56 Coffey DJ, Derynck R, Wilcox JN *et al.* Production and auto-induction of transforming growth factor-α in human keratinocytes. *Nature* 1987; **328**: 817–20.

57 Partridge M, Green MR, Langdon JD, Feldman M. Production of TGF-α and TGF-β by cultured keratinocytes, skin and oral squamous cell carcinomas – potential autocrine regulation of normal and malignant epithelial cell proliferation. *British Journal of Cancer* 1989; **60**: 542–8.

58 Barrandon Y, Green H. Cell migration is essential for sustained growth of keratinocyte cultures: the roles of transforming growth factor α and epidermal growth factor. *Cell* 1987; **50**: 1131–7.

59 Vassar R, Fuchs E. Transgenic mice provide new insights into the role of TGF α during epidermal development and differentiation. *Genes and Development* 1991; **5**: 714–27.

60 Todd R, Chou MY, Matossian K, Gallagher GT, Donoff RB, Wong DTW. Cellular sources of transforming growth factor alpha in human oral cancer. *Journal of Dental Research* 1991; **70**: 917–23.

61 Ishitoya J, Toriyama M, Oguchi N *et al.* Gene amplification and overexpression of EGF receptor in squamous cell carcinomas of the head and neck. *British Journal of Cancer* 1989; **59**: 559–62.

62 Bergler W, Ganzer U. The expression of epidermal growth factor receptors in the oral mucosa of patients with oral cancer. *Archives of Otorhinolaryngology* 1989; **246**: 121–5.

63 Derynck R, Goeddel DV, Ullrich A *et al.* Synthesis of messenger RNAs for transforming growth factors α and β and the epidermal growth factor receptor by human tumours. *Cancer Research* 1987; **47**: 702–12.

64 Lyons M, Keski-Oja J, Moses H. Proteolytic activation of latent transforming growth factor-β from fibroblast conditioned medium. *Journal of Cell Biology* 1988; **106**: 1659–64.

65 Shipley GD, Pittelkow MR, Willie JJ, Scott RE, Moses HL. Reversible inhibition of normal prokeratinocyte proliferation by type β transforming growth factor inhibitor in serum-free medium. *Cancer Research* 1986; **46**: 2068–71.

66 Roberts AB, Thompson NL, Heine U, Flanders C, Sporn MB. Transforming growth factor beta: possible roles in carcinogenesis. *British Journal of Cancer* 1988; **57**: 594–600.

67 Stoker M, Gherardi E, Perryman M, Gray J. Scatter factor is a fibroblast derived modulator of epithelial mobility. *Nature* 1987; **327**: 239–42.

68 Gottesman M. The role of proteases in cancer. *Seminars in Cancer Biology* 1990; **1**: 97–160.

69 Stetler-Stevenson WG, Brown PD, Onisto M, Levy AT, Liotta LA. Tissue inhibitor of metalloproteinase-2 (TIMP) mRNA expression in cell lines and human tumours. *Journal of Biological Chemistry* 1990; **265**: 13933–8.

70 Khokha R, Waterhouse P, Yagel S *et al.* Antisense RNA-induced reduction in metalloproteinase in-

hibitor causes mouse 3T3 cells to become tumourigenic. *Science* 1989; **243**: 947–50.

71 Edwards DR, Murphy G, Reynolds JJ *et al.* Transforming growth factor beta modulates the expression
of collagenase and metalloproteinase inhibitor. *European Molecular Biology Organisation Journal* 1987; **6**:
1899–904.

72 Johnson NW. The role of histopathology in diagnosis
and prognosis of oral squamous cell carcinoma. *Proceedings of the Royal Society of Medicine* 1976; **69**:
740–6.

73 Scully C. Immunology of cancer of the head and neck
with particular reference to oral cancer. *Oral Surgery,
Oral Medicine, Oral Pathology* 1982; **53**: 157–67.

74 Lundy J, Wanebo H, Pinsky C, Strong E, Oettgen
H. Delayed hypersensitivity reactions in patients with
squamous cell carcinoma of the head and neck.
American Journal of Surgery 1974; **128**: 530–3.

75 Vetto RM, Burger DR, Vandenbark AA, Finke PE.
Changes in tumour immunity during therapy determined by leukocyte adherence inhibition and dermal
testing. *Cancer* 1978; **41**: 1034–9.

76 Scully C, Barkas T, Boyle P, McGregor IA. Circulating immune complexes detected by binding of ra-
diolabeled protein A in patients with oral cancer and
oral premalignant lesions. *Journal of Clinical and Laboratory Immunology* 1982; **8**: 113–15.

77 El-Hakim IE, Langdon J. Arachidonic acid cascade
and oral squamous cell carcinoma. *Clinical Otolaryngology* 1991; **16**: 563–73.

78 Rosenberg SA. Immunotherapy of cancer by the systemic administration of lymphoid cells plus interleukin 2. *Journal of Biological Response Modifiers*
1984; **3**: 501–11.

79 Rosenberg SA, Lotze MT, Muul LM *et al.* A progress
report on the treatment of 157 patients with advanced
cancer using lymphokine activated killer cells and
interleukin 2 or high dose interleukin 2 alone. *New
England Journal of Medicine* 1987; **316**: 889–905.

80 Carswell EA, Old LJ, Kassel RJ, Green S, Fiore N,
Williamson B. An endotoxin-induced serum factor
that causes necrosis of tumours. *Proceedings of the
National Academy of Sciences USA* 1975; **72**:
3666–70.

3 Premalignant lesions

JD Langdon

The association of oral carcinoma and other oral mucosal lesions has been recognised for many years. Often these lesions are in the form of white plaques ('leukoplakia') or bright red velvety plaques ('erythroplakia'). They may be present for periods of months to years prior to the onset of malignant change and often they will be present together with the carcinoma at presentation. Because of this association the assumption was made that such lesions led directly to invasive carcinoma and hence were themselves premalignant.

Some white plaques do undoubtedly have a potential to undergo malignant transformation and an examination of established carcinomas will show many to exist in association with white plaques. However, the majority of oral carcinomas are not preceded by or are associated with leukoplakia.

Although historically oral 'leukoplakia' has been recognised as premalignant, the risk of malignant transformation is not as great as was previously thought. Early literature suggested a 30 per cent or higher incidence of malignant transformation of these lesions[1] whereas more recent authors quote an incidence of between 3 per cent and 6 per cent.[2–9] This difference is due to many factors. The most important of these factors is the many different criteria used by these authors to define leukoplakia. Some authors include any white patch on the oral mucosa whilst others define specific histological criteria for making such a diagnosis. However, despite this, many of these differences in the potential for leukoplakia to undergo malignant change are due to the decline in tobacco chewing and pipe smoking and also to the reduction in syphilitic glossitis.[10]

The following oral lesions are now definitely considered to carry a potential for malignant change:

Leukoplakia
Erythroplakia
Chronic hyperplastic candidiasis.

A further group of conditions, although not themselves premalignant, are associated with a higher than normal incidence of oral cancer:

Oral submucous fibrosis
Syphilitic glossitis
Sideropenic dysphagia.

The following lesions have in the past been mistakenly considered premalignant. There is, in fact, no such relationship:

Stomatitis nicotina (leukokeratosis nicotina palati)
Habitual cheek biting (pathomimia, morsicatio buccorum)
White sponge naevus (white folded gingivostomatitis, leukoedema exfoliativa).

There remains a further group of oral conditions about which there is still some doubt as to whether their association with oral cancer is causal or casual:

Oral lichen planus
Discoid lupus erythematosus
Dyskeratosis congenita.

Leukoplakia (Fig. 3.1)

Using the term leukoplakia either in a histological or clinical context is a matter of defining what one means by the term. The World Health Organization (WHO) have defined leukoplakia as 'any white patch or plaque that cannot be characterised clinically or pathologically as any other disease'.[11] This definition has no histological connotation.

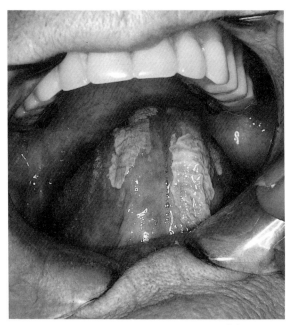

Fig. 3.1 Leukoplakia of the ventral aspect of the tongue in an 81 year old female.

Classifications

Attempts have been made to classify leukoplakia on the basis of clinical features, histological criteria and presumed aetiological factors. Banoczy[9] classified these lesions using clinical criteria as leukoplakia simplex (56 per cent), leukoplakia verrucosa (27 per cent) and leukoplakia erosiva (speckled leukoplakia). It is recognised that speckled leukoplakia, although comprising only 17 per cent of all leukoplakias, has the greatest potential for malignant change.

A histological classification was proposed in 1958 dividing the lesions into four groups:[12]

I   Epithelial hyperplasia (15 per cent)
II Superficial keratosis (31 per cent)
III A combination of hyperplasia and keratosis (18 per cent)
IV Epithelial dysplasia (36 per cent)

It is the final group which is associated with malignant change.

In 1977 Burkhardt and Seifert[13] proposed another histological classification dividing the lesions into flat, papillary–endophytic and papillomatous–exophytic at a microscopic level. A study by Hornstein in 1977[14] suggested a classification based upon aetiological considerations dividing the group into hereditary and endogenous–irritative lesions and into exogenous–irritative and precancerous lesions. These classifications have only limited clinical value.

Clinical features

Clinically leukoplakia may vary from a small circumscribed white plaque to an extensive lesion involving wide areas of the oral mucosa. The surface may be smooth or it may be wrinkled and many lesions are traversed by cracks or fissures. The colour of the lesion may be white, yellowish or grey with some being homogenous whilst others are nodular or speckled on an erythematous base. Many lesions are soft whereas other thicker lesions feel crusty. Induration suggests malignant change and is an indication for immediate biopsy. It is important to recognise that it is the speckled or nodular leukoplakias which are the most likely to undergo malignant change.[9,15,16]

Potential for malignant change

It has been shown that the incidence of ultimate malignant change in oral leukoplakia increases with the age of the lesion.[4] In their study Einhorn and Wersall[4] showed a 2.4 per cent malignant transformation rate at 10 years which increased to 4 per cent at 20 years. They also showed that as the age of the patient increases so does the risk of malignant transformation: for patients younger than 50 years it was 1 per cent whereas for those between 70 and 89 years it was 7.5 per cent during a 5 year observation period. It was conspicuous, incidentally, that in this very large study the rate of malignant change in oral leukoplakias was 10-fold higher in non-smokers than in smokers.

In a study of 257 patients with oral leukoplakia, Silverman *et al.*[17] reported a higher incidence – 17.5 per cent – of malignant change occurring at a mean time of 8.1 years, although half of these patients (8.7 per cent) showed epithelial dysplasia in their original biopsies. The study showed that non-smokers with the clinical presence of erythroplakia and verrucous/papillary pattern leukoplakia were particularly at risk of malignant transformation. It also confirmed that the duration of leukoplakia progressively increased the risk of malignant change. Banoczy[9] has shown that leukoplakia of the tongue showed the highest incidence of carcinomatous change. Kramer *et al.*[18] have shown that in southern England, leukoplakia of the floor of the mouth and ventral surface of the tongue has a particularly high incidence of malignant change. This study suggested that this occurrence was due to pooling of soluble carcinogens in the 'sump' of the floor of the mouth.

Aetiology

Tobacco smoking or chewing are undoubtedly important aetiological factors. Roed-Petersen *et al.*[19] showed that in Indians who smoked or chewed tobacco (often as a component of the betel quid) the incidence of leukoplakia in those of 60 years of age was 20 per cent whereas in those who neither smoked nor chewed tobacco the incidence was 1 per cent. A similar association was shown in Papua New Guinea by Pindborg *et al.*[15] Gupta *et al.*[10] have shown in a population of 36471 in India that if tobacco consumption can be reduced, the incidence of leukoplakia is also dramatically reduced.

The role of alcohol in the development of oral leukoplakia is difficult to assess. Few studies have been reported, but Wilsch *et al.*[20] found that in patients with leukoplakia the incidence of excessive alcohol consumption was greater than in those free of leukoplakia.

Bogdanowicz *et al.*[21] have demonstrated a high incidence of oral leukoplakia in a group of Polish workers in the rubber industry. In the former USSR, Smolyar and Granin[22] have shown a more than two-fold increase in the incidence of oral leukoplakia in workers exposed to soot dust.

Histology

The epithelium may or may not be hyperplastic and is often thinner than normal. The surface usually shows keratosis (although this may be slight), usually in the form of parakeratosis.

The plaque may show both hyperortho- and parakeratosis in different parts, and the two may alternate along the length of the specimen. A chronic inflammatory cellular infiltrate of highly variable intensity is usually present in the corium. In addition, the epithelium itself is characterised by any of the cytological changes of dysplasia. Such changes are as follows:

(1) *Nuclear hyperchromatism*. The nuclei stain more densely due to increased nucleic acid content.
(2) *Nuclear pleomorphism and altered nuclear/cytoplasmic ratio*. The nuclei vary in size but are out of proportion to the size of the cell; there

may then be little cytoplasm surrounding the nucleus.
(3) *Mitoses*. Mitoses may be frequent and may be at superficial levels.
(4) *Loss of polarity*. The basal cells in particular may lie higgledy-piggledy at angles to one another.
(5) *Deep cell keratinisation*. Individual cells may start to degenerate long before the surface is reached and show the characteristic eosinophilic change deeply within the epithelium. Strictly speaking, the term 'dyskeratosis' applies only to this particular cellular change.
(6) *Differentiation*. The organisation of the individual cell layers becomes lost and no clearly differentiated basal and spinous cell layers can be identified.
(7) *Loss of intercellular adherence*. The boundaries of the cells may become separated.

Management

In any patient presenting for the first time with oral leukoplakia a careful history – particularly looking for aetiological factors – and a detailed clinical examination should precede the histological examination of biopsies of any suspicious areas. The toluidine blue dye test is a guide in determining which areas to biopsy. Otherwise, suspicion is aroused by any areas of ulceration, induration or where the underlying tissues are bright red and hyperaemic.

If there is a history of tobacco consumption then the patient should be persuaded to stop immediately. It has been shown that if the patient stops smoking entirely for 1 year the leukoplakia will disappear in 60 per cent of the cases.[10,23,24]

Whenever severe epithelial dysplasia, or carcinoma-*in-situ* is present, surgical excision or CO_2 laser excision of the lesions is mandatory. Small lesions may be excised, the margins of the adjacent mucosa undermined and the defect closed by advancing the margins. For larger defects the area should be left to epithelialise spontaneously or alternatively the area can be skin grafted. On the tongue the graft is quilted onto the raw area[25] whereas on the cheek, floor of mouth or palate the graft can be retained in place by suturing a suitable pack overlying it.

When only mild to moderate epithelial dysplasia is present the patient should be followed up at 4 monthly intervals and the lesions recorded in the notes either photographically or diagramatically.

In those patients who already have had an oral carcinoma very careful follow up of any remaining leukoplakia is particularly important.[26]

Several authors have advocated cryosurgery in the treatment of oral leukoplakia.[27–29] Certainly in the short term the lesions heal with an apparently normal mucosa. However, Sako *et al.*[30] have shown a 33 per cent recurrence rate. More important are the anecdotal reports of the appearance of invasive carcinomas at the sites of previous leukoplakias treated by cryosurgery. It would seem that in those patients who develop an oral cancer there is often a widespread field change, and although the original leukoplakia may be totally destroyed by cryosurgery, the rapid proliferation of adjacent epithelial cells to resurface the cryolesion may be the very stimulus that turns an already unstable cell into a frankly neoplastic state.[31,32]

High doses of retinoids have been advocated for the treatment of oral leukoplakia and may achieve complete resolution of the lesions.[33–35] However, after discontinuing the retinoid therapy the lesions tend to recur.[36,37]

Koch in 1978[38] reported on a series of 75 patients treated for their oral leukoplakia with various analogues of retinoic acid. Initially more than 60 per cent of the cases treated showed some early improvement; however, over a 1 to 6 year follow up period only 45 per cent of the patients showed partial or complete remission. The remainder showed either relapse or progression of the leukoplakia. All the derivatives of retinoic acid tested showed undesirable side effects which either resulted in the discontinuation of treatment or a reduction in dosage.

Peto *et al.*[39] have reviewed the mounting evidence which suggests that retinoids and perhaps also carotenoids can be anticarcinogenic. It is as yet unclear whether these dietary substances are themselves active as cancer protecting agents or whether such diets as contain them are themselves cancer protecting.

In this respect it is interesting to note that Bichler *et al.*[40] have shown that in patients with established malignant tumours of the head and neck, the serum levels of retinol, retinol binding protein and prealbumin are significantly low. Several prospective studies are underway which should demonstrate whether retinoids are effective in reversing premalignant lesions and in preventing multiple cancers in patients who have already developed an index oral cancer.

Erythroplakia (Fig. 3.2)

Erythroplakia is defined as 'any lesion of the oral mucosa that presents as bright red velvety plaques which cannot be characterised clinically or pathologically as any other recognisable condition'.[11] Such lesions are usually irregular in outline although clearly demarcated from adjacent normal epithelium. The surface may be nodular. In some cases erythroplakia co-exists with areas of leukoplakia. Work by Waldren and Shafer[41] and Shafer and Waldren[42] has shown that the incidence of malignant change in erythroplakias is seventeenfold higher than in leukoplakia. These studies showed that in every case of erythroplakia there were areas of epithelial dysplasia, carcinoma-*in-situ* or invasive carcinoma. Clearly all erythroplakic areas must be completely excised either surgically or with a CO_2 laser and the specimens submitted for careful pathological examination.

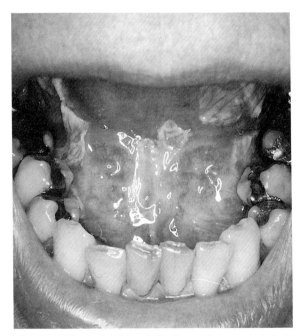

Fig. 3.2 Erythroplakia of the floor of the mouth in a 58 year old male.

Chronic hyperplastic candidiasis (Fig. 3.3)

Candida albicans is a normal oral commensal. Under certain circumstances the organism may be-

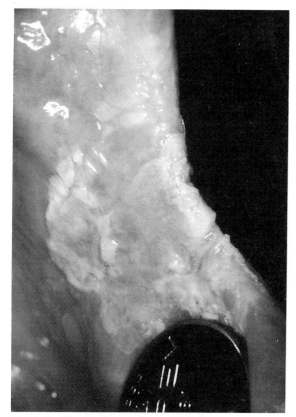

Fig. 3.3 Chronic hyperplastic candidiasis.

come pathogenic producing both acute and chronic infection. Acute oral candidiasis (thrush) is seen most commonly in the malnourished, the severely ill, the immunosuppressed, in patients taking broad-spectrum antibiotics or cytotoxic drugs, and in some denture wearers. The infected lesions may be localised or extremely widespread, the mucosa appearing red with white-yellow plaques that may be wiped off to reveal a haemorrhagic base. The plaques consist of a tangled web of *Candida* hyphae.

In chronic hyperplastic candidiasis, dense chalky plaques of keratin are formed, the plaques being thicker and more opaque than in non-candidal leukoplakia. Such candida-infected leukoplakias were described in 1965 by Cernea *et al.*[43] and Jepsen and Winther.[44] Such lesions are particularly common at the oral commissures extending onto the adjacent skin of the face.

In 1969 Cawson[45] drew attention to the high incidence of malignant transformation in these candidal leukoplakias, suggesting that the invasive candidal infection is the cause of the leukoplakia, and not merely a superimposed infection. It has also been suggested that in such patients there may be an immunological defect which allows the *Candida albicans* to invade the epithelium and may render the patient susceptible to malignant change.[46]

Burkhardt and Seifert[13] have shown that in areas of candidal leukoplakia there is an increased severity of epithelial dysplasia.

It is thought that treatment with nystatin, amphotericin or miconazole to eliminate the candidal infection will reduce the risk of malignant change. However, treatment may be necessary for many months to eliminate the organisms and re-infection is a constant problem.[47]

Oral submucous fibrosis (Fig. 3.4)

Oral submucous fibrosis is a progressive disease in which fibrous bands form beneath the oral mucosa. These bands progressively contract so that ultimately mouth opening is severely limited. Tongue movements may also be limited. The condition is almost entirely confined to Asians. Histologically it is characterised by juxta-epithelial fibrosis with atrophy or hyperplasia of the overlying epithelium which also shows areas of epithelial dysplasia.[48] Paymaster in 1956[49] first discussed the precancerous nature of submucous fibrosis. He noted the

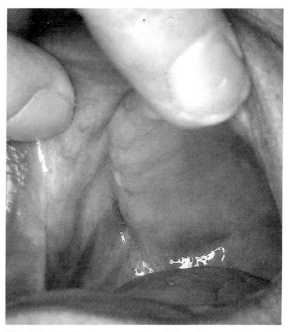

Fig. 3.4 Oral submucous fibrosis in a 47 year old female from India.

onset of a slowly growing squamous cell carcinoma in one-third of such patients. Pindborg in 1972[50] confirmed this observation. The aetiology is obscure. Hypersensitivity to chilli, betel nut, tobacco and vitamin deficiencies have been implicated. Canniff[51] has investigated the various enzyme components of the constituents of the 'betel quid' and has characterised some alkaloids and collagenases that may be responsible for the connective tissue changes which lead to epithelial atrophy and ultimate malignant degeneration. More recently Canniff *et al.*[52] have demonstrated a genetic predisposition to the disease involving the human leucocyte antigens (HLAs) A10, DR3, DR7 and probably B7 and the haplotypic pairs A10/DR3, B8/DR3 and A10/B8. Their tissue culture experiments have shown that alkaloids in the betel nut – particularly arecoline – stimulate collagen synthesis and the proliferation of buccal mucosal fibroblasts.[53] Tannins also present in the betel nut stabilise the collagen fibrils and render them resistant to degradation by collagenase.[54]

The scar bands of submucous fibrosis which result in difficulty in mouth opening can be treated either by intralesional injection of steroids or by surgical excision and grafting but this has little effect in preventing the onset of squamous cell carcinoma in the generally atrophic oral mucosa. Any aetiological factors should, of course, be eliminated.

Syphilitic glossitis

Prior to the antibiotic era, syphilis was an important predisposing factor in the development of oral leukoplakia and oral cancer.[1] Nielsen[55] showed a 19 per cent incidence of syphilis in patients with tongue cancer. This relation was later confirmed by Wynder *et al.*[56] The syphilitic infection produces an interstitial glossitis with an endarteritis which results in atrophy of the overlying epithelium. This atrophic epithelium appears to be more vulnerable to those other irritants which cause oral cancer or oral leukoplakia. As these changes are irreversible there is no specific treatment although active syphilis must be treated. Regular follow up is essential. It should be noted that squamous cell carcinomas may arise in syphilitic glossitis even in the absence of leukoplakia.

Sideropenic dysphagia (Plummer–Vinson syndrome, Paterson–Kelly syndrome)
(Fig. 3.5)

In 1936 Ahlbom[57] showed the relation between sideropenic dysphagia and oral cancer. Sideropenic dysphagia is particularly common in Swedish women, and this accounts for the high incidence of cancer of the upper alimentary tract in this group[58] and the higher incidence of women with oral cancer in Sweden.[59] Of women with oral cancer in Sweden, 25 per cent were sideropenic.

The pathogenesis of oral cancer in such patients may be similar to that of syphilitic glossitis. The sideropenic dysphagia leads to epithelial atrophy which in itself is excessively vulnerable to carcinogenic irritants. Although the anaemia will respond to treatment with iron supplements, it is not known whether such treatment reduces the risk of subsequent malignant change.

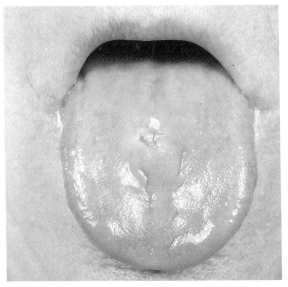

Fig. 3.5 Atrophic tongue in sideropenic dysphagia.

Oral lichen planus (Fig. 3.6)

There have been some reports that in erosive or atrophic lichen planus there is a risk of malignant transformation.[60] However, other authors have questioned the precancerous nature of oral lichen planus.[61,62] Krutchkoff *et al.*,[62] in their critical review of the literature, could only find 15 cases of

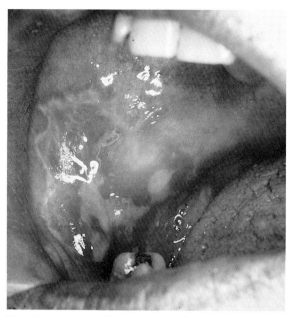

Fig. 3.6 Atrophic lichen planus of the buccal mucosa.

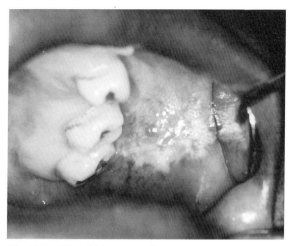

Fig. 3.7 Discoid lupus erythematosus.

oral cancer arising unequivocally from a pre-existing lichen planus. Silverman *et al.*[63] have shown a 1.2 per cent incidence of malignant change in a series of 570 patients with oral lichen planus followed up for a mean of 5.6 years.

Andreasen and Pindborg[64] consider that if there is an association between lichen planus and oral cancer the relation only exists with atrophic or erosive lichen planus. This view is confirmed by case reports from Tyldesley[65] and Marder and Deesen.[66] All patients with erosive or atrophic lichen planus should be carefully reviewed. Erosive lichen planus should be treated with topical steroids, and in severe cases systemic steroids may be necessary. Murti *et al.*[67] followed up a series of 722 patients with lichen planus over a 10 year period (mean observation time, 5.1 years). Three of their patients (0.4 per cent) developed carcinoma. All three patients had atrophic lesions and all were tobacco users.

Discoid lupus erythematosus
(Fig. 3.7)

The oral lesions of discoid lupus erythematosus consist of circumscribed, somewhat elevated white patches usually surrounded by a telangiectatic halo. Epithelial dysplasia may be seen on histological

examination and this may lead to malignant transformation. Andreasen[68] has quoted a 0.5 per cent incidence. Malignant change usually occurs in those lesions of the labial mucosa adjacent to the vermilion border and more often in men than in women. Such patients with discoid lupus erythematosus should be advised to avoid bright sunlight and when in the open air to apply an ultraviolet barrier cream to the lips. Acute exacerbations of the rash respond to the local application of steroids.

Dyskeratosis congenita (Fig. 3.8)

This syndrome is characterised by reticular atrophy of the skin with pigmentation, nail dystrophy and oral leukoplakia.[69] Eventually the oral mucosa becomes atrophic and the tongue loses its papillae. Finally the mucosa becomes thickened, fissured and white. Cannell[70] described carcinomatous changes in the palate of a patient with dyskeratosis congenita. He also warned that areas of erythroplakia may be present in such patients.

Stomatitis nicotina (leukokeratosis nicotina palati)
(Fig. 3.9)

Tobacco chewing or smoking can produce leukoplakia with a malignant potential as previously described. In addition to this a specific lesion may

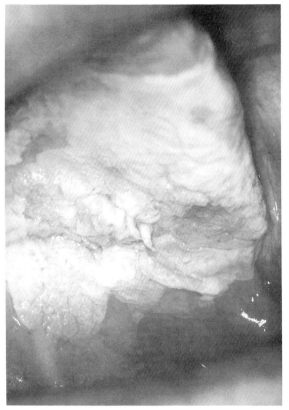

Fig. 3.8 Dyskeratosis congenita.

occur in the palates of very heavy smokers of cigars and pipes. Initially the palatal mucosa is reddened but subsequently becomes grey and wrinkled. In the mature lesion white umbilicated nodules with red centres appear at the sites of minor salivary glands. Where the palate is shielded by a denture these changes do not occur. There is no evidence that this lesion is precancerous. It resolves spontaneously if the patient stops smoking.

Habitual cheek biting (pathomimia, morsicatio buccorum) (Fig. 3.10)

In this condition areas of mucosal thickening with small irregular white flakes alternating with small red erosive areas occur on the buccal mucosa at the occlusal plane. The condition is usually bilateral, but one side may be predominantly involved. The lesions are usually more pronounced posteriorly. Occasionally the lower lip may be affected. This condition has no potential for malignant transformation. Its significance lies in the fact that it may readily mimic an ulcerative leukoplakia or erythroplakia.

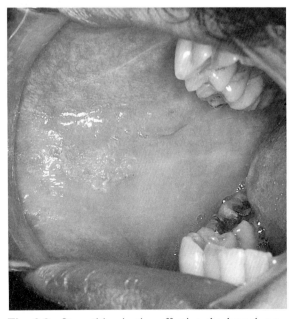

Fig. 3.9 Stomatitis nicotina affecting the buccal mucosa.

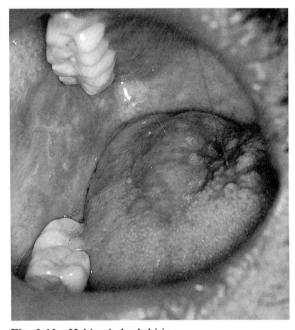

Fig. 3.10 Habitual cheek biting.

White sponge naevus (white folded gingivostomatitis, leucoedema exfoliativa) (Fig. 3.11)

This is an autosomal dominant hereditary condition. The oral lesion may be present at birth or it can appear during infancy, childhood or adolescence. The oral mucosa may be completely or partially involved. The lesion is white or grey and is seen as thickened, folded and spongy areas within the oral cavity. Again it is important to recognise the condition and reassure the patient as it has no malignant potential.

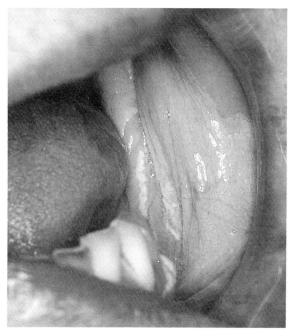

Fig. 3.11 White sponge naevus.

References

1 Hobaek A. Leukoplakia oris. *Acta Odontologica* 1946; **7**: 61–91.
2 Skach M, Svoboda O, Kubat S. A note on the question of leukoplakia. *Acta Universitatis Carolinae Medica* 1960; **10**: 363–71.
3 Mela F, Mongini F. Contributo cafistico allo studio delle leucoplachie orali. *Minerva Stomatologica* 1966; **15**: 502–7.
4 Einhorn J, Wersall J. Incidence of oral carcinoma in patients with leukoplakia of the oral mucosa. *Cancer* 1967; **20**: 2189–93.
5 Silverman S, Rozen RD. Observations on the clinical characteristics and natural history of oral leukoplakia. *Journal of the American Dental Association* 1968; **76**: 772–7.
6 Kramer IRH, Lucas RB, El-Labban N. A computer-aided study on the tissue changes in oral keratosis and lichen planus and an analysis of case groupings by subjective and objective criteria. *British Journal of Cancer* 1970; **24**: 407–26.
7 Mehta FS, Gupta PC, Daftary KK. An epidemiologic study of oral cancer and precancerous conditions among 101,761 villagers in Maharashtra, India. *International Journal of Cancer* 1972; **10**: 134–41.
8 Silverman, S, Bhargava K, Mani NJ. Malignant transformation and natural history of oral leukoplakia in 57,518 industrial workers in Gujarat, India. *Cancer* 1976; **38**: 1790–5.
9 Banoczy J. Follow-up studies in oral leukoplakia. *Journal of Maxillofacial Surgery* 1977; **5**: 69–75.
10 Gupta PC, Mehta FS, Pindborg JJ et al. Intervention study for primary prevention of oral cancer among 36,000 Indian tobacco users. *Lancet* May 1986; **31**: 1235–8.
11 WHO. Collaborating centre for oral precancerous lesions. Definition of leukoplakia and related lesions: an aid to studies in oral precancer. *Oral Surgery* 1978; **46**: 518–39.
12 Fasske E, Hahn W, Morgenroth K. Die leukoplakie der menschlichen mundschleimhaut. *Mittelungsdienst der Gesellschaft Bekampfen Krebsranke Nordrhein – Westfalen* 1958; **2**: 1–35.
13 Burkhardt A, Seifert G. Morphologische klassifikation der oralen leukoplakien. *Deutsche Medizinische Wochenschrift* 1977; **102**: 223–9.
14 Hornstein OP. Orale leukoplakien. 1. Klassifikation, differentialdiagnose, atiologische bedingungen der kanzensierung, prognose. *Deutsche Zahnaerztliche Zertschrift* 1977; **32**: 497–505.
15 Pindborg JJ, Barnes D, Roed-Petersen B. Epidemiology and histology of oral leukoplakia and leukoedema among Papuans and New Guineans. *Cancer* 1968; **22**: 379–84.
16 Silverman NA, Alexander JC, Hollinshead AC, Chretian PB. Correlation of tumour burden with *in-vitro* lymphocyte reactivity and antibodies to herpes virus tumour-associated antigens in head and neck squamous carcinoma. *Cancer* 1976; **37**: 135–40.
17 Silverman S, Gorsky M, Lozada F. Oral leukoplakia and malignant transformation. A follow-up study of 257 patients. *Cancer* 1984; **53**: 563–8.
18 Kramer IRH, El-Labban N, Lee KW. The clinical features and risk of malignant transformation in sublingual keratosis. *British Dental Journal* 1978; **144**: 171–80.
19 Roed-Petersen B, Gupta PC, Pindborg JJ. Association between oral leukoplakia and sex, age and tobacco habits. *Bulletin of the World Health Organization* 1972; **47**: 13–19.

20 Wilsch L, Hornstein OP, Bruning H. Orale leuko-plakie. II. Ergebnisse einer 1 jahrigen poliklinischen pilot studie. *Deutsche Zahnaerztliche Zeitschrift* 1978; **33**: 132–42.

21 Bogdanowicz W, Sebastyariska Z, Wajtuszkiewicz J. Wptyw czynnikow chemicznych na jame vitra u pra-cownikow spoldzielni 'chemi' W. Szizecinie. *Czasop-ismo Stomatologiczne* 1969; **22**: 705–8.

22 Smolyar MY, Granin AV. Precancerous lesions of the oral mucosa after contact with soot dust. *Stomatologia* 1971; **50**: 16–20.

23 Pindborg JJ. *Oral Cancer and Precancer*. Bristol: John Wright, 1980.

24 Mehta FS, Gupta MB, Pindborg JJ, Bonsle RB, Jal-nawalla PN, Sinor PN. An intervention study of oral cancer and precancer in rural Indian populations. *Bulletin of the World Health Organization* 1982; **60**: 441–6.

25 McGregor IA. 'Quilted' skin grafting in the mouth. *British Journal of Plastic Surgery* 1975; **28**: 100–2.

26 Moertel CG, Foss EL. Multicentric carcinomas of the oral cavity. *Surgery, Gynaecology and Obstetrics* 1958; **106**: 652–4.

27 Goode RL, Spooner TR. Office cryotherapy for oral leukoplakia. *Transactions of the American Academy of Ophthalmology and Otolaryngology* 1971; **75**: 968–73.

28 Hausamen JE. Kryochirurgische behandlung von leukoplakien der mundschleimhaut. *Deutsche Zahna-erztliche Zeitschrift* 1973; **28**: 1032–6.

29 Poswillo DE. Electrosurgery and cryosurgery. In: Cohen B, Kramer LHR eds. *Scientific Foundations of Dentistry*. London: Heinemann, 1976: 630–7.

30 Sako K, Marchetto FC, Hayes RL. Cryotherapy of intraoral leukoplakia. *American Journal of Surgery* 1972; **124**: 482–4.

31 Seward GR. The cryoprobe versus the surgical scalpel in the treatment of benign and malignant disease. *Annals of the Royal College of Surgeons of England* 1981; **63**: 311–12.

32 MacDonald DG, Shepherd DE, Critchlow HA. Influence of partial excision of carcinogen treated hamster cheek pouch on subsequent tumour develop-ment. *British Journal of Oral and Maxillofacial Surgery* 1986; **24**: 342–8.

33 Esser E, Tetsch P. Klinik and therapie der intraoralen leukiplakie. *Deutsche Zahn Mund und Keiferheilkunde mit Zentralblatt* 1973; **60**: 378–91.

34 Schettler D, Koch H. Langzeitbeobachtungen nach vitamin-A-saure-therapie bei leukoplakien der mundschleimhaut. In: Suchuchardt K, Pfeiffer G eds. *Grundlagen, Entwicklung und Fortschritte der Mund-Keifer-und Gesichts-Chirurgie*. Volume 21. Stuttgart: George Thieme, 1976: 179–80.

35 Schrey M, Esser E. Exfoliativzytologie im verlauf der lokalbehandlung der intraoralen leukoplakie mit vit-amin-A-saure. *Deutsche Zahnaerztliche Zeitschrift* 1978; **33**: 143–5.

36 Johnson JE, Ringsdorf WM, Chevaskin E. Relation-ship of vitamin A and oral leukoplakia. *Archives of Dermatology* 1963; **88**: 607–12.

37 Silverman S, Renstrup G, Pindborg JJ. Studies in oral leukoplakias. Ill effects of vitamin A comparing clinical, histopathologic, cytologic and haematologic responses. *Acta Odontologica* 1963; **21**: 271–92.

38 Koch HF. Biochemical treatment of precancerous oral lesions: the effectiveness of various analogues of retinoic acid. *Journal of Maxillofacial Surgery* 1978; **6**: 59–63.

39 Peto R, Doll R, Buckley JD, Sporn MB. Can dietary beta-carotene materially reduce human cancer rates? *Nature* 1981; **290**: 201–8.

40 Bichler E, Daxenbichler G, Marth C. Vitamin A status and retinoid-binding proteins in carcinomas of the head and neck region. *Oncology* 1983; **40**: 336–9.

41 Waldron CA, Shafer WG. Leukoplakia revisited. A clinico pathologic study of 3,256 oral leukoplakias. *Cancer* 1975; **36**: 1386–92.

42 Shafer WG, Waldron CA. Erythroplakia of the oral cavity. *Cancer* 1975; **36**: 1021–8.

43 Cernea P, Crepy C, Kuffer R. Aspects peu connus des candidoses buccales, les candidoses a foyers mul-tiples de la cavite buccale. *Revue de Stomatologie* 1965; **66**: 103–38.

44 Jepsen H, Winther JE. Mycotic infection in oral leu-koplakia. *Acta Odontologica* 1965; **23**: 239–56.

45 Cawson RA. Leukoplakia and oral cancer. *Proceed-ings of the Royal Society of Medicine* 1969; **62**: 610–15.

46 Lehner T, Wilton JMA, Shillitoe EJ. Cell-mediated immunity and antibodies to herpes virus hominis type 1 in oral leukoplakia and carcinoma. *British Journal of Cancer* 1973; **27**: 351–61.

47 Samaranayake LP, MacFarlane JW. A retrospective study of patients with recurrent chronic atrophic can-didosis. *Oral Surgery, Oral Medicine, Oral Pathology* 1981; **52**: 150–3.

48 Pindborg JJ, Sirsat SM. Oral submucous fibrosis. *Oral Surgery* 1966; **22**: 764–79.

49 Paymaster JC. Cancer of the buccal mucosa: a clinical study of 650 cases in Indian patients. *Cancer* 1956; **9**: 431–5.

50 Pindborg JJ. Is submucous fibrosis a precancerous condition in the oral cavity. *International Dental Journal* 1972; **22**: 474–80.

51 Canniff JP. *Factors influencing the persistence of in-traoral scar tissue*. Paper at British Association of Oral Surgeons, London, 1982.

52 Canniff JP, Harvey W, Harris M. Oral submucous fibrosis: its pathogenesis and management. *British Dental Journal* 1986; **160**: 429–34.

53 Harvey W, Scutt A, Meghji S, Canniff JP. Stimu-lation of human buccal mucosa fibroblasts *in vitro* by betel nut alkaloids. *Archives of Oral Biology* 1986; **31**: 45–9.

54 Kuttan R, Donnelly PV, Di Ferrante N. Collagen treated with catechin becomes resistant to the action

of mammalian collagenase. *Experientia* 1981; **37**: 221–3.

55 Nielsen J. Om cancer; de ovre luft-og spieseveje. *Tandlaegebladet* 1942; **46**: 1–23.

56 Wynder EL, Bross IJ, Feldman RM. A study of the aetiological factors in cancer of the mouth. *Cancer* 1957; **10**: 1300–23.

57 Ahlbom HE. Simple achlorhydric anaemia, Plummer Vinson syndrome and carcinoma of the mouth, pharynx and oesophagus in women. *British Medical Journal* 1936; **2**: 331–3.

58 Wynder EL, Hultberg S, Jacobsson F. Environmental factors in cancer of the upper alimentary tract. A Swedish study with special reference to Plummer–Vinson (Paterson–Kelly) syndrome. *Cancer* 1957; **10**: 470–82.

59 Larsson LG, Sandstrom A, Westling P. Relationship of Plummer–Vinson disease to cancer of the upper alimentary tract in Sweden. *Cancer Research* 1975; **35**: 3308–16.

60 Fulling HJ. Cancer development in oral lichen planus. *Archives of Dermatology* 1973; **108**: 667–9.

61 Shklar G. Lichen planus as an ulcerative disease. *Oral Surgery* 1972; **73**: 376–88.

62 Krutchkoff DJ, Cutler L, Laskowski S. Oral lichen planus: the evidence regarding potential malignant transformation. *Journal of Oral Pathology* 1978; **7**: 1–7.

63 Silverman S, Gorsky M, Lozada-Nur F. A prospective follow-up study of 570 patients with oral lichen planus: persistence, remission and malignant association. *Oral Surgery* 1985; **60**: 30–4.

64 Andreasen JO, Pindborg JJ. Cancerudirkling i oral-licken planus. *Nordisk Medicin* 1963; **70**: 861–6.

65 Tyldesley WR. Malignant transformation in oral lichen planus. *British Dental Journal* 1982; **153**: 329–30.

66 Marder MZ, Deesen KC. Transformation of oral lichen planus to squamous cell carcinoma. *Journal of the American Dental Association* 1982; **105**: 55–60.

67 Murti PR, Daftary DK, Bhonsle RB, Gupta PC, Mehta FS, Pindborg JJ. Malignant potential of oral lichen planus: observations in 722 patients from India. *Journal of Oral Pathology* 1986; **15**: 71–7.

68 Andreasen J. Oral manifestations in discoid and systemic lupus erythematosus. *Acta Odontologica Scandinavica* 1964; **22**: 295–310.

69 Gorlin RJ, Pindborg JJ, Cohen MM. *Syndromes of the Head and Neck*, 2nd edn. New York: McGraw-Hill, 1976.

70 Cannell H. Dyskeratosis congenita. *British Journal of Oral Surgery* 1971; **9**: 8–20.

4 Classification and staging

4a Mouth cancer and jaw tumours

JD Langdon

Introduction

A universally acceptable classification system for cancer of the oral cavity is essential for clinical research and prognostic determination. The aim of such a classification is to obtain homogenous statistically equivalent groups of patients for the purpose of assessing, evaluating and comparing various therapeutic approaches.[1] Another equally important purpose is the comparison of the efficacy of any given method of treatment in patients attending different hospitals.[2-4]

The first acceptable classification for malignant tumours was developed by Pierre Denoix.[5,6] This classification was based on the extent of the primary tumour (T), the regional node status (N) and the presence or absence of distant metastases (M). This TNM classification has been the basis for all later systems. In 1950 the Union Internationale Contre le Cancer (UICC) appointed a Committee on Tumour Nomenclature and Statistics. In the subsequent years meetings were held with various national groups and in 1958 the Committee published its first recommendations for clinical staging and classification (of breast and larynx). Between 1960 and 1967, nine further brochures were prepared covering twenty-three anatomical sites.

In 1968 the first 'livre de poche' summarizing the TNM classification of all sites was published.[7] Further editions were published in 1974 and 1978 containing site reclassifications and amendments.[8,9] The most recent edition – the fourth – was published in 1987.[10] The rules of classification and stage grouping now correspond exactly with those appearing in the third edition of the American Joint Committee on Cancer (AJCC) Manual for staging of cancer.[11]

Clearly for any classification system to be accepted it must have international recognition, thus the following organisations were consulted:

[AJCC]	The American Joint Committee on Cancer.
[BIJC]	The British Isles Joint TNM Classification Committee.
[CNC]	The Canadian National TNM Committee.
[CNU-TNM]	Comité Nacional Uruguayo TNM.
[DSK]	Deutschsprachiges TNM Komittee.
[EORTC]	The European Organization for Research on Treatment of Cancer.
[FIGO]	Fédération Internationale de Gynecologie et d'Obstetrique.
[FTNM]	The French TNM Group.
[ICC]	The Italian Committee for TNM Cancer Classification.
[JJC]	The Japanese Joint Committee.
[SIOP]	La Société International d'Oncologie Pediatrique.

The practice of dividing cancer cases into groups according to so-called 'stages' arose from the fact that survival times were longer for patients in which the disease was localised than for those in which the disease had extended beyond the organ of origin. Subsequent observation suggested that even for a tumour confined to its origin, the dimensions of the tumour also influenced the prognosis of the patient. These groups are often referred to as 'early cases' and 'late cases', implying some regular progression with time.

There are many bases for classification, such as the anatomical site and size of the tumour found on clinical examination, the reported duration of symptoms or signs, the gender and age of the patient and the histological type and grade. All of these variables are known to influence the outcome of the disease. Classification by anatomical extent of disease as determined clinically is the basis of TNM classification. By definition a TNM classification is a clinical classification and as such the information provided is entirely dependent upon the personal experience, opinions and skills of the examining clinician. When originally introduced the TNM classification had as its primary aim the provision of information regarding tumours affecting various sites accessible to clinical observation without additional diagnostic aids. This was achieved by recording the size and degree of infiltration of the primary tumour (T), the presence and condition of the associated regional lymph nodes (N) and the presence or absence of distant metastases (M). When carefully evaluated, these variables should give an indication of the prognosis and help the clinician in the choice of treatment.

After more than 10 years of research in this field the TNM classification, although extensively modified, faces the same essential problems that were inherent in the original method.[12] Is the examining clinician able to evaluate objectively the available clinical information with sufficient accuracy to describe the dimensions of the primary tumour and the presence and significance of the regional lymph nodes, and detect any possible metastases? Are these criteria sufficient to formulate a prognosis and, if so, how accurately? As much clinical cancer research is based upon retrospective rather than prospective studies, is the data recorded in traditional files sufficiently detailed and reliable?

Need for classification

Before the start of treatment for a patient with oral cancer, the patient's disease must be carefully evaluated. Clinical assessment includes an exhaustive history, physical examination and laboratory and radiological studies, the purposes of which are to determine the extent of the tumour and the presence or absence of demonstrable regional lymph nodes or distant metastases.

Every tumour should be biopsied and a histopathological diagnosis must be determined before the initiation of treatment.[13] Because cancers arising from different sites in the oral cavity have distinctive clinical features, courses and prognoses, an individual therapeutic approach must be tailored

for each patient.[14] The many therapeutic strategies that have been used in cancer of the head and neck suggest that a universally applicable form of treatment for a particular tumour in a specific stage of advancement in an individual patient is entirely dependent upon a meaningful comparison of the end results of similar cases reported from different centres.[1,15] For these reasons a classification system is essential, although at present an ideal system does not exist.

Every classification system has the same basic concept of grouping together homogenous and comparable elements for subsequent analysis. For reporting purposes it is desirable to group together those permutations of T, N and M for which there is a similar survival rate. The prime purpose of such staging is to determine what forms of treatment will most favourably alter the natural course of the disease and any staging procedure must correlate with the actual survival of the patients. The coordination of the data with particular TNM categories is based upon the clinical observation that patients with less extensive primary tumours have a longer survival time than those with extensive tumours.[16] Statistical surveys have emphasised the need for a more precise staging system for oral cancer, which if it could be applied universally to a large number of patients would be invaluable.[4,11,17]

Existing TNM classification and its limitations

In the most recent UICC-TNM classification two classifications are described for each tumour:[10]

(1) *Pretreatment Clinical Classification* (cTNM). This is based on evidence acquired prior to the decision as to definitive treatment. Such evidence arises from clinical, radiological and other investigations.
(2) *Postsurgical Histopathological Classification* (pTNM). This is based on the evidence given in point 1 above supplemented by the surgical findings and the examination of the therapeutically resected specimen. This presupposes that all treatment will be surgical!

As applied to the oral cavity, the TNM pretreatment classification is as follows:

T – Primary Tumour
TX Primary tumour cannot be assessed
TO No evidence of primary tumour

T1S Pre-invasive carcinoma (carcinoma-*in-situ*)
T1   Tumour 2 cm or less in its greater dimension
T2   Tumour more than 2 cm but no more than 4 cm in its greatest dimension
T3   Tumour more than 4 cm in its greatest dimension
T4   Tumour invades adjacent structures, e.g. through cortical bone, into deep (extrinsic) muscles of tongue, maxillary sinus, skin

N – Regional Lymph Nodes

NX   Regional lymph nodes cannot be assessed
N0   No regional lymph node metastasis
N1   Metastasis in a single ipsilateral lymph node 3 cm or less in its greatest dimension
N2   Metastasis in a single ipsilateral lymph node more than 3 cm but not more than 6 cm in its greatest dimension, or in multiple ipsilateral lymph nodes, none more than 6 cm in its greatest dimension
N2a Metastasis in a single ipsilateral lymph node more than 3 cm but not more than 6 cm in its greatest dimension
N2b Metastasis in multiple ipsilateral lymph nodes, none more than 6 cm in its greatest dimension
N2c Metastasis in bilateral or contralateral lymph nodes, none more than 6 cm in its greatest dimension
N3   Metastasis in a lymph node more than 6 cm in its greatest dimension

M – Distant Metastases

MX   Presence of distant metastasis cannot be assessed
M0   No distant metastases
M1   Distant metastases

The postsurgical histopathological classification uses the same categories for pT, pN and pM.

In addition a Histopathological Grading (G) has now been introduced:

GX   Grade of differentiation cannot be assessed
G1   Well differentiated
G2   Moderately differentiated
G3   Poorly differentiated
G4   Undifferentiated

The absence or presence of residual tumour after treatment is described by the symbol R:

RX   Presence of residual tumour cannot be assessed
R0   No residual tumour

R1   Microscopic residual tumour
R2   Macroscopic residual tumour

The stage grouping in this current UICC classification is as follows:

Stage 0	TIS	N0	M0
Stage I	T1	N0	M0
Stage II	T2	N0	M0
Stage III	T3	N0	M0
	T1, T2, T3	N1	M0
Stage IV	T4	N0, N1	M0
	Any T	N2, N3	M0
	Any T	Any N	M1

No account is taken of histopathological grading.

This most recent UICC-TNM classification, although a development of earlier systems, has now become so complicated that its value is in doubt. Many of the specific criteria are confusing. For example, no importance is attached to fixation of lymph nodes. Carcinomatous deposits in the regional lymph nodes from the primary lesion commonly occur in patients with oral cancer. Successful treatment of such spread requires a knowledge of lymphatic drainage and an awareness of the difficulties in the clinical assessment of the regional nodes. Considerable difficulty arises in making a clinical distinction between those palpable nodes considered to contain neoplasm and those considered to be enlarged due to reactionary hyperplasia or secondary infection. Where clinically involved nodes are present, the object is to devitalise or extirpate the neoplastic tissue in the knowledge that if these nodes remain untreated they will have an unfavourable influence upon the ultimate course of the disease. An understanding of the influence on prognosis of the site and size of the primary lesion, or homolateral or contralateral lymph node involvement, provides important guidelines for therapy.[18,19]

The variation between different individual clinicians' ability to assess the neck in terms of the TNM classifications adds further confusion.[20] The accuracy of clinical examination of the neck is between 70 and 80 per cent.[21-23] Three anatomical groups of lymph nodes appear to be important: the submental, the submandibular and the jugular chain. Cady and Catlin[21] evaluated the accuracy of detecting nodal involvement at various levels of the neck and found that the accuracy of physical examination of the jugular chain was 70 per cent but that it fell to 44 per cent when the submandibular and submental triangles were involved. This increased difficulty in the evaluation of nodal involvement in these areas is probably responsible for the higher incidence of clinical inaccuracy that Sako et al.[24] found (35 per cent) when only lesions of the mobile tongue and floor of the mouth were considered.

Staging

All graduations of prognosis can be demonstrated by grouping the patients on the basis of the size of the primary tumour (T), the presence or absence of involved nodes (N) and the presence or absence of distant metastases (M) into groups with a similar survival rate. In certain studies, when large numbers of patients are available for review, it may be desirable to subdivide the case material by these criteria. However, this can result in as many as thirty different permutations, with too few cases in any one group to allow statistical analysis. For reporting purposes it is desirable to group together those combinations of T, N and M for which there is a similar survival rate in order to restrict the total number of categories. The prime purpose of staging is that by knowing the prognosis, appropriate treatment can be selected which will most favourably alter the natural course of the disease. Any staging procedure must correlate with a reasonable spread of survival data.[2,4,15]

Development of a new classification and staging system

In an attempt to overcome the deficiencies of TNM classifications, their modifications and the present system of staging whereby various permutations of T, N and M are grouped together, an expanded classification applicable primarily to tumours of the oral cavity has been developed. An entirely new staging system which circumvents the problem of having large subgroups of the permutations of T, N and M and provides a more accurate indication of the prognosis is also suggested.

Clinical experience supported by statistical surveys shows that in order to make any reasonable assessment of a tumour in terms of its treatment and prognosis it is necessary to take into account the site of the lesion and its histology in addition to the more conventional TNM criteria.[4,12,15–17,25–30] Because of variations in local anatomy, the signifi-

cance of the size of the tumour differs according to the site. A lesion arising in the posterior third of the tongue will have a graver prognosis than a lesion of similar dimensions arising from the anterior third of the tongue. The majority of investigators recognise this as an important element and state that the TNM classification should be modified according to the anatomical site.[12,17,28–31] Others do not differentiate between lesions of similar size arising at different sites.[11,13,14,16,32] Hoopes,[15] and Anneroth et al.[33] have stated that it is desirable in individual studies to include information based upon histological study of the surgical specimen.

A new classification for intra-oral carcinomas is proposed consisting of S (site), T (tumour dimension), N (lymph node involvement), M (distant metastases) and P (histopathology).[34–36] The anatomical site of the primary tumour (S) has been subdivided into nine different categories as shown in Table 4a.1. As the depth of the infiltration of a tumour cannot be assessed clinically, T is based on a measurement of the maximum diameter of the tumour, plus its extension to involve adjacent structures (Table 4a.2). A new category of N has been introduced (Table 4a.3), which applies to those clinical cases where, although there is a palpable node, doubt remains as to whether this represents an extension of malignant disease. It is considered important to distinguish between suspected and proven metastases (M) (Table 4a.4). The histopathology (P) of the primary lesion is considered to be of great importance in the formation of a prognosis, and Table 4a.5 shows the subgroups utilised.

A new method of staging was developed on the basis of a retrospective analysis of 136 cases of squamous cell carcinoma (SCC) which were followed up for at least 5 years or until death. As a result of this analysis it was possible to estimate an arithmetic value for each of the variables, S, T, N,

Table 4a.1 STNMP: S Category

S (Site)	
S1	Lip – skin
S2	Lip – mucous membrane
S3	Tongue
S4	Cheek
S5	Palate
S6	Floor of mouth
S7	Alveolar process
S8	Antrum
S9	Central carcinoma of bone

Table 4a.2   STNMP: T Category

T (Tumour)

T1	Tumour less than 20 mm in diameter
T2	Tumour between 20 mm and 40 mm in diameter
T3	Tumour between 40 mm and 60 mm in diameter and/or extending beyond the primary region and/or through adjacent periosteum
T4	Any tumour greater than 60 mm in diameter and/or extending to involve adjacent structures

Table 4a.3   STNMP: N Category

N (Node)

N0	No palpable nodes
N1	Equivocal node enlargement
N2	Clinically palpable homolateral regional node(s) – not fixed
N3	As N2 but fixed
N4	Clinically palpable contralateral or bilateral node (s) – not fixed
N5	As N4 but fixed

Table 4a.4   STNMP: M Category

M (Metastases)

M0	No distant metastasis
M1	Clinical evidence of distant metastasis without definite histological and/or radiographic confirmation
M2	Proven evidence of metastases beyond the regional nodes

Table 4a.5   STNMP: P Category

P (Pathology)

P0	Hyperkeratotic lesion showing atypia
P1	Carcinoma-*in-situ*
P2	Basal cell carcinoma
P3a	Verrucous carcinoma
P3b	Well differentiated squamous cell carcinoma
P3c	Moderately differentiated squamous cell carcinoma
P3d	Poorly differentiated squamous cell carcinoma

Table 4a.6   STNMP weighting and stages

S		T		N		M		P	
S1	4	T1	0	N0	0	M0	0	P0	0
S2	6	T2	10	N1	10	M1	30	P1	5
S3	8	T3	20	N2	20	M2	40	P2	5
S4	10	T4	35	N3	30			P3a	5
S5	12			N4	40			P3b	10
S6	14			N5	40			P3c	15
S7	16							P3d	20
S8	18								
S9	20								

Stage I	0–30
Stage II	31–50
Stage III	51–70
Stage IV	70–155

nosis than a patient with a high score. For convenience and to enable direct comparison with TNM staging, the scores have been 'banded' to form equivalent stages, i.e. Stage I: 0–30; Stage II: 31–50; Stage III: 51–70 and Stage IV: 71–155. As a result of analysing the material it was found that the presence or absence of nodes (N) and distant metastases (M) carried the greatest prognostic significance. The site, histology and tumour dimension (S, P and T) carried equal but less significance than the presence or absence of enlarged nodes and/or metastases. By applying this staging system to the pilot study material it has been shown that this system offers many advantages and is better able to predict those patients whose prognosis is good. The information is important in planning the management of the primary lesion.

The STNMP classification has since been applied to a larger series of patients in comparison to the TNM classification. Table 4a.7 shows the distribution of this sample by stages together with the *crude* 5 year survival figures for each stage. Using

M and P (Table 4a.6). By summating the figures for each of these variables for a particular tumour a figure is arrived at which falls on a scale 0–155, a patient with a low total score having a better prog-

Table 4a.7   Distribution and *crude* 5 year survival figures comparing TNM and STNMP classifications

	TNM		STNMP	
	% of sample	*% 5 year survival*	*% of sample*	*% 5 year survival*
Stage I	17.7	50.0	30.8	51.5
Stage II	12.9	50.0	25.3	40.7
Stage III	61.3	26.3	32.7	21.6
Stage IV	8.1	20.0	11.2	8.3

STNMP it is apparent that nearly 31 per cent of the patients fall into Stage I, compared with approximately 18 per cent using TNM. Despite this difference the survival figures are similar, suggesting that when using TNM many patients are unnecessarily relegated to Stage II. Similarly, using STNMP many patients previously classified by TNM as Stage III are reclassified as Stage II and are seen to have better 5 year survival figures (Stage II, STNMP) than would be expected (Stage III, TNM).

Stage I (0–30 score) had a crude 5 year survival of 51.5 per cent; Stage II (31–50 score) a crude 5 year survival of 40.7 per cent; Stage III (51–70 score) a crude 5 year survival of 21.6 per cent and Stage IV (71–155 score) a crude 5 year survival of 8.3 per cent (Table 4a.7). These computations for survival were not corrected for the important influences of age and gender, and were based on all patients in the study irrespective of whether or not oral cancer was considered as the primary cause of death. A further study was undertaken to make these corrections, using appropriate statistical approaches and, on the basis of corrected figures, analyse the relative importance of the components of the STNMP system in predicting survival.[37] The predictive value of velocity of tumour growth was also assessed. The opportunity to update the original data by a further 2 years was taken and is included in the analysis.

The series of oral cancer patients on which the study is based have been described elsewhere,[38] together with the variables recorded and the way in which they were measured.

An entirely different statistical approach, utilising life tables, was used which allows the application of actuarial methods to the analysis of time of survival. The essential problem lies in the handling of incomplete survival times which arise for two reasons: first, the patient may still be alive at the time the analysis is performed; and second, the patient may have been alive when last seen but subsequently lost to follow up.

There have been two important advances in the analysis of data in this form; those described by Cox[39] and those by Peto and Peto.[40] The Cox method was employed here, in which incomplete survival times are known as 'censored' observations, the life tables in this context being known as 'clinical life tables'.[41] More details of the methods and their applications, together with reasons for preferring them to 5 year survival percentages are discussed by Evans.[42]

The method employed is able to use several different variables simultaneously as predictors of survival, hence the effect of, say, STNMP score, may be computed correcting for the effect of age. The method is analogous to that of multiple regression, but does not make many assumptions about the shape of the survival curves themselves. Regression co-efficients are computed, together with approximate standard errors which may be used to assess both the practical and statistical significance of the predictor variables.

Survival curves by Stage, utilising all causes of death including unknown causes, are illustrated in Fig. 4a.1. This shows the good separation achieved by the STNMP system.

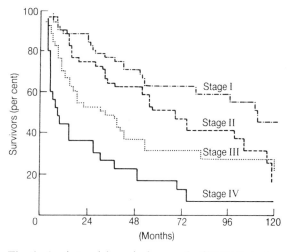

Fig. 4a.1   Actuarial survival curves by STNMP staging.

Velocity of tumour growth

In addition to the S, T, N, M and P variables a further variable, V, for velocity of tumour growth, was computed by dividing the area of the lesion by the time elapsed since symptoms were first noted. The area taken was three-quarters of length times breadth, a rough estimate of the area of an ellipse.

In the original study,[38] one of the variables recorded was the delay between onset of symptoms and the patient presenting at hospital for a definitive diagnosis. Even when this delay is not added to the survival time since diagnosis, the co-efficient for delay is always negative. This would suggest that a long delay is advantageous! A likely explanation for this observation is that a long delay is only possible when the velocity of growth is low and that a slowly growing tumour carries a better prognosis. The velocity of growth can be taken as the area of the tumour at presentation divided by the delay. This derived velocity of growth is more important than size at presentation or delay alone.

Discussion

The STNMP system is clearly a good indicator of prognosis and the present results make possible some weighting of the scores in order to further improve the system. However, it is suggested that before such changes are made, the STNMP system should be applied to a much larger, perhaps national, group of patients in a prospective study.

Although estimates of the delay between the first onset of symptoms and a definitive diagnosis being made are highly subjective (relying on the 'memory' of the patient), the velocity of a tumour shows some prognostic significance and a further study of this with a view to incorporating it in a STNMP*V* score may be worthwhile. Feinstein,[43] emphasises that it is more important to analyse relevant variables that may be difficult to measure reliably than it is to analyse reliable data that are irrelevant. 'The investigators who have neglected or abandoned this information [derived from talking to the patient] because it is scientifically "soft" have created the hazard of a clinical science that is "hard" but often irrelevant or erroneous'.

It is also important to remember that survival time is the only outcome variable studied; the quality of life may be at least as important to the patient and is a major factor in the clinician's decision making. The measurement of survival is easier than that of quality of life and it is tempting to ignore factors that are difficult to measure whatever their relevance.[42] However, even with this reservation the STNMP scoring system is an important predictor of survival and is a significant improvement over the TNM system of Schwab[44] (Table 4a.8).

Table 4a.8 Actuarial 5 year survival figures by Stage (oral cancer deaths only)

	TNM (%)	STNMP (%)
Stage I	77	78
Stage II	76	67
Stage III	44	36
Stage IV	20	20

Interestingly, Prime *et al.*[45] have recently shown that in cell lines established from oral cancers, data concerning the nuclear cytoplasmic ratio and serum dependence of the cell lines correlated with the STNMP grading of the original tumours.

Continuing efforts are being made to further refine these classifications and staging systems. Spiro *et al.*[46] and Urist *et al.*[47] have shown that tumour thickness is a more useful guide than conventional T stage in predicting subsequent nodal metastasis and survival. Several authors have demonstrated a worse prognosis for those tumours demonstrating aneuploidy in their DNA content and have suggested using DNA analysis as a prognostic factor.[48,49] Another approach used by Chauvel *et al.*[50] has been to use the thymidine labelling index to measure cells in the DNA synthesis phase. This has shown that tumours with a labelling index greater than 15.5 per cent have a significantly lower survival rate.

Great advances have been made in molecular biology in recent years and attempts have been made to link the expression of various oncogenes and tumour suppressor genes to tumour behaviour and outcome (see Chapter 2). To date, the most likely indicator is the presence of p53 (the product of a mutant tumour suppression gene) which seems to predict recurrence, nodal involvement and poor survival.[51]

References

1 Voss R. The importance of consistency in the classification of malignant tumours, illustrated by oral cancer material. *Journal of Maxillofacial Surgery* 1985; **13**: 154–7.

2 Black RJ, Gluckman JL. Staging systems for cancer of the head and neck region – comparison between AJC and UICC. *Clinical Otolaryngology* 1983; **8**: 305–12.

3 Schwab W, Schmeisser KJ, Steinhoff HJ, Mang WL. Directions for documentation of malignant tumours of the head and neck using the TNM system: a contribution to the validity of the TNM system. *HNO* 1985; **33**: 337–48.

4 Platz H, Fries R, Hudec M. *Prognosis of Oral Cavity Carcinomas: Results of a Multicentric Observational Study*. Munich: Carl Hanser, 1986.

5 Denoix PF. *Bulletin of the Institute of National Hygiene (Paris)* 1944; **1**: 1–69.

6 Denoix PF. *Bulletin of the Institute of National Hygiene (Paris)* 1944; **5**: 52–82.

7 Union Internationale Contre le Cancer. *TNM Classification of Malignant Tumours*, 1st edn. Geneva: UICC, 1968.

8 Union Internationale Contre le Cancer. *TNM Classification of Malignant Tumours*, 2nd edn. Geneva: UICC, 1974.

9 Union Internationale Contre le Cancer. *TNM Classification of Malignant Tumours*, 3rd edn. Geneva: UICC, 1978.

10 Union Internationale Contre le Cancer. *TNM Classification of Malignant Tumours*, 4th edn. Berlin: Springer-Verlag, 1987.

11 American Joint Committee for Cancer Staging and End Results Reporting. *Manual for Staging of Cancer*. Philadelphia, PA: Lippincott, 1992.

12 Spiessl B, von Albert J, Bitter K *et al*. Clinical examination on value determination of the TNM classification of the carcinoma of the buccal cavity. *Zeitschrift fur Krebsforsch I* 1973; **80**: 83–95.

13 Vermund H, Gollin RG. Role of radiotherapy in the treatment of cancer of the tongue. A retrospective analysis on TNM staged tumours treated between 1958 and 1968. *Cancer* 1973; **32**: 333–5.

14 Wang CC. The role of radiation therapy in the treatment of carcinoma of the oral cavity. *Otolaryngologic Clinics of North America* 1972; **5**: 357–63.

15 Hoopes JE. The TNM staging system. In: *Symposium on Cancer of the Head and Neck. Total Treatment and Reconstructive Rehabilitation*. St Louis, MO: CV Mosby, 1969.

16 Fries R, Grabener H, Langer H *et al*. Comparative investigation on the classification of carcinoma of the oral cavity. *Journal of Maxillofacial Surgery* 1973; **1**: 222–35.

17 Binnie WH, Cawson RA, Hill GB, Soaper AE. *Oral Cancer in England and Wales. A National Study of Morbidity, Mortality, Curability and Related Factors*. London: HMSO, 1972.

18 DiTrioa JF. Nodal metastases and prognosis in carcinoma of the oral cavity. *Otolaryngolic Clinics of North America* 1972; **5**: 333–42.

19 Snow GB, Annyas AA, van Slooten EA, Bartelink H, Hart AAM. Prognostic factors of neck node metastasis. *Clinical Otolaryngology* 1982; **7**: 185–92.

20 Maw RA. An assessment of treatment methods for carcinoma of the larynx presenting with cervical lymph nodes. *Proceedings of the Royal Society of Medicine* 1975; **63**: 80–3.

21 Cady B, Catlin D. Epidermoid carcinoma of the gum: a 20 year survey. *Cancer* 1969; **23**: 551–69.

22 Spiro RJ, Frazell EL. Evaluation of radical surgical treatment of advanced cancer of the mouth. *American Journal of Surgery* 1968; **116**: 571–7.

23 Ali S, Tiwari RM, Snow GB. False positive and false negative neck nodes. *Head and Neck Surgery* 1985; **8**: 78–82.

24 Sako L, Pradier RN, Marchetto FC, Pickren JW. Fallibility of palpation in the diagnosis of metastases to cervical nodes. *Surgery, Gynaecology and Obstetrics* 1964; **118**: 989–90.

25 Fayos JV, Lampe I. Treatment of squamous cell carcinoma of the oral cavity. *American Journal of Surgery* 1972; **124**: 493–500.

26 Fayos JV, Lampe I. The therapeutic problem of metastatic neck adenopathy. *American Journal of Roentgenology* 1972; **114**: 65–75.

27 Skolnik EM, Campbell JM, Meyers RM. Carcinoma of the buccal mucosa and retromolar area. *Otolaryngologic Clinics of North America* 1972; **5**: 327–31.

28 Sakai S, Masaki N. Proposals for the TNM classifications and its extended application for malignant tumours of the head and neck regions. *Acta Otolaryngologica* 1971; **72**: 370–6.

29 Sakai S, Shigematzu Y, Fuchihate H. Diagnosis and TNM classification of maxillary sinus carcinoma. *Acta Otolaryngologica* 1971; **74**: 123–9.

30 Westbrook KC. Evaluation of patients with head and neck cancer. In: *Neoplasia of Head and Neck*. Chicago, IL: Yearbook Medical Publishers, 1974.

31 Moss TW, Brand WN, Battifora N. *Radiation Oncology: Rationale, Technique, Results*, 4th edn. St Louis, MO: CV Mosby, 1973.

32 Vermund H, Rappaport I, Nethery WJ. Role of radiotherapy in the treatment of cancer. *Journal of Oral Surgery* 1974; **32**: 690–5.

33 Anneroth G, Hansen LS, Silverman S. Malignancy grading in squamous cell carcinoma. *Journal of Oral Pathology* 1986; **15**: 162–8.

34 Rapidis AD, Langdon JD, Patel MF, Harvey PW. Clinical classification and staging in oral cancer. *Journal of Maxillofacial Surgery* 1976; **4**: 219–26.

35 Rapidis AD, Langdon JD, Patel MF, Harvey PW. STNMP a new system for the clinico-pathological classification and identification of intra-oral carcinomata. *Cancer* 1977; **39**: 204–9.

36 Langdon JD, Rapidis AD, Harvey PW, Patel MF. STNMP – a new classification for oral cancer. *British Journal of Oral Surgery* 1977; **15**: 49–54.

37 Evans SJW, Langdon JD, Rapidis AD, Johnson NW. Prognostic significance of STNMP and velocity of tumour growth in oral cancer. *Cancer* 1982; **49**: 773–6.

38 Langdon JD, Harvey PW, Rapidis AD, Patel MF, Johnson NW, Hopps R. Oral cancer: the behaviour and response to treatment of 194 cases. *Journal of Maxillofacial Surgery* 1977; **5**: 221–37.

39 Cox DR. Regression models and life tables. *Journal of the Royal Statistical Society* 1972; **34**: 187–220.

40 Peto R, Peto J. Asymptotically efficient rank in varient test procedures. *Journal of the Royal Statistical Society (A)* 1972; **135**: 185–206.

41 Peto R, Pike MC, Armitage P *et al*. Design and analysis of randomised clinical trials requiring prolonged observation of each patient. *British Journal of Cancer* 1977; **34**: 586–612.

42 Evans SJW. *Survival of patients with oral cancer*, MSc thesis. University of London, 1978.

43 Feinstein AR. *Clinical Biostatistics*. St Louis, MO: CV Mosby, 1977.

44 Schwab W. Zur klassifizierung und dokumentation bosartiger geschwulste im hals-nasen-ohrenbe-reich unter beruckichtigung der richtlinien der UICC (TNM system). *Zeitschrift fur Laryngologie und Rhinologie* 1968; **47:** 21–41.

45 Prime SS, Nixon SVR, Crane IJ *et al.* The behaviour of human squamous cell carcinoma in cell culture. *Journal of Pathology* 1990; **160:** 259–369.

46 Spiro RH, Huvos AG, Wong GY, Spiro JD, Gnecco CA, Strong EW. Predictive value of tumour thickness in squamous cell carcinoma confined to the tongue and floor of mouth. *American Journal of Surgery* 1986; **152:** 345–50.

47 Urist MM, O'Brien CJ, Soong SJ, Visscher DW, Maddox A. Squamous cell carcinoma of the buccal mucosa: analysis of prognostic factors. *American Journal of Surgery* 1987; **154:** 411–14.

48 Kokal WA, Gardine RL, Sheibani K *et al.* Tumour DNA content as a prognostic indicator in squamous cell carcinoma of the head and neck region. *American Journal of Surgery* 1988; **156:** 276–80.

49 Ogden GR, Cowpe JG. Quantitative cytophotometric analysis as an aid to the detection of recurrent oral cancer. *British Journal of Oral and Maxillofacial Surgery* 1989; **27:** 224–8.

50 Chauvel P, Courdi A, Gioanni J, Valliconi J, Santini J, Dermard F. The labelling index: a prognostic factor in head and neck carcinoma. *Radiology and Oncology* 1989; **14:** 231–7.

51 Langdon JD, Partridge M. Expression of the tumour suppressor gene p53 in oral cancer. *British Journal of Oral and Maxillofacial Surgery* 1992; **30:** 214–20.

4b   World Health Organization classification and staging – salivary tumours

JW Eveson

The first World Health Organization (WHO) Histological Typing of Salivary Gland Tumours was published in 1972[1] and received widespread acceptance by surgical pathologists and clinicians (Table 4b.1). Although this classification has the merit of simplicity, since its publication much has been learnt about new tumour entities and the behaviour of various tumour subtypes. In order to incorporate the advances in knowledge into an updated, but hopefully practical tumour classification, a new international group of pathologists with particular interests and expertise in salivary gland tumours was established in 1987 on the initiative of Dr Sobin, Head of the WHO Collaborating Centre for International Histological Classification of Tumours. The co-ordinator was Dr Seifert/Germany and the group included Dr Batsakis/USA; Dr Brocheriou/France; Dr Dardick/Canada; Dr Ellis/USA; Dr Eveson/UK; Dr Gusterson/UK in collaboration with Dr Cardesa/Spain; and Dr Shanmugaratnam/Singapore (Head of WHO Collaborating Centre for the Histological Classification of Upper Respiratory Tracts Tumours).

As a result of the deliberations of this panel, the

Table 4b.1   First World Health Organization classification of salivary gland tumours (1972)

I EPITHELIAL TUMOURS

A   ADENOMAS
  1   Pleomorphic adenoma (mixed tumour)
  2   Monomorphic adenomas
    (a) Adenolymphoma
    (b) Oxyphilic adenoma
    (c) Other types

B   MUCOEPIDERMOID TUMOUR

C   ACINIC CELL TUMOUR

D   CARCINOMAS
  1   Adenoid cystic carcinoma
  2   Adenocarcinoma
  3   Epidermoid carcinoma
  4   Undifferentiated carcinoma
  5   Carcinoma in pleomorphic adenoma (malignant mixed tumour)

II NON-EPITHELIAL TUMOURS

III UNCLASSIFIED TUMOURS

IV ALLIED CONDITIONS

A   BENIGN LYMPHOEPITHELIAL LESION

B   SIALOSIS

C   ONCOCYTOSIS

---

proposed revision of the WHO classification was published in 1990.[2]

The official classification was published in the series *International Histological Classification of Tumours* by Springer-Verlag in 1991.[3]

One of the principles behind the revised classification was that clearly defined entities, even though uncommon or rare, should be included. This has inevitably meant that the new classification is considerably longer. However, it was considered that the wider range of diagnostic options, many of which have prognostic implications, would aid rather than hinder pathologists and also reflect the morphological diversity of this difficult but fascinating group of tumours. It was hoped that the classification would thus be useful to practising surgical pathologists who will have limited experience with this group of tumours due to their relative rarity.

The classification was divided into six main groups:

(1) Adenomas
(2) Carcinomas
(3) Non-epithelial tumours
(4) Lymphomas
(5) Secondary tumours
(6) Tumour-like conditions

The opportunity was taken to rationalise some of the terminology, particularly in the intermediate tumours such as acinic and mucoepidermoid which are now classified as carcinomas, albeit of variable degrees of malignancy. Several other minor modifications in terminology were instituted and there were major reviews of the monomorphic adenoma and carcinoma subtypes.

The revised classification is shown in Table 4b.2.

In the first WHO classification the major division in the benign tumours was between pleomorphic adenoma and monomorphic adenomas. However, many monomorphic adenomas are neither monomorphic nor monocellular and the all-embracing term 'other monomorphic adenomas' was considered to be unsatisfactory.

Thus, in the new classification clearly defined

Table 4b.2 Revised World Health Organization classification of salivary gland tumours (1991)

1	**Adenomas**	
1.1	Pleomorphic adenoma	8940/0*
1.2	Myoepithelioma (myoepithelial adenoma)	8982/0
1.3	Basal cell adenoma	8147/0
1.4	Warthin's tumour (adenolymphoma)	8561/0
1.5	Oncocytoma (oncocytic adenoma)	8290/0
1.6	Canalicular adenoma	
1.7	Sebaceous adenoma	8410/0
1.8	Ductal papilloma	8503/0
1.8.1	Inverted ductal papilloma	8503/0
1.8.2	Intraductal papilloma	8503/0
1.8.3	Sialadenoma papilliferum	8260/0
1.9	Cystadenoma	8440/0
1.9.1	Papillary cystadenoma	8450/0
1.9.2	Mucinous cystadenoma	8470/0
2	**Carcinomas**	
2.1	Acinic cell carcinoma	8550/3
2.2	Mucoepidermoid carcinoma	8430/3
2.3	Adenoid cystic carcinoma	8200/3
2.4	Polymorphous low grade adenocarcinoma (terminal duct adenocarcinoma)	
2.5	Epithelial–myoepithelial carcinoma	8562/3
2.6	Basal cell adenocarcinoma	8147/3
2.7	Sebaceous carcinoma	8410/3
2.8	Papillary cystadenocarcinoma	8450/3
2.9	Mucinous adenocarcinoma	8480/3
2.10	Oncocytic carcinoma	8290/3
2.11	Salivary duct carcinoma	8500/3
2.12	Adenocarcinoma	8140/3
2.13	Malignant myoepithelioma (myoepithelial carcinoma)	8982/3
2.14	Carcinoma in pleomorphic adenoma (malignant mixed tumour)	8941/3
2.15	Squamous cell carcinoma	8070/3
2.16	Small cell carcinoma	
2.17	Undifferentiated carcinoma	
2.18	Other carcinomas	
3	**Non-epithelial tumours**	
4	**Malignant lymphomas**	
5	**Secondary tumours**	
6	**Unclassified tumours**	
7	**Tumour-like lesions**	
7.1	Sialadenosis (sialosis)	71000
7.2	Oncocytosis	73050
7.3	Necrotising sialometaplasia (salivary gland infarction)	73220
7.4	Benign lymphoepithelial lesion	72240
7.5	Salivary duct cysts	33400
7.6	Chronic sclerosing sialadenitis of submandibular gland (Kuttner tumour)	45000
7.7	Cystic lymphoid hyperplasia in AIDS	

*Morphology code of the International Classification of Diseases for Oncology (ICD-O) and the Systematised Nomenclature of Medicine (SNOMED). AIDS, acquired immune deficiency syndrome.

tumours were categorised separately. Although 'myoepithelioma' is somewhat controversial and similar areas can be seen in pleomorphic adenomas, it was felt that myoepithelioma was a universally recognised variant and should be considered separately.[4] The term Warthin's tumour was adopted in preference to adenolymphoma as some of these tumours have ended up coded as lymphomas in tumour registries. Within the other adenomas it should be stressed that typical oncocytomas are extremely uncommon and many tumours diagnosed as such are merely oncocytic variants of other tumour types.[5,6] The basal cell adenoma group is heterogeneous[2] and canalicular adenomas are a distinctive tumour of minor salivary glands, particularly the upper lip.[7]

In the carcinomas there have been changes in terminology and a considerable expansion of the various subtypes. The most important recently recognised of these are the polymorphous low-grade adenocarcinoma,[8] epithelial–myoepithelial carcinoma[9] and salivary duct carcinoma.[10,11]

The polymorphous low-grade adenocarcinoma has also been called a terminal duct carcinoma,[12] and lobular carcinoma.[13] It is essentially a tumour of minor glands and is characterised by cytological uniformity and morphological diversity. The epithelial cells are isomorphic, with pale, uniform nuclei and faintly eosinophilic cytoplasm. Mitoses are infrequent. The tumour is usually clearly infiltrative and shows a variety of morphological patterns including theques, small duct-like structures, cribriform and papillary areas. There is often a striking tendency to show perineural and sometimes periductal whorling which, together with some of the other features, leads to an erroneous diagnosis of adenoid cystic carcinoma. The distinction is important as the polymorphous adenocarcinoma has a particularly good prognosis and the perineural involvement which appears alarming, rarely spreads far beyond the main tumour mass.

The epithelial–myoepithelial carcinoma,[9] also known as an intercalated duct carcinoma, is an important tumour as in the past it was thought to be an adenoma and was given a variety of names including clear cell adenoma and glycogen rich adenoma. It consists of two cell types in varying proportions. There is an inner dark-staining duct cell and outer clear cells which have been shown to be myoepithelial in type.[14] Sometimes the duct lining cells are extremely scanty and an initial diagnosis of a clear cell tumour is made. Despite the rather bland cytology of these tumours perineural

and vascular invasion, together with recurrence and metastasis, are not uncommon.

The salivary duct carcinoma appears to arise from large ducts and morphologically resembles duct carcinoma of the breast. A variety of appearances have been described, the most common being comedo necrosis, cribriform patterns or papillary areas. A striking desmoplastic stromal response is common. Nuclear and cytoplasmic atypia are variable but can be extreme. Intra- and extrasalivary gland spread and regional metastases are common and the prognosis is extremely poor.

Other named carcinomas are rare and include basal cell adenocarcinoma (the malignant counterpart of basal cell adenoma),[15] sebaceous carcinoma,[16] oncocytic carcinoma[6] and papillary cystadenocarcinoma. It is worthwhile emphasising that most papillary salivary gland tumours apart from Warthin's tumour, even when cytologically bland, turn out to be adenocarcinomas. Myoepithelial carcinoma is very rare.[17]

TNM classification

The anatomical distribution and extent of salivary gland carcinoma has a significant impact on the clinical outcome. The TNM classification is a system which enables at least a semiquantitative recording of cases and monitoring of the extent of disease and provides a basis for comparing data.[18]

Rules of the TNM classification

In the salivary glands the TNM classification applies only to carcinomas of the major glands (1CD-0C07, C08); the parotid (C07) submandibular (C08.0) and sublingual (C08.1) glands. The tumour size (T), regional (cervical) lymph nodes (N) and distant metastases (M) can be assessed by physical examination or by imaging (computed tomography or magnetic resonance imaging scans).

In addition it is possible to use a postsurgical histopathology based classification (pTNM) with measurements based on resected specimens with equivalent categories, i.e. pT, pN and pM.

Staging is based on defined grouping of the TNM categories:

TNM clinical classification
T – Primary Tumour
TX Primary tumour cannot be assessed
T0 No evidence of primary tumour

T1 Tumour 2 cm or less in its greatest dimension
T2 Tumour more than 2 cm but not more than 4 cm in its greatest dimension
T3 Tumour more than 4 cm but not more than 6 cm in its greatest dimension
T4 Tumour more than 6 cm in its greatest dimension

All the above categories are subdivided into:

(a) no local extension;
(b) evidence of local extension such as clinical or macroscopical evidence of invasion into skin, soft tissue, bone or nerves. Microscopical evidence of local invasion is not utilised in this part of the classification.

N – Regional Lymph Nodes

NX Regional lymph node cannot be assessed
N0 No regional lymph node metastasis
N1 Metastasis to a single ipsilateral lymph node, 3 cm or less in its greatest dimension
N2 Metastasis in a single ipsilateral lymph node, more than 3 cm but not more than 6 cm in its greatest dimension, or in multiple ipsilateral nodes, none more than 6 cm in its greatest mension, or in bilateral or contralateral lymph nodes, none more than 6 cm in its greatest dimension
N2a Metastasis in a single ipsilateral lymph node, more than 3 cm but not more than 6 cm in its greatest dimension
N2b Metastasis in multiple ipsilateral lymph nodes, none more than 6 cm in its greatest dimension
N2c Metastasis in bilateral or contralateral lymph nodes, none more than 6 cm in its greatest dimension
N3 Metastasis in a lymph node more than 6 cm in its greatest dimension

Midline lymph nodes such as the submental and prelaryngeal nodes are considered to be ipsilateral.

M – Distant Metastases

MX Presence of distant metastases cannot be assessed
M0 No distant metastases
M1 Distant metastases

Stage grouping

Stage I	T1a	N0	M0
	T2a	N0	M0
Stage II	T1b	N0	M0
	T2b	N0	M0
	T3a	N0	M0
Stage III	T3b	N0	M0
	T4a	N0	M0
	Any T (except T4b)	N1	M0
Stage IV	T4b	Any N	M0
	Any T	N2,N3	M0
	Any T	Any N	M1

Possibly because of the large range of histological diversity in salivary gland tumours and the fact that some of the benign tumours can end with a clinically aggressive course, the usefulness and use of the TNM classification has been limited. However, in some of the tumour types criteria such as size have been shown to have prognostic significance and application of the TNM system to the salivary tumours may have more practical merit than is generally appreciated.

Jaw tumours

A similar problem arises with malignant jaw tumours. The suggested TNM classification is that applied to bone tumours in general and takes no account of odontogenic and non-odontogenic types. It cannot usefully be applied to jaw tumours.

References

1 Thackray AC, Sobin LH. *Histological Typing of Salivary Gland Tumours*. Geneva: World Health Organization, 1972.
2 Seifert G, Brocheriou C, Cardesa A, Eveson JW. WHO International Histological Classification of Tumours. Tentative histological classification of salivary gland tumours. *Pathology Research and Practice* 1990; **186**: 555–81.
3 Seifert G. *WHO International Histological Classification of Tumours. Histological Typing of Salivary Gland Tumours*. Berlin: Springer-Verlag, 1991.
4 Mori M, Ninomiya T, Okada Y, Tsukitani K. Myoepithelioma and myoepithelial adenomas of salivary gland origin. *Pathology Research and Practice* 1989; **184**: 168–78.
5 Palmer TJ, Gleeson MJ, Cawson RA, Eveson JW. Oncocytic adenomas and oncocytic hyperplasia of salivary glands. A clinicopathological study of 26 cases. *Histopathology* 1990; **16**: 487–93.

6 Brandwein MS, Huvos AG. Oncocytic tumors of major salivary glands. A study of 68 cases with follow-up of 44 patients. *American Journal of Surgical Pathology* 1991; **15**: 514–28.

7 Daley TD, Gardner DG, Smout MS. Canalicular adenoma: not a basal cell adenoma. *Oral Surgery, Oral Medicine, Oral Pathology* 1984; **57**: 181–8.

8 Gnepp DR, Chen JC, Warren C. Polymorphous low-grade adenocarcinoma of minor salivary gland: an immunohistochemical and clinicopathologic study. *American Journal of Surgical Pathology* 1988; **12**: 461–8.

9 Hamper K, Brugmann M, Koppermann R *et al*. Epithelial–myoepithelial duct carcinoma of salivary glands: a follow-up and cytophotometric study of 21 cases. *Journal of Oral Pathology and Medicine* 1989; **18**: 299–304.

10 Hui KK, Batsakis JG, Luna MA, Mackay B, Byers RM. Salivary duct adenocarcinoma: a high grade malignancy. *Journal of Laryngology and Otology* 1986; **100**: 105–14.

11 Batsakis JG, Luna MA. Low-grade and high-grade adenocarcinomas of the salivary duct system. *Annals of Otology, Rhinology and Laryngology* 1989; **98**: 162–3.

12 Batsakis JG, Pinkston GR, Luna MA *et al*. Adenocarcinoma of the oral cavity: a clinicopathologic study of terminal duct carcinomas. *Journal of Laryngology and Otology* 1983; **97**: 825–35.

13 Freedman PD, Lumerman H. Lobular carcinoma of intraoral minor salivary gland origin. Report of twelve cases. *Oral Surgery, Oral Medicine, Oral Pathology* 1983; **56**: 157–65.

14 Palmer RM. Epithelial–myoepithelial carcinoma: an immunocytochemical study. *Oral Surgery, Oral Medicine, Oral Pathology* 1985; **59**: 511–15.

15 Ellis GL, Wiscovitch JG. Basal cell adenocarcinomas of the major salivary glands. *Oral Surgery, Oral Medicine, Oral Pathology* 1970; **69**: 461–9.

16 Gnepp DR, Brannon R. Sebaceous neoplasms of salivary gland origin. Report of 21 cases. *Cancer* 1984; **53**: 2155–70.

17 Singh R, Cawson RA. Malignant myoepithelial carcinoma (myoepithelioma) arising in a pleomorphic adenoma of the parotid glands. *Oral Surgery, Oral Medicine, Oral Pathology* 1988; **66**: 65–70.

18 Hermanek P, Sobin LH. *TNM Classification of Malignant Tumours*, 4th edn. Union Internationale Contre le Cancer. Berlin: Springer-Verlag, 1987; 30–2.

5 Clinical presentation and diagnosis of oral cancer

JD Langdon

Early diagnosis of oral cancer should lead to better treatment results and ideally the clinical diagnosis of oral cancer should be easy. Also, a high proportion of the population in the Western hemisphere are regular attenders at the dentist, and the oral cavity is readily examined and requires no special facilities. Oral lesions, unlike those at many other sites, give rise to early symptoms. In general patients become aware of and usually complain about minute lesions within the mouth and biopsy may be carried out under local analgesia. Yet, despite all the above, between 27 per cent and 50 per cent of patients present for treatment with late lesions.[1,2] This delay in diagnosis and treatment has been analysed by Cooke and Tapper-Jones[3] and Scully *et al.*[4] They cite the fact that many of these patients are elderly and frail and, therefore, delay the effort of visiting their doctor or dentist. Many of this group of patients wear dentures and are accustomed to discomfort and ulceration in the mouth and thus see no urgency in seeking treatment. Furthermore, the practitioner himself is often not suspicious that a lesion may be malignant and the lesion is often treated initially with anti-fungal therapy, antibiotics, steroids and mouthwashes thus contributing to further delay in the ultimate diagnosis and treatment. Another factor is that oral cancer is not usually painful until such time as either the ulcer becomes secondarily infected or the tumour invades sensory nerve fibres.

It has been widely stated that general medical practitioners are more likely to fail to make the correct diagnosis on the first visit than dental practitioners, but Scully *et al.*[4] have refuted this. It is only by being constantly suspicious that the 'front-line' practitioner will avoid overlooking oral cancer. This awareness should be instilled during the undergraduate medical and dental courses as part of a screening philosophy for malignant disease. It is essential that every clinician should use a thorough and methodical technique for examining the oral cavity so as not to overlook any suspicious lesion.

The tongue (Fig. 5.1)

The majority of tongue cancers occur on the middle third of the lateral margins, extending early in the course of the disease onto the ventral aspect and floor of the mouth. Approximately 25 per cent occur on the posterior third of the tongue, 20 per cent on the anterior third and rarely (4 per cent) on the dorsum.[5] Those rare cases occurring on the dorsum of the tongue are usually associated with a history of syphilitic glossitis.

Early tongue cancer may manifest in a variety of ways. Often the growth is exophytic with areas of ulceration. It may occur as an ulcer in the depths of a fissure or as an area of superficial ulceration with unsuspected infiltration into the underlying muscle. Leukoplakic patches may or may not be associated with the primary lesion. A minority of tongue cancers may be asymptomatic, arising in an atrophic depapillated area with an erythroplakic patch with peripheral streaks or areas of leukoplakia.

There is increasing evidence that carcinoma can arise in areas of atrophic lichen planus particularly in the lateral borders of the tongue. Indeed Silverman *et al.*[6] reported a 1–2 per cent incidence of malignant change in a series of 570 patients with oral lichen planus followed up for a mean period of 5–6 years. Thus any atrophic lesions on the lateral

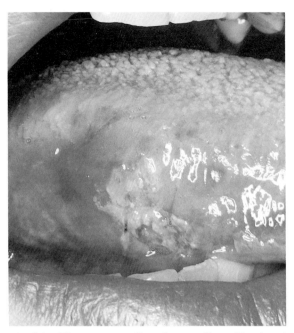

Fig. 5.1   T2 squamous cell carcinoma of lateral border of the tongue.

border of the tongue, and particularly those with any suspicion of induration or areas of red granulations, should be viewed with suspicion.

Later in the course of the disease a more typical malignant ulcer will usually develop, often several centimetres in diameter. The ulcer is hard in consistency with heaped-up and often everted edges. The floor is granular, indurated and bleeds readily. Often there are areas of necrosis. The growth infiltrates the tongue progressively causing increasing pain and difficulty with speech and swallowing. By this stage pain is often severe and constant, radi-

ating to the neck and ears. Lymph node metastases at this stage are common – indeed 50 per cent may have palpable nodes at presentation. Because of the relatively early lymph node metastasis of tongue cancer, 12 per cent of patients may present with no symptoms other than 'a lump in the neck'.[5]

The floor of the mouth (Fig. 5.2)

The floor of the mouth is the second most common site for oral cancer.[7,8] It is defined as the U-shaped area between the lower alveolus and the ventral surface of the tongue; carcinomas arising at this site involve adjacent structures very early in their natural history. Most tumours occur in the anterior segment of the floor of the mouth to one side of the midline.

The lesion usually starts as an indurated mass which soon ulcerates. At an early stage the tongue and lingual aspect of the mandible become involved. This early involvement of the tongue leads to the characteristic slurring of the speech often noted in such patients. The infiltration is deceptive but may extend to reach the gingivae, tongue and genioglossus muscle. Subperiosteal spread is rapid once the mandible is reached. Lymphatic metastasis, although early, is less common than with tongue cancer. Spread is usually to the submandibular and jugulodigastric nodes and may be bilateral.[9,10]

Floor of mouth cancer is associated with a pre-existing leukoplakia more commonly than at other sites. Kramer *et al.*[11] have shown that leukoplakia in the floor of the mouth has a much greater frequency of malignant transformation than at other sites. They have suggested that the floor of the

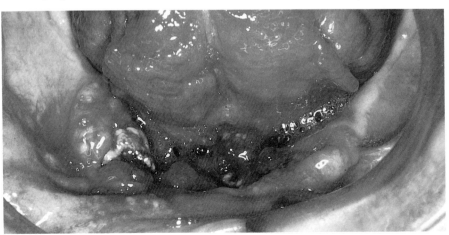

Fig.   5.2 Carcinoma arising in the anterior floor of mouth. Such tumours very rapidly extend to involve both the lower alveolus and root of the tongue as seen here.

mouth may act as a 'sump' into which the various carcinogens collect.

The gingiva and alveolar ridge

(Fig 5.3)

Carcinoma of the lower alveolar ridge occurs predominantly in the premolar and molar regions.[12] The patient usually presents with proliferative tissue at the gingival margins or superficial gingival ulceration. Diagnosis is often delayed because there is a wide variety of inflammatory and reactive lesions which occur in this region in association with the teeth or dentures. Indeed there will often be a history of tooth extraction with subsequent failure of the socket to heal prior to definitive diagnosis. Another common story is that of sudden difficulty in wearing dentures which may previously have been comfortable for many years.[13]

Dental infection, such as an apical or periodontal abscess, may present as a swelling in the alveolar ridge with an ulcerated area surrounding a discharging sinus. Chronic infection of the periodontal tissues may produce a pyogenic granuloma. Peripheral giant cell granuloma, pregnancy granuloma and polypoid and sessile fibro-epithelial lesions all occur in this region and may closely mimic a carcinoma with resulting confusion in the correct diagnosis of the latter. In the edentulous alveolus the so-called denture granuloma – an area of reactive hyperplasia which forms in response to ill-fitting dentures – can cause confusion with subsequent delay in diagnosis.

In the dentate patient there is often associated loosening of the adjacent teeth due to early proliferation of the growing tumour along the periodontal ligament. Together these signs may closely mimic dental sepsis and periodontal disease, and even when radiographs reveal some bony destruction the diagnosis may not be apparent.[14] On the edentulous alveolar ridge the carcinoma commonly presents as an area of indolent superficial ulceration often adjacent to or within an area of leukoplakia. Occasionally the lesion may be proliferative and again mimic classical 'denture hyperplasia'. Because of this clinical presentation gingival and alveolar carcinomas are the most frequently misdiagnosed oral cancers,[15] and often there is a preceding history of a tooth extraction in an attempt to resolve 'dental sepsis'.[13] Even in the absence of radiographic changes, invasion of the underlying bone occurs in 50 per cent of cases and this has important consequences for treatment.[16,17]

Regional nodal metastasis is common at presentation, varying from 30 per cent to 84 per cent,[12,18,19] although false positive and false negative clinical findings are common.[12]

The buccal mucosa (Fig. 5.4)

The buccal mucosa extends from the upper alveolar ridge down to the lower alveolar ridge and

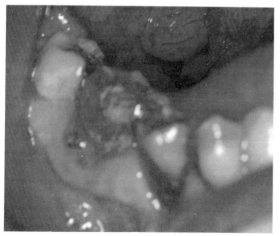

Fig. 5.3 Lower alveolar carcinoma. A granulating tooth socket can be seen. This patient presented 6 weeks following a tooth extraction when the socket failed to heal.

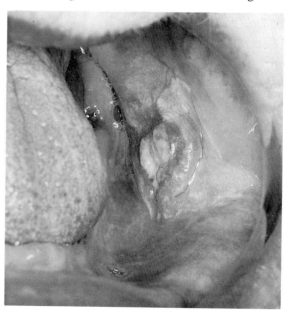

Fig. 5.4 Buccal carcinoma arising in an area of preexistent leukoplakia.

from the commissure anteriorly to the mandibular ramus and retromolar region posteriorly. Squamous cell carcinomas mostly arise either at the commissure or along the occlusal plane to the retromolar area, the majority being situated posteriorly. Exophytic, ulcero-infiltrative and verrucous types occur. They are subject to occlusal trauma with consequent early ulceration and often become secondarily infected. The onset of the disease may be insidious, the patient sometimes presenting with trismus due to deep neoplastic infiltration into the buccinator muscle. Extension posteriorly involves the anterior pillar of the fauces and soft palate with consequent worsening of the prognosis. Ulcero-infiltrative lesions will often involve the overlying skin of the cheek resulting in multiple sinuses. Lymph node spread is to the submental, submandibular, parotid and lateral pharyngeal nodes.

Verrucous carcinoma occurs as a superficial proliferative exophytic lesion with minimal deep invasion and induration. Often the lesion is densely keratinised and presents as a soft white velvety area mimicking benign hyperplasia.[20,21] Lymph node metastasis is late and the tumour behaves as a low grade squamous cell carcinoma.

Another relatively slow growing lesion arising on the buccal mucosa is the carcinoma associated with candidal leukoplakia. This lesion occurs usually at the commissure and presents as a speckled leukoplakia.[22,23]

In the Indian subcontinent buccal cancer arises characteristically in betel chewers. The tumours occur below the occlusal line of the cheek mucosa and also involve the lower buccal sulcus arising in that part of the oral mucosa in direct contact with the betel quid. Furthermore, the tumour usually arises at a site of pre-existing leukoplakia. Oral submucous fibrosis, also associated with betel chewing (see Chapter 3), by severely limiting mouth opening often results in delayed diagnosis of buccal carcinoma.

The hard palate, maxillary alveolar ridge and floor of antrum (Fig. 5.5)

These three sites are anatomically distinct, but a carcinoma arising from one site soon involves the others. Consequently it can be difficult to determine the exact site of origin. Except in countries where reverse smoking is practised,[24,25] cancer of

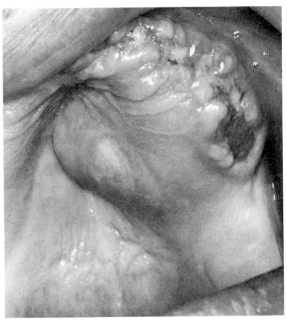

Fig. 5.5 This carcinoma, arising in the floor of the antrum, presented with loose teeth in the area and swelling in the palate so that the patient could no longer wear his previously comfortable denture.

the palate is uncommon.[13] The majority of squamous cancers arise in the antrum and later ulcerate through to involve the hard palate.[26,27] The majority of malignant tumours arising from the palatal mucosa are of minor salivary gland origin. Palatal cancers usually present as sessile swellings which ulcerate relatively late. A finding in contrast to mandibular alveolar tumours is that deep infiltration into the underlying bone is uncommon.[28]

The presenting symptom is often a complaint that a previously comfortable denture has become painful or ill-fitting. Carcinomas arising in the floor of the maxillary antrum often present as palatal tumours. Although the fully established picture of antral carcinoma is difficult to miss, the early symptoms are non-specific and may mimic chronic sinusitis. Tumours of the lower half of the antrum below Ohngren's line usually present with 'dental' symptoms because of early alveolar invasion. The commonest presenting feature is pain, swelling or numbness of the face. Later symptoms of nasal obstruction, discharge or bleeding and dental symptoms such as painful or loose teeth, ill-fitting dentures, oro-antral fistula or failure of an extraction socket to heal soon follow.

In the edentulous patient carcinoma may present as a painful or loose denture. In the dentate patient often painless loose teeth may be the presenting sign and these teeth are sometimes extracted with a consequent failure of the sockets to heal. Occasionally localised or referred pain in the premolar or molar teeth will occur due to early infiltration of the posterior superior dental nerve. Swelling may also occur in the mucogingival fold. Trismus may occur when these tumours extend backwards into the pterygoid region.[29] Lymph node metastasis from carcinomas of the palate and floor of the antrum occurs late but carries a poor prognosis. Lymph node spread is initially to the submandibular nodes and then to the deep cervical chain. Posterior antral tumours and tumours involving the pterygoid region metastasise first to the posterior pharyngeal nodes making detection of nodal disease very difficult.

Diagnosis

The diagnosis of intra-oral carcinoma is primarily clinical and a high index of suspicion is necessary for all those clinicians seeing and treating patients with oral symptoms. A careful and detailed history with particular attention to recording the dates of the onset of particular signs and symptoms precedes the clinical examination. All areas of the oral mucosa are carefully inspected and any suspicious lesion palpated for texture, tethering to adjacent structures and induration of underlying tissue. The World Health Organization (WHO) *Oral Mucosa Manual*[30] suggests a systematic technique.[30] If such a systematic approach is used there will be little risk of overlooking any suspicious lesion.

The clinical notes are of particular importance, not only as a record for an individual patient but also for use in prospective and retrospective analyses of treatment methods and results.[31] The notes must include a detailed description of the presenting lesion including its appearance, extent, texture, fixation and induration. Precise measurements of the lesion should be recorded. Whenever facilities are available, a photographic record is useful. Currently there are moves towards the use of standard proformas suitable for transfer to computer data bases. Such computerised records are not only useful for audit but contribute an invaluable record for prospective studies.

It is important to realise that this initial record is the basis upon which treatment should be planned and progress assessed; as soon as even a biopsy is performed the presenting lesion is irrevocably changed.

Investigation

Surgical biopsy

A clinical diagnosis of oral cancer should always be confirmed histologically. Within the oral cavity a surgical biopsy can nearly always be obtained using local anaesthesia. It is often tempting to remove small lesions *in toto* by an excisional biopsy. However, this can be dangerous – without histological confirmation of the malignant nature of the lesion it is difficult to justify an excision with wide margins, whereas if the lesion is excised locally subsequent management is compromised. Also it may be difficult to persuade patients to undergo further treatment for a lesion which as far as they are concerned has been eliminated. Once the primary lesion has been excised, the surgeon no longer has a guide as to the extent of further excision and the radiotherapist cannot define accurately what field to treat.

For these reasons an incisional biopsy is recommended in all cases. Whenever possible the patient should be seen at a combined clinic by a surgeon and radiotherapist before even the biopsy is carried out, but provided careful records are made an initial incisional biopsy is acceptable and may indeed save time in the planning and execution of subsequent therapy. The biopsy should include the most suspicious area of the lesion and include some normal adjacent mucosa. Areas of necrosis or gross infection should be avoided as they may confuse the diagnosis. If a combination of radiotherapy followed by surgical resection is contemplated it is useful to tattoo the margins of the primary lesion with India ink at the time of initial biopsy or at least prior to the start of radiotherapy. Surgical resection must be planned according to the original dimensions of the tumour and not to the dimensions following radiotherapy. As the tumour volume shrinks, the surgeon may be tempted to perform less radical surgery. The tattoo marks help to record the initial dimensions.

Exfoliative cytology

Following the widespread introduction by Papanicolou of staining of cervical smears as a screening method for detecting early cancers attempts have been made to apply this technique to the examination of suspicious oral lesions. Folsom *et al.*,[32] in an excellent 3 year study reported on a series of 158 996 patients on whom exfoliative cytology was performed. They found a total of 148 lesions proved malignant by conventional biopsy. Of these 148 lesions there was a false negative rate of 31 per cent for exfoliative cytology. Banoczy[33] found a similar incidence of false negatives. Folsom *et al*[32] concluded that oral cytology should be used as an adjunctive measure in the evaluation of visible oral lesions but should not be used in preference to, or as a substitute for, biopsy unless biopsy is specifically contra-indicated.

Flow cytometry based on exfoliative scrapes has been advocated. In this technique it is possible to measure the nuclear DNA and demonstrate the ratios of haploid, diploid and aneuploid nuclei and to use this as a guide to imminent malignant change. However, this technique is far from being a simple chair-side investigation and is not widely available.[34]

Toluidine blue test

Richart[35] described an *in vitro* method of vital staining for delineating malignant and dysplastic lesions of the cervix. The technique has been applied to oral lesions. The suspicious area is painted with a 1 per cent aqueous solution of toluidine blue for 10 seconds. The mouth is then thoroughly rinsed with a 1 per cent solution of acetic acid. The toluidine blue binds to DNA present in the superficial cells and resists decolouration by the acetic acid. Dye binding is, therefore, proportional to the amount of DNA present and the number and size of superficial nuclei in the tissues. Several authors have found this test valuable,[36-38] but Sabes *et al.*[39] criticise the technique and condemn its use on the grounds that false negatives occur so frequently as to render the test unreliable. They reported, for an experimentally induced carcinoma in the hamster cheek pouch, 65.6 per cent false positive and 21.4 per cent false negative in early carcinomas and 12.1 per cent false positive and 39.6 per cent false negative in late tumours. At best the technique may be used as a guide as to which areas should be formally biopsied.[40]

Acridine-binding test

Roth *et al.* in 1972[41] described a technique in which the DNA content of desquamated buccal squames was estimated by measuring their acridine binding. They compared the acridine uptake in patients both with and without oral cancer and suggested that there were sufficient differences between the two groups to make the test clinically useful. Unfortunately no further follow up studies have been published to date.

Fine needle aspiration biopsy

This technique is applicable mainly to lumps in the neck, especially suspicious lymph nodes in a patient with a known primary carcinoma. It consists of the percutaneous puncture of the mass with a fine needle and aspiration of material for cytological examination. The method of aspiration needs no specialised equipment and is fast, almost painless and without complications. Despite this the technique is often performed incorrectly and very little tissue aspirated. The technique depends on two aspects; the successful puncture of the node and the transfer of cells and stroma from the needle onto the microscope slide. The node is fixed between finger and thumb and then punctured by a 21 or 23 gauge needle on a 10 ml syringe, the gauge of the needle depending on the size of the node. Important points to note are that the needle is properly pushed onto the syringe to prevent air leaking in when the plunger is withdrawn and that a small amount of air is already in the syringe (about 2 ml) before the node is punctured in order subsequently to expel the aspirate from the needle onto the slide. Aspiration should be forcible and accompanied by moving the needle around different parts of the node for 10–30 seconds; the plunger is then released and the needle withdrawn through the skin. The needle contents are then expelled onto a glass slide using the 2 ml of air previously drawn into the syringe. To do this the tip of the needle must touch the slide to prevent splashing of the material, which can be gelatinous or sticky. Blobs of material can be deposited on several slides and then smeared with a second slide to provide a thin film for staining and microscopy. Some pathologists prefer wet fixed material, which must be sprayed with an alcoholic 'spray fix' immediately; others prefer thinner films which can be left to air dry. Strong[42] has recently described a variation on this technique that eliminates the risk of losing the biopsy material within the needle. After performing the aspiration, instead of making a smear directly onto the microscope slide, he aspirates 2 ml of 95 per cent ethanol as fixative into the same syringe. The syringe containing fixative and biopsy material is then sent off to the laboratory where the contents are centrifuged and a smear prepared from the deposit. Frable and Frable[43] and Young[44] have reported on the results of 516 fine needle aspiration biopsies and have reported 94.5 per cent accuracy with head and neck lesions. Both papers advocate this technique as it may avoid the need for open biopsy and the risk of spreading malignant cells into the surrounding tissues where they cannot be detected at the time of radical surgical excision but are at the same time rendered anoxic, and, therefore, relatively resistant to radiotherapy.

Although tumour implantation into the needle track has been described, it has been reported only when large gauge needles have been used. Puigvert *et al.*[45] describe six cases of prostatic carcinoma spreading to the perineum following aspiration biopsy. Ackerman and Wheat[46] describe one case of squamous carcinoma and one of malignant melanoma where the tumour spread along the needle track following biopsy. Crile and Hazard[47] describe a single case of thyroid carcinoma behaving in a similar manner. All of these occurred following the use of the Vim Silverman biopsy needle. At present there appears to be no authentic documented case of needle track dissemination of cancer following aspiration using 21 or 23 gauge needles.[48]

Aspiration biopsy is a most useful technique for examining equivocal masses in the submental and submandibular areas and also the neck in patients who, having received treatment for their primary tumour, are found to have masses at later follow up. However, although usually there is little doubt that such a mass represents lymph node recurrence it is sometimes difficult to distinguish such a mass from a chronically enlarged submandibular salivary gland. Certainly if the aspiration biopsy confirms either the presence of tumour or salivary tissue the cause of the mass is known. Failure to find tumour or salivary gland leaves all the doubts of a negative biopsy – did the aspiration needle miss the mass?

Radiography (Fig. 5.6)

Plain radiography is of limited value in the investigation of oral cancer. At least 50 per cent of the calcified component of bone must be lost before any radiographic change is apparent. Furthermore, the facial bones are of such a complexity that confusion from overlying structures makes X-ray diagnosis more difficult. However, rotational pantomography of the jaws can be helpful in as-

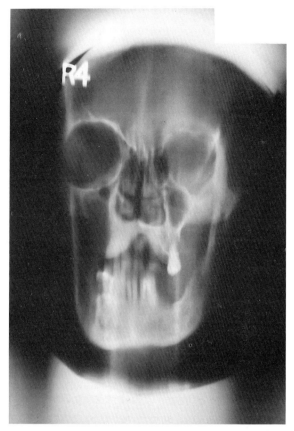

Fig. 5.6 Conventional tomography used to visualise an antral carcinoma. There is clear evidence of destruction of the lateral wall of the antrum.

sessing alveolar and antral involvement provided that the above limitations are understood.

Conventional tomography can be used particularly in assessing bony involvement of antral lesions and in the pterygoid region where posterior extension at this site may render the lesion inoperable. Radiography is, of course, important in assessing secondary deposits in the lungs and skeleton.

Computerised tomography (Fig. 5.7)

The increasing availability of computerised tomography (CT) scanning has undoubtedly been of great benefit in the investigation of head and neck tumours.[49-52] However, for intra-oral tumours its value is more limited. Larsson *et al.*[52] have described the role of CT in tongue lesions. For the evaluation of antral tumours, particularly assessment of the pterygoid regions, CT has superseded

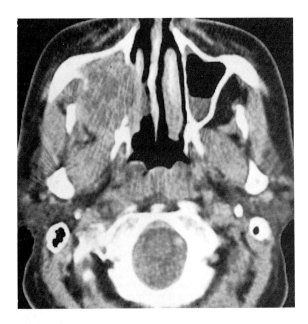

Fig. 5.7   An axial CT (computed tomography) scan gives an accurate and clear image of the extent of this antral carcinoma. There is destruction of both the medial and lateral walls with posterior extension of the tumour. The pterygoid plates remain intact.

plain radiography and conventional tomography. CT is also of value in the investigation of metastatic disease in the lungs, liver and skeleton.

Radionuclide studies

Technetium pertechnetate bone scans of the facial skeleton are of little value in the diagnosis of primary oral cancers. There will be obvious clinical disease long before bone changes are visible on a technetium scan. Furthermore, such scans are not specific and will show increased uptake wherever there is increased metabolic activity in the bone.

Radionuclide scans for bone and liver metastases have been used but currently CT scanning or ultrasound scans have displaced this technique. They are both less invasive and more sensitive techniques. However, routine bone and liver scanning is not advocated as a screening technique. Belson *et al.*[53] performed routine bone and liver scans as part of the initial evaluation of 169 patients with head and neck cancer. No true positive liver scans were found, but there were two false positives. There were two true positive and four false positive bone scans. The likelihood of detecting distant metastases is so low that these techniques are not worthwhile in the initial assessment of the patient with oral cancer.

Magnetic resonance imaging (Fig. 5.8)

McLay,[54] working in Aberdeen, has investigated the role of nuclear magnetic resonance imaging (MRI) in the diagnosis of head and neck cancer. He demonstrated the presence of metastatic oral cancer in clinically negative necks and also the absence of disease in suspicious necks, apparently with a high degree of accuracy. Unfortunately this early promise has not been fulfilled by subsequent experience. However, MRI remains the technique of choice for imaging bone invasion by tumour although of course the presence of bone can only be inferred by its negative image as bone itself is not imaged by MRI, only the marrow being directly visualised.

Ultrasound

Abdominal ultrasound to detect liver metastases is probably as accurate as CT scanning. As it is non-invasive, readily available and cost effective it is probably the most appropriate technique for assessing the liver.

More recently Norer *et al.*,[55] using small flexible transducers attached to the tip of the operator's fingers, have been able to scan intra-oral tumours with a high degree of accuracy, demonstrating the presence of bone invasion at an early stage. Mende

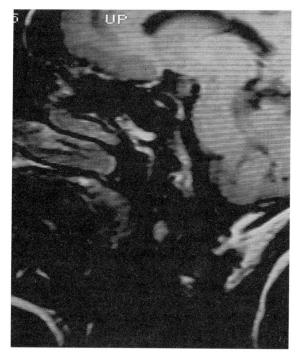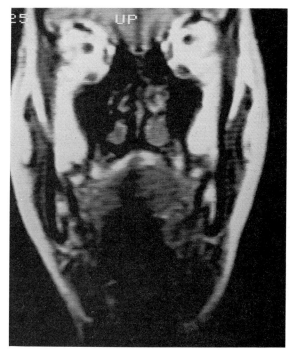

Fig. 5.8 Magnetic resonance imaging is particularly useful for imaging soft tissue extension of tumours adjacent to and involving bone (a situation in which computed tomography is not good).

et al.,[56] in a series of 260 patients, have shown a 92.3 per cent accuracy for T staging (tumour size) by ultrasound compared with 75 per cent accuracy based on clinical staging. For N staging (presence and condition of regional lymph nodes) the diagnostic accuracy was 89.6 per cent and 58.9 per cent, respectively.

References

1 Binnie WH, Cawson RA, Hill GB, Soaper AE. *Oral Cancer in England and Wales. A National Study of Morbidity, Mortality, Curability and Related Factors.* London: HMSO, 1972.

2 Langdon JD, Harvey PW, Rapidis AD, Patel MF, Johnson NW, Hopps R. Oral cancer: the behaviour and response to treatment of 194 cases. *Journal of Maxillofacial Surgery* 1977; **5**: 221–37.

3 Cooke BED, Tapper-Jones L. Recognition of oral cancer, causes of delay. *British Dental Journal* 1977; **142**: 96–8.

4 Scully E, Malamos D, Levers BGH, Porter SR, Prime SS. Sources and patterns of referrals of oral cancer: role of general practitioners. *British Medical Journal* 1986; **293**: 599–601.

5 Frazell EL, Lucas JC. Cancer of the tongue: report of the management of 1,554 patients. *Cancer* 1962; **15**: 1085–99.

6 Silverman S, Gorsky M, Lozada-Nur F. A prospective follow-up study of 570 patients with oral lichen planus: persistence, remission and malignant association. *Oral Surgery* 1985; **60**: 30–4.

7 Shaw HJ, Hardingham M. Cancer of the floor of the mouth: surgical management. *Journal of Laryngology* 1977; **91**: 467–88.

8 Berthelsen A, Hansen HS, Rygard J. Radiation therapy of squamous carcinoma of the floor of the mouth and the lower alveolar ridge. *Journal of Laryngology* 1977; **91**: 489–99.

9 Kolson H, Spiro RH, Rosewit B, Lawson W. Epidermoid carcinoma of the floor of the mouth. *Archives of Otolaryngology* 1971; **93**: 280–3.

10 Lindberg R. Distribution of cervical lymph node metastasis from squamous cell carcinoma of the upper respiratory and digestive tracts. *Cancer* 1972; **29**: 1446–9.

11 Kramer IRH, El-Labban N, Leek KW. The clinical features and risk of malignant transformation in sublingual keratosis. *British Dental Journal* 1970; **144**: 171–80.

12 Cady B, Catlin D. Epidermoid carcinoma of the gum: a 20 year survey. *Cancer* 1969; **23**: 551–69.

13 Ackerman LV, del Regato JA. *Cancer: Diagnosis, Treatment and Prognosis*, 4th edn. St Louis, MO: CV Mosby, 1976.

14 Schreiber HR, Waldron CA. Carcinoma of the gingiva simulating gingival hyperplasia. *Journal of Periodontology* 1958; **29**: 196–8.

15 Thoma KH. Development and dissemination of oral cancer. *New York State Dental Journal* 1950; **16**: 366–71.

16 Whitehouse GH. Radiological bone changes produced by intraoral squamous carcinomata involving the lower alveolus. *Clinics in Otolaryngology* 1976; **1**: 45–52.

17 Byars LT. Extent of mandibular resection required for treatment of oral cancer. *Archives of Surgery* 1955; **70**: 914–20.

18 Mattick WL, Meehan DJ. Carcinoma of the gum. *Surgery* 1951; **29**: 249–54.

19 Willen R, Nathanson A. Squamous cell carcinoma of the gingiva. *Acta – Oto-Laryngologica* 1973; **75**: 299–300.

20 Duckworth R. Verrucous carcinoma presenting as mandibular osteomyelitis. *British Journal of Surgery* 1961; **49**: 332–7.

21 Kraus FP, Perez-Mesa C. Verrucous carcinoma. Clinical and pathologic study of 105 cases involving the oral cavity, larynx and genitalia. *Cancer* 1966; **19**: 26–38.

22 Cawson RA. Leukoplakia and oral cancer. *Proceedings of the Royal Society of Medicine* 1969; **62**: 610–15.

23 Pindborg JJ. Oral leukoplakia. *Australian Dental Journal* 1971; **16**: 83–93.

24 Pindborg JJ, Mehta FS, Daftary DK. Incidence of oral cancer among 30,000 villagers in India in a 7 year follow-up study of oral precancerous lesions. *Community Dentistry and Oral Epidemiology* 1975; **3**: 86–8.

25 Ramulu C, Prasad CSV, Krishnamurthy K, Reddy CRRM. Benign tumours of the hard palate. *Indian Journal of Surgery* 1974; **36**: 113–17.

26 Ratzer ER, Schweitzer RJ, Frazell EL. Epidermoid carcinoma of the palate. *American Journal of Surgery* 1970; **119**: 294–7.

27 Eneroth CM, Hjertman L, Moberger G. Squamous cell carcinoma of the palate. *Acta Oto-Laryngologica* 1972; **73**: 418–27.

28 Spiessl B. *Plattenepithal Karzinomen Mundhole, Grundlagen der Behandlung*. Stuttgart: George Thieme, 1966.

29 Batsakis JG. *Tumours of the head and neck, clinical and pathological considerations*. Baltimore, MD: Williams & Wilkins Company, 1979.

30 World Health Organization. *Oral Mucosa Manual*. Geneva: WHO, 1982.

31 Langdon JD, Rapidis AD. The importance of accurate records and follow-up in patients with oral cancer. *Journal of Maxillofacial Surgery* 1978; **6**: 226–30.

32 Folsom TC, White CP, Bromer L. Oral exfoliative study. Review of the literature and report of a three year study. *Surgery* 1972; **33**: 61–74.

33 Banoczy J. Exfoliative cytologic examinations in the early diagnosis of oral cancer. *International Dental Journal* 1976; **26**: 398–404.

34 Ogden GR, Cowpe JG. Quantitative cytophotometric analysis as an aid to the detection of recurrent oral cancer. *British Journal of Oral and Maxillofacial Surgery* 1989; **27**: 224–8.

35 Richart RM. A clinical staining test for the *in vivo* delineation of dysplasia and carcinoma-*in-situ*. *American Journal of Obstetrics and Gyneocology* 1962; **86**: 703–12.

36 Shedd DP, Hukill PB, Bahn S *et al.* Further appraisal of *in vivo* staining properties of oral cancer. *Archives of Surgery* 1967; **95**: 16–22.

37 Strong MS, Vaughan CW, Ineze JS. Toluidine blue in the management of carcinoma of the oral cavity. *Archives of Otolaryngology* 1968; **87**: 527–31.

38 Meyers EN. The toluidine blue test in lesions of the oral cavity. *Cancer* 1970; **20**: 134–9.

39 Sabes WR, Singer RE, Kuhn T. Effectiveness of toluidine blue as an aid to biopsy in the diagnosis of DMBA–induced hamster pouch dysplasia and carcinoma. *Cancer* 1972; **29**: 1584–9.

40 Moyer GN, Taybos GM, Pelleu GB. Toluidine blue rinse: potential for benign lesions in early detection of oral neoplasms. *Journal of Oral Medicine* 1986; **41**: 111–13.

41 Roth D, Hayes RT, Ross NM. Effectiveness of acridine-binding method in screening for oral pharyngeal and laryngeal cancer. *Cancer* 1972; **29**: 1579–83.

42 Strong MS. In: Evans PHR, Robin PE, Fielding JWL eds. *Head and Neck Cancer*. Tunbridge Wells: Castle House, 1983: 97–101.

43 Frable WJ, Frable MA. Thin-needle aspiration biopsy: the diagnosis of head and neck tumours revisited. *Cancer* 1979; **43**: 1541–8.

44 Young JEM. Current status of needle aspiration biopsy of the head and neck. *Canadian Journal of Surgery* 1982; **25**: 410.

45 Puigvert A, Elizalde C, Maiz JA. Perineal implantation of carcinoma of the prostate following needle biopsy. *Journal of Urology* 1972; **107**: 821–4.

46 Ackerman LV, Wheat MW. Implantation of cancer an avoidable surgical risk? *Surgery* 1955; **37**: 341–55.

47 Crile G, Hazard JB. Classification of thyroiditis with special reference to use of needle biopsy. *Journal of Clinical Endocrinology* 1951; **11**: 1123–7.

48 Trott PA. *Personal communication*. 1982.

49 Clausson C, Singer R. Progress in the diagnosis of craniofacial injuries and tumours by computer tomography. *Journal of Maxillofacial Surgery* 1979; **7**: 210–17.

50 Rapidis AD, Angelopoulos AP, Langdon JD, Skouteris CA. Computerized axial tomography in the diagnosis of head and neck tumours. *International Journal of Oral Surgery* 1980; **9**: 387–93.

51 North AF, Rice J. Computed tomography in oral and maxillofacial surgery. *Journal of Oral Surgery* 1981; **39:** 199–207.

52 Larsson SG, Mancuso A, Hanafee W. Computed tomography of the tongue and floor of mouth. *Radiology* 1982; **43:** 493–500.

53 Belson TP, Lehman RH, Chobanian SL, Malin TC. Bone and liver scans in patients with head and neck carcinoma. *Laryngoscope* 1980; **90:** 1291–6.

54 McLay L. *Preliminary report on nuclear magnetic resonance imaging of tumours of the head and neck*. Paper read at the Academic Meeting of the Association of Head and Neck Oncologists of Great Britain, Cambridge, 1982.

55 Norer B, Stobl V, Bertram S. Sonography within the oral cavity. *Journal of Cranio-Maxillo-Facial Surgery* 1992; **20:** (suppl.): 26 (abstract).

56 Mende U, Zoller J, Maier H, Born IA. The sonographic staging of head and neck tumours. *Journal of Cranio-Maxillo-Facial Surgery* 1992; **20:** (suppl.): 26 (abstract).

6 Basic principles of management

JD Langdon and JM Henk

Objectives

Before treatment is started for a patient with oral cancer, two important factors must be considered: first, the precise objectives of treatment – exactly what it is we are trying to achieve for a particular patient; and second, the limitations of treatment and how to reconcile such limitations with objectives.

Whenever patients are treated a balance must be achieved between the overall length of survival and the quality of life remaining. It is worth repeating in this context the advice of the Arabian physician and philosopher Avicenna: 'The cure of a disease must never be worse than the disease itself.'

With current surgical techniques it is virtually possible to resect any tumour in the head and neck region. Thus the vast majority of patients with head and neck cancers are potentially treatable by surgery, but many of them should not be, because of advanced age, general disability or the mutilating effects of surgery. Many of our patients are elderly and it is more important to consider the quality of life in their remaining years.

The clinician must be willing to tailor treatment to a particular patient even though on occasions this may compromise the chances of 'cure'. In general the younger the patient at presentation the more aggressive should be the treatment – there is so much more to gain by achieving a cure at whatever the cost. The underlying principle must be that if treatment is to be embarked upon it must prolong the patient's life as a reasonable human being. As Gardham wrote in 1964:[1] 'How often by prolonging life do we really add to its sum of happiness, and how often do we prolong the quantity of life at the expense of its quality?'

The radical excisions necessary for successful surgical treatment of maxillofacial cancers have been technically possible for many years, but before the decision to operate for cure is made, three principles must be considered:[2]

(1) The whole tumour must be removed. To leave some of the tumour behind after cancer surgery invalidates the whole procedure and leaves the patient worse off than before: 'I do not think that any of us enjoyed explaining that we had done the wrong operation because the patient would not stand the right one.'[1] If one is going to operate then it must be with a reasonable prospect of cure.
(2) Although normal anatomy and function should be retained or restored whenever possible, this consideration should *never* be allowed to compromise the excision.
(3) To the patient, probably the most important factor is that the end result should be cosmetically and functionally acceptable. Above all else the patient must be able to maintain his or her dignity upon completion of treatment. What the patient will accept is often very different from what the surgeon might accept, and this observation must be carefully considered when defining the objectives of any proposed treatment.

Importance of team work

Tumours of the head and neck will often respond to irradiation. In many cases surgical excision or irradiation may be equally successful. The availability of alternative methods of treatment makes a team approach to the problem of management mandatory.[3]

The best possible surgery and radiotherapy should be made available to the patient, even if this means referral to another clinician or another hospital some distance away. In some countries oral cancer is now not a common disease and not every surgeon or radiotherapist can claim to be expert in its management. Side issues, such as which surgical subspeciality should operate on the mouth, must never be allowed to influence a decision as to what treatment a particular patient receives.

The head and neck is one of the most complex regions of the human body and no other part is affected by such a wide variety of different tumours, although the majority are squamous cell carcinomas. Patients who present with malignant tumours of the head and neck require accurate diagnosis and thorough evaluation of their presenting condition, comprehensive treatment planning, coordination of the appropriate therapeutic modalities, careful reconstruction; and rehabilitation and supportive psychological and social care to expedite their return as integrated members of society.[4] Especially when dealing with oral cancer, we should have as a basic aim the eradication of the tumour with satisfactory physiological function as regards mastication, phonation, facial expression and an acceptable cosmetic appearance (see also Chapter 7).[5]

It is therefore clear that the management of maxillofacial cancer is beyond the capabilities of any single specialist. No one individual or discipline can be expected to anticipate all the problems arising during or after the treatment of the 'cancer patient'.

Patients with maxillofacial cancer are referred to hospital from many sources. A patient with a lesion in the mouth, jaws or salivary glands will seek advice from general dental or medical practitioners; general surgeons; ear, nose and throat surgeons and oral surgeons. When a biopsy has confirmed the diagnosis the patient should be seen at a joint clinic. A combination of approaches should be considered and a definitive treatment plan agreed by the team. After treatment the patient's progress should be reviewed at the joint clinic from time to time.

However, it should always be borne in mind that patients prefer to deal with a single doctor and therefore it is important that someone assumes responsibility for leading the team and acts as the main source of information for the patient.

The surgeon

Many surgical specialties deal with the treatment of patients with maxillofacial cancer. Historically general surgeons, otorhinolaryngologists and plastic surgeons had the major responsibility.

A new specialty, that of head and neck surgery, has developed and has advanced rapidly, particularly in the USA and Canada. The head and neck surgeon has been gaining responsibility for the treatment of maxillofacial tumours in these countries. In Europe the development of maxillofacial surgeons from the medically qualified dentists of the postwar era has given the dental profession an important role in this field. Whoever the designated surgeon is, adequate training and surgical ability in the specialised field of maxillofacial oncology are more important than his or her title.[6]

The radiotherapist

Surgery and radiotherapy are the two forms of treatment which have a curative role in oral cancer. These should be regarded as complementary rather than rivals. In some patients one or the other treatment method may be preferable, while in others both may be needed to give the best chance of cure. In recent years there has been a steady increase in our knowledge of basic biological mechanisms underlying the action of ionising radiation, and of its early and late effects on tumours and normal tissues. An understanding of these basic principles is essential if radiotherapy is to be used to the best advantage, so a radiotherapist must be present at the time a decision is made regarding the treatment strategy for each patient.

The medical oncologist

Chemotherapy in cancer of the head and neck had until recently been mainly palliative, usually given only after failure of surgery and radiotherapy. In the past few years there has been increasing interest in the use of chemotherapy as an adjuvant to surgery or radiotherapy in curative treatment. To date results have been conflicting, with little effect on overall survival rates. Further developments in this field may occur and it is possible that in future the medical oncologist will be a significant member of the team.

The pathologist

There is a strong association between the histology of a malignant tumour of the head and neck and its subsequent behaviour. No treatment should be started for a patient suffering from oral cancer before the tumour's histology has been evaluated by the pathologist and discussed by the team. Regular clinicopathological meetings where the pathologists and clinicians can discuss cases together are essential. Postoperatively the status of neck nodes and surgical margins must again be discussed when considering postoperative irradiation.

The supportive team

The role of the supportive team is to facilitate the prompt application of the selected therapeutic regimen and also to help the patient overcome the physical, psychological and social problems that will arise during or after treatment.

The family medical and dental practitioners will help the primary team by providing useful information about the patient's general condition and about the family environment, and will facilitate communication between the team and the patient.

The role of the nurse in the team is very important. Skilled nursing care is essential to the recovery of the patient. Ideally, in the postoperative period and during and after radiotherapy, the patient should be cared for by nurses specially trained in the care of head and neck cancer patients. The nurse's responsibilities not only include postoperative care, dressings, care of skin grafts and flaps but also maintaining morale. For all these aspects of care special training is necessary.

Other members of the supportive team such as the maxillofacial prosthetist, the speech therapist, the dietician, the psychiatrist and the social worker can provide great help in selected cases. Proper understanding of the disease and its consequences by any member of the patient's own family and friends will help him or her to re-adjust within the family environment and help to maintain morale.

Approach to the patient

The disease should always be discussed with the patient. It is only by achieving a rapport with the patient from an early stage that he or she can be given the support and courage to face what may well be a long, protracted and perhaps deforming and distressing course of treatment. Furthermore, if local recurrence and lymph node metastases develop later, the patient must be able to retain faith and confidence in those providing advice and treatment. Some facile story at the start leads ultimately to an embarrassed and suspicious relationship at a later stage.

A few patients will want to know everything, a few will want to know no details – the great majority will be between these two extremes. How we explain the condition varies similarly. Indeed, it is only as the relationship with a patient develops that information is fed little by little to the patient. If this relationship is genuine and trusting, the patient will gradually feel able to ask, even if not overtly, for details.

It is of course right and proper that the truth should be given in a positive manner, in the sense that favourable aspects are discussed at greater length than unfavourable aspects. We should, however, always answer the patient's questions with the truth and never with a lie. The fact that a patient's 'doctor' has lied will almost invariably become apparent at some stage, and from then on the chances of maintaining confidence and a rapport are gone. However, the truth should be told with kindness and understanding, and where necessary tempered with hope and a positive approach to the patient's difficulties. Language appropriate to the particular patient should always be used. The patient must not be overawed by the erudition of the doctors. The aim at all times should be to develop an optimistic but realistic partnership with the patient in order to face the ensuing battle against the disease. These considerations apply equally to the relatives. Both patient and doctor will require the support and understanding of the patient's family in the weeks, months and years to follow. One of the cruellest of decisions is to tell the patient's relatives of the diagnosis while withholding that information from the patient. This act creates an ever-increasing barrier between the patient and family, so that a loving and supporting relationship becomes increasingly more difficult.

Preparation for treatment

It is important to prepare both the patient and the relatives prior to surgery or radiotherapy. Unfortunately in head and neck cancer, surgery is very often, to a greater or lesser extent, cosmetically damaging and temporarily or permanently inhibits speech or swallowing. It is therefore only right that, without going into unnecessarily gruesome details, the patient be warned of the consequences of surgery. Similarly the patient must be told that he or she may wake up in the intensive care unit and in this context it is often helpful to take the patient on a visit to the intensive care unit pre-operatively in order to see the environment and meet the staff.

If secondary corrective surgery is envisaged, or a two-stage procedure is planned, it is wise to inform the patient of this before starting. Inevitably the patient's morale will be low immediately following surgery and this is not the time to start speaking of 'further surgery'.

Particular care should be taken following surgery to prepare relatives for what they will see on visiting the patient. Any abhorrence expressed in the faces of visitors during this sensitive postoperative phase will do untold damage to the patient's morale and make subsequent rehabilitation much more difficult.

Similarly the patient should be prepared for radiotherapy. Many myths are attached to 'radium treatment' and many patients expect to be very ill as a result of treatment. Furthermore, much of the hardware employed in administering radiotherapy is frightening. The radiotherapist should therefore explain what the treatment will involve and what complications might arise and how they will be managed. It is particularly valuable to tell the patient how short treatment times are with modern megavoltage equipment. Patients should be warned of the temporary loss or alteration of taste, loss of hair and dry mouth.

General medical care

For a condition which is invariably fatal if left untreated, there can be few absolute medical contraindications.

Surgery would be very unwise within 6 to 8 weeks of myocardial infarction, although with modern anaesthetic techniques a history of ischaemic heart disease is not a contra-indication. Similarly chronic respiratory disease, although adding to the risk of surgery, is not an absolute contra-indication. Obviously any remediable underlying diseases must be controlled prior to surgery.

Any obvious causes of infection should be dealt with before surgery. The general dental status should be assessed and any dental or periodontal infection controlled. Dental care is especially important if radiotherapy is envisaged (see Chapter 8).

Nutrition

Many patients with oral cancer will have feeding difficulties. This may be due to pain or fixation of the tongue, or may be the result of surgical resection or radiotherapy. In addition to this the general loss of morale and depression may further suppress appetite.

Recently attention has been turned to the effects of poor nutrition on the response to surgery or irradiation, with subsequent delay in healing. Brookes and Clifford[7] studied a series of 53 patients with head and neck cancer to determine the relation between nutritional status and immune competence. They showed a highly significant correlation between nutritional status and a variety of tests for suppressed immunocompetence; they speculated that nutritional deficiency might be the primary adverse prognostic factor in patients with head and neck cancer and that immuno-incompetence may be a secondary phenomenon (see also Chapter 7).

Nutritional support for a malnourished patient with malignant disease may also improve the response to treatment by conferring greater tolerance to radiotherapy or cytoxic chemotherapy, thus allowing more treatment to be given; or alternatively may reduce morbidity following surgery. The correction of malnutrition by intravenous alimentation is slow, difficult and expensive but may be a very worthwhile aspect of pre-operative preparation which will improve prognosis. Consideration should be given to the establishment pre-operatively of a feeding gastrostomy if it is anticipated that feeding problems will be experienced post-treatment.

Postoperatively, long-term feeding may be a problem. It is not always possible to restore good function as part of reconstruction and rehabilitation. For the relatively short term a nasogastric Ryle's tube is commonly used, but this is irritating and unsightly and has a tendency to make aspiration pneumonia more likely. The introduction of microbore Clinifeed® tubes has made tube feeding more comfortable for the patient and practicable for medium-term feeding. However, there is a limit to the viscosity of the material that can be passed down such tubes, and this necessitates the production of special synthetic feeds with ensuing electrolyte problems. It is often impossible to administer drugs through these fine tubes.

Long-term feeding may sometimes be a problem, particularly for those patients who have undergone extensive mandibular resections or for maxillectomies when soft palate function has been disturbed. Similarly, those with total or subtotal glossectomies, even when soft tissue reconstruction has been achieved, will have difficulties with swallowing at least initially. As some of these disabilities may be permanent it is important that an acceptable feeding regimen be established. It is no help to a patient facing a lifetime of liquid or semi-solid diet just to be given a prescription for one of the high calorie dietary supplements.

Food must be as palatable and tempting as possible and must involve the minimum of inconvenience to prepare. Ideally the patient should be encouraged to eat whatever the rest of the family has at any meal, even if this involves modifying the texture in some way. A common mistake is to recommend putting the meal through a liquidiser. This in fact renders the most tempting food unpalatable and indeed many patients find a liquid diet more difficult to swallow. It is often better to mince or finely chop meat and vegetables, and then combine them in a thick sauce or gravy. Such a semi-solid diet is often easier to swallow successfully. The intake of calories, protein, vitamins and minerals must all be adequate, so some dietary supplements may also be needed. A sympathetic and imaginative dietician can be very helpful.

For permanent nutrition in patients unable to learn to swallow, it may be wiser to create a gastrostomy which allows the removal of the feeding tube, reduces oral secretions and may allow the patient to return home. The technique of percutaneous endoscopic gastrostomy first described in 1980 has made long-term enteral nutrition for patients unable to tolerate oral feeding an acceptable alternative.[8] In experienced hands the procedure takes only 15 to 30 minutes and can be undertaken using intravenous sedation. Effective nutritional support and weight gain is consistently better with a feeding gastrostomy than with a nasogastric tube.[9,10] Wood[11] has described a simple technique of cervical oesophagostomy for long-term nutrition. In this technique an oesophagostomy tube passes through the pyriform sinus into the oesophagus. However, complications, even fatalities, have been described with this technique.[12]

Records

Anyone who has attempted retrospective or prospective analyses based upon hospital and clinic records of patients treated by a multiplicity of different clinicians at a variety of institutions will have realised the importance of complete, accurate and comprehensible records.

Many authors have commented on the difficulties of undertaking research on large groups of patients when many clinicians are involved over many years.[13-19] Unfortunately traditional clinical notes, although excellent in many cases, can often be incomplete and omit vital details, particularly dates. One missing detail during perhaps a 5 year follow up may invalidate all the otherwise useful information concerning one particular patient.

With this in mind Langdon and Rapidis[20] proposed a universal record chart to be inserted into the records of all patients with oral cancer. It is important to realise that the use of such a data sheet does not replace conventional clinical records, but rather is an aide memoire to ensure that the examining clinician does not forget essential factual data. With the current emphasis on clinical audit it is more important to maintain accurate clinical records. Several computer based systems are currently under development.

Rehabilitation and follow up

The goal of rehabilitation following treatment of cancer is to achieve the maximum level of emotional, physical, social and mental function. This will of course involve integrating the patient back into his or her family and community, and whenever possible a return to the previous occupation.

The basis of a rehabilitation programme must be built before the start of definitive treatment. The trusting relationship between patient and doctors must be established from the earliest time and this relationship will remain the bedrock for all attempts at rehabilitation. To maintain the relationship the patient should be seen whenever possible at each attendance by those doctors with whom this relationship exists. It is not satisfactory for follow up appointments to be delegated to a variety of different junior staff.

Prosthetic rehabilitation of facial and intra-oral defects produced by the surgical eradication of malignant disease has improved tremendously in recent years (see Chapter 19). This is due to improvements both in surgery and laboratory technique. Indeed, it is important that the surgeon works closely with the prosthetist. There are many situations in which small therapeutically insignificant changes in surgical techniques reap great benefits for the ultimate fit and retention of a subsequent prosthesis. Materials research has developed, as has our knowledge of their application. New materials are far more stable and their texture both kinder to the underlying tissues and cosmetically closer to normal tissues. Similarly, pigment technology has advanced, and now stable colour systems are available for most facial prosthetic materials.

The restoration of facial and intra-oral defects, such as single unit areas (e.g. orbital, nasal, facial or maxillary structures) does not usually present major difficulties relative to satisfactory functional and prosthetic restoration. More difficult is the prosthetic restoration of combination defects (e.g. maxilla and orbit, nose and lip) but these problems are not usually insurmountable given some ingenuity on the part of the prosthetist. Indeed, such is the state of the art that it behoves the surgeon in many situations not to attempt surgical reconstruction. Often better results are achieved both functionally and cosmetically by the use of a prosthesis. Examples of this are maxillary obturators, prosthetic noses and prosthetic eyes following orbital exenteration. The development of osseo-integrated implants has made a significant contribution (see Chapter 19).

The social worker's role is to assist the patient and his or her family in dealing with the emotional and social problems which so often accompany illness, hospitalisation and possible deformity. Initial contact with the patient and family helps to identify underlying psychological problems and factors such as interpersonal relationships within the family, emotional responses to treatment and deformity (from both patient and family), and social resources. The social worker must liaise closely with the general practitioner, hospital team and social services.

The services of a speech therapist may be needed. Not only can he or she help the patient with speech problems, but also he or she can give great assistance in re-establishing swallowing patterns. This may also aid Eustachian tube function and improve hearing.

Psychiatric help may be required in specific cases where the primary health care team establishes such a need. Some of these patients will 'by chance' have underlying psychiatric disorders. Many will go through a period of depression following therapy and may require both psychotropic drugs and professional psychiatric counselling. Locally or nationally organised 'support groups' can be of great benefit to some patients. Examples of such groups include 'Lets Face It' (10 Wood End, Crowthorne, Berkshire, RG11 6DQ) and 'Changing Faces' (27 Cowper Street, London EC2A 4AP).

Rehabilitation continues throughout the remaining life span of the patient following primary treatment. Those in regular contact with the patient at follow up clinics must be ever vigilant in detecting psychological and social problems as they arise. The relationship should be such that the patient can turn to his doctors as soon as a problem arises in the knowledge that help and sympathy will be forthcoming.

Continuing care

Another aspect to be faced by the surgeon or radiotherapist is the patient with incurable cancer, who will probably need more help and support than the potentially curable. To tell such a patient that 'nothing more can be done' and to add 'I don't need to see you again' is as helpful as throwing a drowning man both ends of a rope. Regular concerned follow up and symptomatic and palliative treatment is essential. Such patients often find great inner strength and courage and have inwardly come to terms with their disease. It is not death which they fear but the process of dying and the fear of being abandoned at this stage.

This aspect of patient care becomes particularly important when the patient is admitted for terminal care. Inevitably the 'doctor' under whose care the patient is admitted is embarrassed by having to face a 'failure'; but the doctor must *not* hurry by on a ward round and avoid stopping by that patient's bed. Dunphy[21] has put this very clearly:

'The one patient in the service who wants most to be seen, examined and talked to is the patient who is or may be dying. One need not hold lengthy discussions over such a patient, the entire retinue should not crowd into the room; but a sympathetic visit on the part of the responsible doctor can be more beneficial than an extra dose of narcotic. One should ask the patient about his pain, listen to his chest, do a gentle examination, and then make the recommendations for changes in management. Attention to little details, such as food, drink, bowels, position in bed, and air in the room bring great emotional dividends. Above all, touch the patient, shake hands, take the pulse and gently palpate the areas of pain'.

At this stage the patient should not be submitted to any treatment or investigation unless that treatment will relieve some specific symptom without exacting too heavy a price. An example of this is so-called palliative chemotherapy. Tracheostomy is in much the same position as colostomy in that it is tolerable when it is the necessary conclusion to a radical operation for an operable carcinoma; but it may be the last straw if it is added to the trials of a growth that cannot be removed.[1]

When finally we reach the end, it is the doctor's last duty to see that the patient dies without pain and distress and with dignity. It may well be that the very act of relieving symptoms will hasten death. There comes a time when it is a final act of kindness to withdraw active treatment. This cannot be a committee decision but one made in all humility by the doctor with whom the patient at earlier times has formed that special relationship. There is no place in this final scene for parenteral nutrition or a last desperate cut-down to find a vein to correct dehydration. There is no value at this moment in knowing the electrolyte or haemoglobin levels. The course of terminal head and neck malignancy is always prolonged and uniquely difficult for the patient and doctor, and especially for the nursing staff and family and friends.

For further details of continuing care the reader is referred to 'The Management of Terminal Malignant Disease' edited by Cicely Saunders.[22]

The development of the Hospice movement in the UK has done much to improve the lot of incurable patients. Unfortunately such facilities are not available throughout the UK and are not acceptable to all patients, but when available they offer a more suitable environment than a busy surgical ward for the terminal patient. Most health authorities in the UK now have 'home support teams' with special expertise in symptom control and many patients with their support are able to remain at home until they die.

References

1 Gardham J. Palliative surgery. *Proceedings of the Royal Society of Medicine* 1964; **57**: 123–8.
2 Stell PM, Maran AGD. *Head and Surgery*. London: William Heineman Medical Books, 1972: 2–3.
3 Bryce DP. Unique features of head and neck malignancies which relate to their management. *Journal of Otolaryngology* 1981; **10**: 3–9.
4 Sandler HC. A retrospective study of head and neck cancer program. *Cancer* 1970; **25**: 1153–61.
5 Lindberg RD. Present day role of radiation therapy in the treatment of head and neck cancer. In: Chambers RG *et al.* eds. *Cancer of the Head and Neck*. Amsterdam: Excerpta Medica, 1975.
6 Rapidis AD, Angelopoulos AP, Langdon JD. The team approach in the management of oral cancer. *Annals of the Royal College of Surgeons of England* 1980; **62**: 116–19.
7 Brookes GB, Clifford P. Nutritional status and general immune competence in patients with head and neck cancer. *Journal of the Royal Society of Medicine* 1981; **74**: 132–9.
8 Gauderer MWL, Ponsky JL, Izant RJ. Gastrostomy without laparotomy: a percutaneous endoscopic technique. *Journal of Paediatric Surgery* 1980; **15**: 872–5.
9 Forgacs I, Macpherson A, Tibbs C. Percutaneous endoscopic gastroscopy. *British Medical Journal* 1992; **304**: 1395–6.
10 Park RHR, Allison MC, Lang J *et al.* Randomised comparison of percutaneous endoscopic gastrostomy and nasogastric tube feeding in patients with persisting neurological dysphagia. *British Medical Journal* 1992; **304**: 1406–9.
11 Wood G. Cervical oesophagostomy and the use of a fine bore tube. *British Journal of Oral Surgery* 1983; **21**: 16–20.
12 Edge C, Langdon JD. Complications of pharyngostomy. *British Journal of Oral and Maxillofacial Surgery* 1991; **29**: 237–40.
13 Batley F. The dilemma of cancer statistics. *Archives of Surgery* 1964; **88**: 163–6.
14 Hoopes JE. *Symposium on Cancer of the Head and Neck: Total Treatment and Reconstructive Rehabilitation*. St Louis, MO: CV Mosby, 1969.
15 Binnie WH, Cawson RA, Hill GB, Soaper AE. *Oral Cancer in England and Wales. A National Study of Morbidity, Mortality, Curability and Related Factors*. London: HMSO, 1972.
16 Fries R, Grabner H, Langer H *et al.* Comparative investigation on the classification of carcinoma of the oral cavity. *Journal of Maxillofacial Surgery* 1973; **1**: 222–35.
17 Moss TW, Brand WN, Battifora H. *Radiation Oncology: Rationale, Technique, Results*, 4th edn. St Louis, MO: CV Mosby, 1973.
18 Speissl B, von Albert J, Bitter K *et al.* A clinical examination on value determination of the TNM-classification of the carcinoma of the buccal cavity. *Zeitschrift fur Kresforschung* 1973; **80**: 83–95.
19 Langdon JD, Rapidis AD, Harvey PW, Patel MF. STNMP. A new classification for oral cancer. *British Journal of Oral Surgery* 1977; **15**: 49–54.
20 Langdon JD, Rapidis AD. The importance of accurate records and follow-up in patients with oral cancer. *Journal of Maxillofacial Surgery* 1978; **6**: 226–30.
21 Dunphy JE. On caring for the patient with cancer. *Bulletin of the American College of Surgeons* 1976.
22 Saunders CM. *The Management of Terminal Malignant Disease*. London: Edward Arnold, 1984.

7 Surgery

DS Soutar and I Taggart

Introduction

In malignant tumours of the mouth, jaws and salivary glands, mortality is most commonly associated with inability to control the local disease. Difficulties in obtaining local control of malignant disease might suggest a more radical approach to surgery is required, but this has to be balanced against the disability and deformity that such surgery produces. The morbidity of radical surgery can be reduced by alterations in surgical technique, and by reconstructing the defect at the time of surgical excision. For this reason excision and reconstruction go hand in hand and form the basis of surgical management in head and neck malignancy. Furthermore, advances in reconstructive techniques have lifted many of the restrictions previously placed on excisional surgery.

Although the principles of resection and the principles of reconstruction may differ, the two have to be considered together in the overall surgical management of the patient. Excision is directed towards curing or controlling the disease process whereas reconstruction is aimed at minimising the morbidity of surgery. It is important however that reconstruction should not compromise excisional treatment. Knowledge and experience of a wide variety of reconstructive techniques has enhanced the excisional aspects of surgery, a wider clearance of tumours permitted through confidence in our abilities to reconstruct the defect. Pre-operative planning plays an essential role in mapping out both excision and reconstruction and facilitates patient counselling and rehabilitation.

Pre-operative planning

Joint consultation and a team approach is required since surgery may form only part of the overall treatment of the patient with malignant disease. Consideration has to be given to adjuvant or combined treatment in the form of radiotherapy and/or chemotherapy and general treatment strategies, discussed previously, have to be considered. From a surgical point of view there are a variety of parameters that must be fully assessed pre-operatively.

General medical condition

A full medical history and examination is an essential part of any pre-operative evaluation. Of particular interest in the head and neck is the association of many tumours, particularly intra-oral and upper aerodigestive squamous carcinoma, with smoking and alcohol intake. Certain malignant diseases are associated with an advanced age group of patients who often suffer from other generalised conditions affecting the respiratory, cardiovascular, genito-urinary and digestive systems. For example, it is estimated that 40 per cent of patients with head and neck cancer are malnourished when first seen;[1,2] Any nutritional deficiencies should be corrected prior to undertaking major surgery.

The risks for major surgery have to be assessed on an individual patient basis. General medical examination and investigation is therefore directed towards assessing the suitability of the patient to undergo major surgery. This is a key decision since if the patient is deemed unfit for surgery then alternative methods of treatment such as chemotherapy and/or radiotherapy, or palliative care aimed at controlling symptoms, should be instituted. If the patient is fit to undergo major surgery subsequent planning and execution of surgery is carried out without further concessions to the general medical condition of the patient. Where this involves simple excision and reconstruction and a short operation, this is a relatively easy concept to accept. It is with the more difficult complex cases which require a lengthy and complicated surgical procedure that a dilemma may arise. Any compromise should be avoided by proper pre-operative planning. Limitation in surgery results in incomplete excision of otherwise curable tumours and poor and ineffective reconstruction. In the present author's practice, once a patient is passed fit for surgery then that patient is scheduled for what appears to be the most radical and best method of excision combined with what is thought to be the best available method of reconstruction. Even adopting this very aggressive policy the mortality from major surgery for intraoral cancer is remarkably low. This is a tribute not only to modern surgical techniques but also to the expertise of physicians, anaesthetists, intensive care specialists and trained nursing staff.

Where general pre-operative medical examination and investigation assess the suitability of the patient to undergo major surgery, more specific clinical examination and further detailed investigations are required to assess the extent and nature of the malignancy.

Examination under anaesthetic

Superficial lesions can often be accurately assessed by the standard techniques of palpation and inspection. Deeper lesions, or those that are difficult to see from the surface, or those in close proximity to muscle or associated with pain, are often difficult to assess when the patient is awake. In these situations an examination under anaesthetic (EUA) facilitates more accurate staging of the extent of the disease. It renders muscles relaxed which would otherwise naturally constrict due to the pain associated with examination. Assessment of lymph nodes in the neck is also facilitated when the patient is under anaesthetic.

An EUA is certainly mandatory in intra-oral cancer when the pain associated with ulceration makes standard clinical examination extremely difficult. EUA also allows a more detailed examination aimed at mapping out in considerable detail the extent of the tumour, the likely resection, the reconstruction that will be required, and the detection of any second primary tumour. At the same time a careful search should be made for other synchronous tumours in the region (see also Chapter 5).

Radiological investigation

Plain X-rays of facial bones and jaws can provide evidence of gross invasion by tumour or highlight problem areas, e.g. opacity of a maxillary antrum. Orthopantomograms and occlusal views are very useful in pre-operative assessment of the lower jaw, not only to show gross involvement of tumour, but also to assess the dental status of the patient and to help identify any teeth which should be removed at the time of surgical treatment. This is particularly important for patients going on to have post operative radical radiotherapy or for patients in whom dental rehabilitation is planned using a bridge or denture or later osseointegrated implants. Special X-rays such as tomograms of particular facial bones likely to be involved by tumour are also of use.

Tumour involvement of facial bones and the spread of disease to the local regional lymph nodes in the neck have both been associated with a poor prognosis. It is therefore not surprising that considerable effort has been made towards improving the pre-operative assessment of bone invasion and lymph node involvement. Invasion of bone can significantly alter treatment protocols since radiotherapy has proved relatively ineffective in the treatment of tumour within bone. In addition, the surgery that might be required to excise and reconstruct bony defects can often complicate the surgical procedure. It would therefore be advantageous in pre-operative planning to identify cases in which there is bone involvement, and also the extent of this involvement. This assumes great importance where there are possibilities of maintaining some degree of bony continuity, such as in the preservation of the lower border of the mandible.

Computed tomography (CT) scans have proved useful in determining bony invasion, particularly in upper jaw tumours and maxilla extending towards the base of the skull.[3] CT scans however have proved less useful in determining invasion of the mandible. This is because the irregularities of the occlusal surface and the presence of unhealed tooth sockets and residual dentition make the interpretation of these scans exceedingly difficult.[4] The authors have found technetium 99 bone scans to be of use in predicting tumour involvement in the mandible.[5] Other authors have similarly shown the usefulness of bone scans in this area.[6–8]

CT scanning has also been used effectively in determining lymph node involvement in the neck (see Chapter 13).[9–11] Nuclear magnetic resonance imaging (NMR) may prove even more effective than CT scanning in defining soft tissue tumours and in the detection of lymph nodes in the neck.[12] Additional information can be obtained by using contrast medium,[13,14] and with improved software both NMR and CT scanning can provide additional information on both soft tissue and bone.

Ultrasound is another useful investigation that is not routinely used in head and neck malignancy but can be combined with fine needle aspiration biopsy to help localise lesions and ensure biopsy from a tumour mass. Ultrasound is currently being used effectively in lymph node biopsy in the neck[15,16] and can be used equally effectively in fine needle aspiration of salivary glands.

Both clinical and radiological investigations are aimed at determining the extent of the malignancy. Currently in Europe the TNM classification is most commonly used,[17] while in the USA the American Joint Committee of Cancer (AJCC) system is used.[18] Despite the limitations of staging malignant disease, they form an essential part of the pre-operative treatment planning to determine the extent of excision and reconstruction, the likely prognosis and the chances of survival so that patients can be adequately counselled with regard to the proposed treatment.

Pathology

An accurate pre-operative pathological diagnosis is essential in planning surgical management. The tumour may be sampled in an open or closed fashion. Closed tissue sampling includes fine needle aspiration biopsy (see Chapter 5) which is most useful in the diagnosis of salivary gland tumours and masses in the neck.[19,20] The procedure can be carried out in an outpatient clinic and can be combined with ultrasound to aid tumour localisation and improve accuracy of tissue sampling.[15,16]

Needle biopsy can also be used to provide a core of tissue for histological diagnosis as with the tru-cut needle biopsy. This technique can also be performed in the outpatient clinic; most surgeons excise the tract following a tru-cut needle biopsy if the patient comes to surgery. Excision of the needle tract is not required when using fine needle aspiration.

Open biopsies require a minor surgical procedure. The site of incision for the biopsy should not compromise any further surgical intervention that may be required. The site of incision should not pass through tissue that will not be surgically excised should the case come to radical surgery. Similarly a biopsy site should be placed either within the tumour so that it is removed at the time of excision, or in a line of access to the tumour. This is particularly important when performing external biopsies for lumps in the neck which may subsequently require a radical or functional neck dissection. Careful placement of the biopsy site allows it to be excised in continuity with either the incision for access or the excision of the tumour.

Special considerations

(see also Chapter 6)

The planning of surgical treatment is not limited to considerations of the type of malignancy, its extent, the feasibility of resection and reconstruction and the general medical condition of the patient. Of equal importance are considerations of what surgical treatment will mean to the patient in the short or long term. These special considerations include function, cosmesis, and quality of life.

Function

Malignant tumours of the mouth, jaws and salivary glands can in themselves affect important functions, particularly of the oral cavity. These include speech, chewing, swallowing and breathing. Difficulties may arise from the site of the tumour itself, because of swelling associated with the tumour or, most commonly, because of pain. A tumour on the tongue for example may restrict tongue movement leading to alterations in speech and difficulty in swallowing. The pain associated with such tumours also severely restricts dietary intake leading to dramatic weight loss. Tumours affecting the jaws are often painful and severely restrict chewing activity and again dietary intake. It is clear that the patient presenting with this type of malignancy often already shows impaired function.

Most research has concentrated on looking at the functions of speaking and eating. Certainly both surgery and radiotherapy have adverse affects on both these functions and create significant physiological and mechanical problems.[21-23] Our own experience[24] showed that there was significant under-reporting of problems by patients when compared with spouses' reports. Twenty-five per cent of patients however did report problems in the areas of speech, eating and drinking and a concern about their appearance. Our more recent study[25] showed that 21 per cent of patients undergoing surgery and radiotherapy for intra-oral cancer experienced difficulty in swallowing solid foods. Furthermore, 65 per cent of patients were unable to regain their pre-operative weight after 6 months.

Functional problems that patients experience following surgery have proved difficult to evaluate and a variety of different tests and scores have been proposed.[26–31] Assessment of postoperative function cannot be taken in isolation without considering the pre-operative status of the patient. Teichgraeber *et al.*[26] showed that the functional result was in proportion to the size of the primary tumour. Similarly our series[25] showed that patients with small tumours (T1) faired much better postoperatively and were more likely to return to a normal diet and to regain their pre-operative weight. In the assessment of speech a pre-operative assessment by a speech therapist is essential if appropriate and well planned speech therapy is to be instituted.[32,33]

It is only recently that attention has focused on the effects of surgical procedures on the functions of speech, swallowing and chewing. There remain significant problems in the assessment of function, particularly when linked to pre-operative evaluation and postoperative rehabilitation. The majority of swallowing assessments rely on videofluoroscopy or scintography to determine transit times and swallowing patterns.[34–37] This provides an objective assessment that can be repeated at varying intervals during the rehabilitative period.

The assessment of speech however is somewhat less sophisticated and often relies on subjective assessment by speech scientists and speech therapists using a variety of scales and techniques.[32,33,35,38,39] Such investigations, and particularly those considering differing surgical techniques, are still in their infancy.[34,39,40] The majority of tests for the assessment of function are very time consuming and elaborate.[26,27] The authors are currently evaluating a simple scale to assess speech, swallowing and chewing. This scale, known as the Functional Intra-oral Glasgow Scale (FIGS), has shown excellent interobserver reliability. This essentially means that the scores that the patient achieves using this simple scale are virtually the same whether the investigation is carried out by the patient, the patient's relative, a general practitioner, a dietician, a speech therapist or a surgeon. This scale not only provides a base line prior to treatment but can also be used in the follow up period as an aid to patient rehabilitation. With appropriate therapy the patient can identify with an improved functional score and this acts as an incentive. Of equal importance is the early detection of a deterioration in the patient's score in any of the three functions. This serves as a warning that the patient's condition is changing and can be seen long before the appearance of significant signs of problems such as weight loss. Recurrent intra-oral cancer for example has been identified on several occasions from the deterioration in the patient's FIGS scores, before there has been apparent evidence of the tumour or significant symptoms such as pain or loss of weight. The initial results are encouraging and the scale appears to act as a good monitor of the patient's progress (Tables 7.1 and 7.2).

Pre-operative dental impressions and the creation of a dental obturator are required in maxillectomy. Pre-operative planning with regard to prosthodontics is important and the increasing role of osseointegrated implants also requires planning with regard to both excision and reconstruction (see also Chapter 19).[41,42]

Another vital function that can be affected by head and neck cancer is respiration. Many of the patients will present with a history of smoking and chronic obstructive airways disease. Assessment of respiratory function pre-operatively will be part of the general medical assessment. Additionally, however, in the pre-operative planning the surgeon must consider aspiration since this is a major cause of morbidity and mortality. Aspiration may occur pre-operatively and need not be dramatic but is often insidious and results from trickling of small amounts of saliva into the lungs. The after effects of surgery have also to be considered and whether postoperatively the patient will be incompetent, allowing aspiration either as the result of mechanical disruption or as a result of loss of sensation and normal reflex mechanisms. Such a patient may well require the protection of a tracheostomy in the early postoperative phase. It is therefore important in pre-operative planning to accurately assess respiratory function and consider the effects of surgery on the airway so that the question of tracheostomy can be discussed with the patient pre-operatively.

Cosmesis

Patients presenting with head and neck cancer are naturally worried about the scarring and deformity that surgical treatment might inflict. Our own experience has shown that female patients were more

Table 7.1 Functional Intra-oral Glasgow Scale

How to score yourself	
I can chew	
Any food, no difficulty	5
Solid food, with difficulty	4
Semisolid food, no difficulty	3
Semisolids with difficulty	2
Cannot chew at all	1
I can swallow	
Any food, no difficulty	5
Solid food, with difficulty	4
Semisolid food only	3
Liquids only	2
Cannot swallow at all	1
My speech	
Clearly understood always	5
Requires repetition sometimes	4
Requires repetition many times	3
Understood by relatives only	2
Unintelligible	1

concerned about their appearance than male patients.[24] In addition to scarring, excisional surgery can result in functional cosmetic problems. Loss of the facial nerve or loss of facial muscles results in facial paralysis with all its cosmetic sequelae. Surgery that affects oral competence and the control of saliva can result in unsightly drooling.

Modern reconstructive techniques have certainly improved the cosmetic results that can now be achieved in major head and neck cancer surgery (Fig. 7.1). In addition, the surgeon has to consider morbidity of the donor site for any reconstruction and here again there may be significant cosmetic factors.[43]

Advances in reconstruction have brought a freedom with regard to excision facilitating the performance of larger and more extensive resections. This freedom has of course brought additional problems since cases previously deemed inoperable can now be treated surgically. The surgeon must

Table 7.2 Functional Intra-oral Glasgow Scale scorecard

Your monthly score

	Oct	Nov	Dec	Jan	Feb	Mar	Apr	May	June	July	Aug	Sept
Chewing score												
Swallowing score												
Speech score												

Your clinic score

	Oct	Nov	Dec	Jan	Feb	Mar	Apr	May	June	July	Aug	Sept
Chewing score												
Swallowing score												
Speech score												
Your weight												

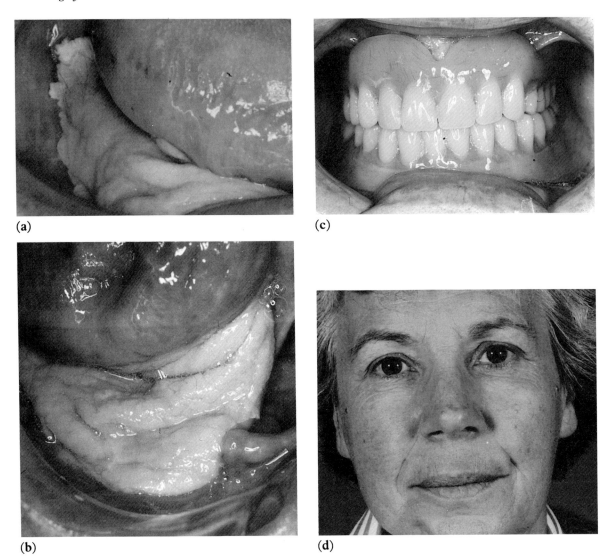

Fig. 7.1 (a) Appearance of a radial forearm flap at 4 years. (b) The thin pliable skin allows good tongue mobility. (c) The patient is able to wear a satisfactory denture over the flap. (d) A good cosmetic and functional result has been achieved in this 51 year old patient.

temper his or her enthusiasm to undertake major surgery with a consideration of what is in the patient's best interests with regard to mortality and morbidity.

Quality of life

This is perhaps the most difficult pre-operative evaluation that the surgeon has to make. It is all too easy for a surgeon to embark upon a major

excision and reconstruction but it is extremely difficult to turn down a patient for surgery and advocate some other treatment. Unfortunately the surgeon cannot confine himself to dealing only with a disease process but has to consider the ethical and financial implications of treatment. The surgical treatment of many forms of head and neck cancer appears to have reached a plateau with very little improvement in overall survival in the last two or three decades. Since surgery does not appear to be altering the pattern of this type of malignancy nor its natural history, then the quality of life of cancer patients assumes increasing importance. Considerable efforts are now being made in this direction.[44-46] Problems remain however in objectively assessing the quality of life.[47]

Patient counselling

The final stage in pre-operative planning is a full and frank discussion with the patient. By this time the pathological diagnosis will be known, the extent of the surgical excision will have been mapped out and the method of reconstruction planned. It is the surgeon's duty to inform the patient of the likely outcome, not only in terms of excision of the tumour, and the deficit that removal of this tissue will cause, but also the reconstruction and the functional and cosmetic results that it is hoped to achieve. Furthermore, the donor sites for tissue used in reconstruction have to be identified and discussed with regard to additional scarring and morbidity. Only then can patient and surgeon move together towards appropriate surgical management, confident in the knowledge of both excision and reconstruction.

The diagnosis of cancer frequently causes considerable psychological morbidity and distress.[48,49] This can be compounded particularly in head and neck cancer because of the functional and cosmetic problems discussed previously.[22-24,49] A study carried out on our own patients[50] demonstrated a need to assess patients pre-operatively and identify patients particularly at risk of developing psychological problems. This study, which reviewed patients who had undergone major intra-oral surgery, showed 41 per cent of patients to have significant levels of psychological distress. Females and younger patients appeared to be more at risk of psychological distress and anxiety problems were more common than depressive states.

Currently patients with intra-oral cancer presenting to our institution undergo assessment using the hospital anxiety depression scale.[51] It has been our impression that those showing high scores, i.e. a degree of anxiety or depression, do not react well to surgery and can pose significant problems for rehabilitation.

It is perhaps surprising that few patients presenting with head and neck cancer enter into discussions about outcome and survival. Perhaps this is only a reflection of their fear and anxiety. However, some patients and the majority of relatives do ask questions about the natural history of the disease and likely outcome.

Despite the voluminous publications on the results obtained in head and neck cancer treatment, predicting the outcome in individual cases remains a major problem. Accepting the deficiencies of the TNM and AJCC staging systems, clinical staging of the disease remains the mainstay in predicting outcome.[52-56] In particular, the significance of regional lymph node metastasis and its association with a poor prognosis has been confirmed.[52-59] Anatomical site also appears to be important since different sites metastasise at different rates.[56,57,60] The significance of site however may not simply be its relationship to lymph node metastasis. The tongue for example shows a poorer prognosis than other sites,[61,62] and even where the same treatment is employed the tumour appears to behave differently with differing anatomical locations.[62,63]

In addition to clinical staging and the anatomical site of the malignancy, the tumour thickness has been implicated.[54,64,65]

In addition to the problems of predicting the natural history of the malignancy, there are equal problems in comparing the results of differing modalities of treatment. Encouraged by the reported improved loco-regional control and survival using combined modality treatment incorporating surgery and radiotherapy,[66-68] our head and neck combined team adopted the policy of surgery followed by radical radiotherapy. Our initial results[69,70] were promising and we have continued this policy to the present day. We have expanded the role of surgery and postoperative radical radiotherapy to include tumours of the upper jaw and maxilla and have again demonstrated improved results.[71] The 5 year survival of advanced maxillary antral tumours treated with radiotherapy alone was only 19 per cent whereas with combined modality treatment comprising radical surgery followed by radical postoperative radiotherapy the 5 year survival has improved to 61 per cent.[71]

When counselling patients who are to undergo surgery for head and neck cancer, it is important to adopt a positive approach: the patient should feel confident in the treatment proposed. During preparation of the patient for surgery a specialised nurse counsellor forms an essential part of the head and neck team: a good relationship between counsellor and patient greatly facilitates pre-operative planning and discussion and has proved to be of great benefit in the rehabilitation of patients undergoing major surgery.

Principles of resection

It is important to identify the main aim of any cancer treatment, whether it be surgery, chemotherapy or radiotherapy. All these modalities can be used singly or in combination to effect a 'cure' or for palliation.

In surgery, the principals of curative and palliative resection differ.

Palliative resection

The main aim of palliative resection is to improve quality of life. The main objectives are to:

(1) Reduce tumour size
(2) Prevent fungation
(3) Minimise pain
(4) Permit additional treatment

Often in palliative resection all of these objectives have to be taken into account. Reduction of the tumour size by an operative procedure can be useful particularly when there is evidence of compression of vital structures. Debulking may also facilitate control of the tumour with subsequent radiotherapy and/or chemotherapy for a longer period of time.

Fungating tumours in the head and neck region terrify patients and relatives, and are often associated with an odour due to secondary infection. The surgical aim is to debulk the tumour and cover the area with a flap of good quality tissue which should prevent subsequent ulceration through the skin surface, although the disease will continue underneath the flap. Residual tumour can be treated with postoperative radiotherapy and/or chemotherapy if appropriate.

Even in cases where there is ulceration following radical radiotherapy, surgery is still a palliative treatment option. Excision and recontruction using a flap with good padding and thickness can be combined with brachytherapy.

One further advantage of palliative surgery is in the relief of pain. This is achieved either by direct excision of tumour and associated nerves or by surgical decompression of an expanding tumour mass. Surgery can be combined with definitive ablation of nerves, particularly the trigeminal nerve or its branches, or the cervical nerves, either by diathermy or chemical agents such as alcohol. Relief of pain in the postoperative period is often dramatic and is much appreciated by patients.

Curative resection

The aim of resection in curable head and neck malignancy is relatively straightforward. Ideally the tumour should be removed in one piece with a margin of microscopically normal tissue appropriate to the pathology being treated. The specimen should be submitted for pathological examination in such a way that the pathologist can orientate the tissue. Any margins of particular interest can be marked with a suture to draw the pathologist's attention to specific regions.

Frozen section can also be used to advantage in determining tumour clearance at difficult parts of the dissection[72] but it should be remembered that there is a considerable sampling error when using frozen sections and that interpretation can be difficult in previously irradiated patients.

For resection to be regarded as curative the margins must be clear of tumour. Looser *et al.*[73] showed a 39 per cent failure to control advanced Stage III and IV disease despite satisfactory resection margins of greater than 5 mm clearance. Unsatisfactory resection margins of less than 5 mm dramatically increased the failure rate to 73 per cent. Zieske *et al.*[74] in a retrospective study demonstrated positive margins in surgical resections in 8.8 per cent of their series. Of these, 60 per cent failed to achieve local regional control despite being treated with radiotherapy. It would appear that on histological examination should any margins show incomplete excision then re-excision is the safest course of action.

Surgeons have had to come to terms with the debilitating effects of surgical excision and the loss of function mentioned previously. This has resulted in a gradual change in attitude away from ultraradical surgery towards accurate excision with preservation of vital structures wherever possible.

In intra-oral cancer, for example, increasing debate has centred around techniques aimed at preserving all or part of the mandible intact.[75–79]

Similarly, in the management of regional lymph nodes, the classical radical neck dissection is gradually being replaced by function-preserving neck dissections aimed at minimising the morbidity (see Chapter 13).[80–83]

These techniques should not be regarded as conservative surgery, but are aimed at increasing the accuracy of excision. Such techniques are often technically more difficult, demanding a greater level of surgical expertise. Most head and neck surgeons would agree that it is simpler to perform a radical neck dissection than a functional neck dissection and similiarly a standard hemimandibulectomy is a much simpler and quicker operation than that preserving a rim of intact mandible.

These techniques are only possible as a result of our increased understanding of the methods of invasion of tumours locally and of the patterns of lymph node spread according to the site of the primary tumour. As a general rule, this type of surgery is only suitable in previously untreated cases and is particularly useful when surgery is the first arm in a combined modality treatment plan. In our practice the majority of cases undergo surgery followed by radical postoperative radiotherapy. Despite combined modality treatment, the 5 year cure rates of advanced tumours in this region have only slightly improved (5–10 per cent).[84] There have however been significant increases in loco-regional control.[53,85,86] We do not use the techniques of preserving a rim of mandible, or selective or functional neck dissections, in patients who have previously undergone radiotherapy and/or chemotherapy. In such cases it is often difficult to define accurately the extent of the disease, which often exhibits a more aggressive pattern both locally and in the regional neck nodes.

Untreated tumours often invade in an advancing line, whereas those that have been treated previously, particularly with radiotherapy, often lose this advancing edge and show a diffuse widespread infiltrating pattern often with skip lesions. This makes the histological diagnosis of adequate clearance of tumour exceedingly difficult. Most surgeons excise more radically when a malignant tumour has previously undergone treatment, particularly radiotherapy.

Case selection therefore becomes vital but in experienced hands such techniques have proved to be as equally effective as the more traditional radical procedures.[77–80,83] It would appear, therefore, that the surgery remains radical enough to treat the local disease, but has the advantage of preserving intact, uninvolved structures that could play an important functional or cosmetic role. Accuracy of excision should be regarded as an important principle of excisional surgery. Surgeons can often delude themselves into thinking they have performed a radical operation by creating a large defect, forgetting that the tumour clearance might only be a few millimetres at certain margins such as the base of skull or carotid vessels. It is the minimum tumour clearance that is important and not the extent of surgery into normal tissue.

The extent of resection should be well defined in those patients who have undergone a full and complete pre-operative work up. The surgeon has to be prepared to adapt both his resection and reconstructive plans if the findings at operation are different from those envisaged in the pre-operative planning. If it becomes clear for example that the tumour cannot be completely excised, then the plan has to change from a curative to a palliative resection and reconstruction.

Certain pathological diseases are notoriously difficult to cure despite apparently clear excision margins. Adenoid cystic carcinoma is a prime example and has led many surgeons to wonder whether the disease is ever curable by surgery.

Local resection

As stated previously the principal aim of resection is to excise the malignancy with a margin of normal tissue appropriate to the pathology of the tumour. The surgical planning has to include surgical access to the tumour as well as the extent of the local excison and the management of the regional lymph nodes in the neck.

Surgical exposure

Visualisation of the tumour is an essential prerequisite for accurate excision and requires a similar approach to the extensile exposure described by Henry.[87] Good access simplifies both excision and reconstruction and may be divided into several levels (listed below), increasing progressively as the tumour becomes less accessible.

Direct cutaneous access
In tumours involving the skin, excision margins can be mapped out on the skin surface. This allows a direct approach to the tumour and excision can proceed deeper and deeper into the facial structures and bone.

Transoral approach
In small mobile tumours, usually situated in the anterior area of the oral cavity, this approach can provide adequate access for resection and reconstruction. A wide sublabial incision for example can allow a cheek flap to be raised in a degloving manoeuvre that can be used effectively in both upper and lower jaw resections.

Even a total maxillectomy can be performed via a wide upper labial incision. Whereas these incisions give adequate access for resection, it is often difficult to adequately reconstruct. The transoral approach should always be considered, but should not be used if assessment, resection or reconstruction is in any way compromised. If this is the case, the surgeon should progress to the next stage which would include a lip split.

Lip split

A lip split is a simple full thickness vertical incision that can be extended laterally along the labial sulcus in either the upper or lower lips. In the upper lip, it is classically used as part of the Weber Fergusson approach for maxillectomy and radical upper jaw surgery.[88] The lower lip can be split vertically through the chin prominence but we prefer a modified lip split (Fig. 7.2) which places the scars in the contour of the chin prominence and gives a superior cosmetic result. Another advantage of the modified

lip split is that the incision overlies the site for a lateral mandibular osteotomy should this be required. A lip split alone only marginally improves access to the oral cavity and is most useful when combined with an access osteotomy.

Access osteotomy

Whereas a lip split only slightly increases access to the oral cavity a mandibular or maxillary osteotomy vastly improves access to all areas of the oral cavity and beyond. This approach has often been described as similar to opening a book. In the upper jaw a wide variety of osteotomies are possible depending on the site of the primary tumour.[88–90] Similarly, in the mandible the position of the osteotomy largely depends on the position of the tumour and whether the mandible is to be resected or not. When performing a mandibular osteotomy purely for improving access, the choices are be-

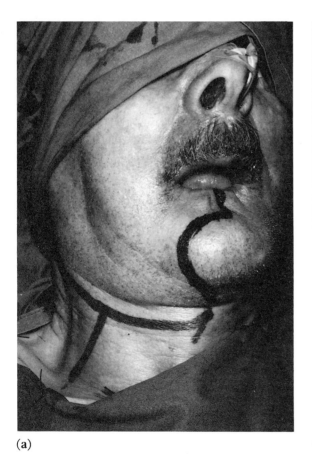

(a)

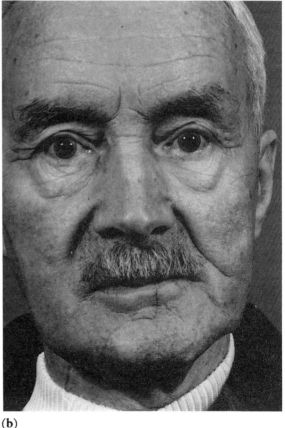

(b)

Fig. 7.2   (a) Skin markings for a lip and chin split combined with a neck dissection. (b) Appearance at 4 weeks following resection and reconstruction with a free radial forearm flap.

tween a midline osteotomy or a lateral osteotomy. The midline or symphyseal osteotomy is the traditional approach originally performed with the classical lip split.[91] It was arguably thought to be the optimum site as symmetrical muscle pull allowed stability and the osteotomy was usually asymptomatic even if only fibrous union was achieved. The lateral osteotomy is performed between the mental foramen and the lateral border of the anterior belly of the digastric preserving the mental nerve (Fig. 7.3). The advantage of the lateral osteotomy is that there is minimal soft tissue stripping especially with the preferred modified lip split.[92,93] The lateral osteotomy also facilitates easy identification of the mental foramen and the mandibular canal. The other advantage is that when performing a mandibular swing to increase access, the only structures requiring division are the mucosa and the mylohyoid. This preserves the anterior belly of digastric, genioglossus and geniohyoid, maintaining their function and the blood supply to the mandible.[92] Having selected the osteotomy site, the type of osteotomy performed can be vertical, oblique or stepped.[94] A straight vertical osteotomy is easy to perform but difficult to re-oppose and maintain position. The oblique osteotomy has the advantages of being quick to perform and easy to oppose for fixation, and with modern titanium plates (two per osteotomy) has the advantage of being extremely stable. This is now our first choice of osteotomy technique. The more traditional stepped osteotomy takes longer to perform and its advantage of stability is less important with plating techniques for fixation.

Although it is possible to preserve teeth and to carry out an osteotomy between tooth roots[93] we have abandoned this procedure and routinely remove a single tooth to enable the osteotomy to be safely performed without risk of damage to the

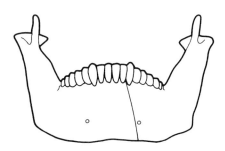

Fig. 7.3 The oblique lateral osteotomy passes between the mental foramen and the insertion of the anterior belly of the digastric.

neighbouring tooth roots. In our practice this has proved to be important since by far the majority of cases undergo postoperative radiotherapy within 6 weeks of surgery.

Mandibular resection

It was once standard practice to resect part of the mandible when excising intra-oral tumours, even when bone involvement was clearly not an issue. This was performed to facilitate access and to allow soft tissue closure. The current techniques for exposure and access and for introducing new tissues for reconstruction have made this approach obsolete. Indeed, maintaining continuity of the mandible by either conservative mandibular resection or bony reconstruction is one of the main objectives in cancer surgery. Mandibular resection should only be performed for sound pathological reasons.

Where limited resection of the mandible is performed parallel to the occlusal surface of the bone, the term 'rim resection' is used. Lower border preservation denotes maintenance of the mandible, inferior to the mental foramen and the inferior dental canal. The resection removes the inferior dental nerve and the contents of the canal from the mental foramen to the base of the skull. Segmental resection of the mandible implies complete removal of a portion of the mandible from its occlusal surface to its lower border for a varying length according to the requirements for tumour clearance (Fig. 7.4). Where there is evidence of periosteal reaction either on radiographs or technetium scan or at the time of operation then a rim resection of the mandible may suffice. Early tumour invasion shown either by pre-operative evaluation or identified at the time of operation in previously untreated cases may also only require limited resection of the mandible with preservation of the lower border. Gross involvement of the mandible demands a segmental resection resulting in discontinuity of the mandible combined with immediate reconstruction.

Surgical management of regional lymph nodes

The presence of a palpable node in the neck makes exploration of the neck and some form of neck dissection mandatory (see Chapter 13). In the authors' practice there has been a gradual tendency towards function-preserving neck dissections, particularly

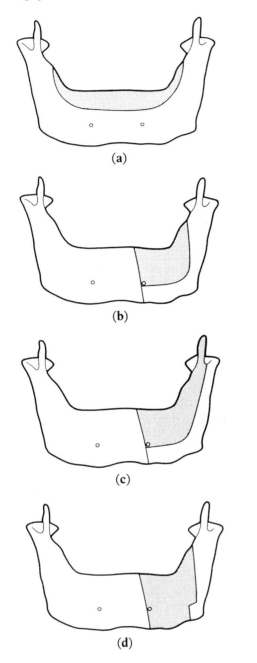

Fig. 7.4 (a) Rim resection of mandible. (b) and (c) Lower border preservation. (d) Segmental excision of mandible.

still favour a radical neck dissection in cases with clinically positive nodes. The aim, wherever possible, is to carry out a neck dissection in continuity with the local resection, although there remains considerable debate as to whether 'en bloc resection' of tumour and nodes is necessary.[95] In certain situations en bloc resection is not feasible, e.g. in lip cancer or in tumours of the upper jaw and maxilla where incontinuity excision is not anatomically possible. From an oncological point of view however the concept of 'en bloc' resection is an important one for the surgeon since it clarifies in his mind the lines of resection.

It is not our surgical practice to carry out prophylactic neck dissections for malignant disease of the mouth, jaws and salivary glands. There are, however, numerous occasions when the neck may be entered as part of the surgical access, either for excision or reconstruction of the primary tumour. In such cases a functional neck dissection is performed. The authors do not favour supra-omohyoid neck dissection, but prefer to remove the whole of the jugular chain and complete the resection and confirm staging of disease.

Neck dissection is also targeted towards the patterns of lymph node spread associated with differing tumour sites and differing pathologies.[95–97] There appears to be a gradual swing towards accuracy of lymph node dissection just as there is towards accuracy of local resection of head and neck malignant tumours. This has resulted in a wide variety of differing classifications and types of neck dissection.[98]

Principles of reconstruction

The first aim of reconstruction is, as far as possible, to replace like with like in terms of quality, quantity and type of tissue. For simplicity this is often divided into soft tissue and bone reconstruction and the latter is often more readily achieved. This is because bone can be replaced with bone from another donor site in the body either as a free graft or as a vascularised bone flap, attached by a pedicle, or as a free tissue transfer using microvascular techniques. Such bone can be fashioned into the required shape and because like tissue is replaced with like the results are surprisingly good.

The replacement of soft tissue, however, is much less successful because of the specialised nature of the tissues involved. In intra-oral reconstruction, for example, some of the commonest techniques

in tumours placed anteriorly, e.g. anterior floor of mouth, symphysis, anterior and anterolateral tongue and lips. For tumours situated more posteriorly, e.g. posterior third of tongue, tonsil, the authors replace oral epithelium with skin. Oral mucosa is, of course, highly specific having secretory and sensory functions as well as providing intra-oral lining. Replacing this specialised tissue with skin results in a non-sensate non-secretory substitute. Patches of jejunum as a mucosal lining replacement are also not ideal since the secretory function is totally dissimilar to that of oral mucosa and again the reconstruction lacks sensation. Replacing skin of the face and neck is equally difficult because of the specialised nature of differing areas of the face and neck and the inability to provide a good colour and texture match for facial skin.

The muscles attached to the mouth and jaw are practically irreplacable following excision or loss. Despite major advances in reconstructive techniques incorporating the transfer of functioning muscles, it has proved impossible to regain normal oral function and facial expression in for example facial paralysis.

Soft tissue reconstruction cannot replace like with like in terms of type of tissue nor in terms of quality. Attention therefore has to be focused on providing the correct quantity of tissue. For external defects this means paying attention to the contour of the face and neck. In intra-oral reconstruction similar attempts should be made to maintain the various anatomical relations within the oral cavity. Intra-oral contour is important and flaps that are too bulky and distort the oral anatomy can have deleterious effects on function.

A second aim of reconstructive surgery is to provide well vascularised tissue to enable wounds to heal by primary intention. Primary wound healing of both soft tissue and bone is essential to produce satisfactory scars and cosmesis and avoid problems such as fistulae, sepsis and wound breakdown. Primary uncomplicated wound healing allows other treatment modalities to be employed in the early postoperative period, minimising the risk of wound breakdown.

In cases where combined treatment is planned, the authors favour a single stage technique and the introduction of well vascularised tissue. This principle applies equally to bone and to soft tissue. Vascularised bone has proved superior to traditional bone grafts in the patient who is to undergo radical postoperative radiotherapy or chemotherapy for example. Flaps with an independent and permanent blood supply are preferred to those that are inset and subsequently divided at a second stage following capilliary link up. This latter group of flaps contributes nothing to the local vascularity and are

therefore less suitable when combined modality treatment is used.

Immediate versus delayed reconstruction

As stated previously the authors believe that excision and reconstruction cannot be dissociated from each other and that morbidity can be significantly decreased if these two aspects are considered within the same surgical operation. For this reason the overriding principle is one of immediate reconstruction.

From a purely technical point of view it is much simpler to reconstruct at the time of creation of the defect. Accurate measurements with regard to size and volume can be made. In particular, bone reconstruction can be carried out very accurately using the resected specimen of bone to provide an accurate template and vital structures can be replaced in the correct anatomical position (Fig. 7.5). This is certainly not true of delayed reconstruction where tissues become distorted by scarring and contracture making it almost impossible to regain the normal functional anatomy.

The patient, moreover, has only one significant

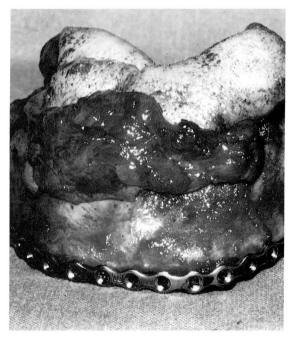

Fig. 7.5 A titanium plate is contoured to the resection specimen. Following resterilisation this acts as a template for mandible reconstruction.

procedure to undergo and postoperative rehabilitation can commence early. Modern methods of reconstruction do not limit adjuvant therapy should this be required and in fact can increase the range of treatment options, particularly the role of brachytherapy.

Reconstructive techniques

A wide variety of surgical techniques are now available for head and neck reconstruction:

(1) Primary closure
(2) Skin grafts
(3) Local flaps
(4) Pedicle flaps
(5) Free flaps

Primary closure

Primary or direct wound closure involves simple approximation of the edges of the defect. This can be achieved at the time of surgery by direct suturing or by leaving the wound open and letting it contract over a period of a few weeks. Some degree of distortion of the tissues must occur, and the technique of primary closure therefore is usually restricted to very small defects.

Skin grafts

Skin grafts whether full thickness or split thickness require a well vascularised bed to ensure their revascularisation and survival. Split thickness grafts will of course contract and the thinner the graft the more contraction that can be expected. They are therefore of limited use in external facial reconstruction but can be used effectively intra-orally.[99] Full thickness grafts can provide a satisfactory cosmetic appearance externally but are not used routinely for intra-oral reconstruction. The main problem with grafts in cancer surgery is that they require revascularisation from the donor defect and contribute nothing to that area. There may very well be delays in primary wound healing due to partial or incomplete graft take and this may delay or render relatively ineffective subsequent modalities of treatment.

Local flaps

Local flaps are most useful for reconstructing cutaneous defects since this method provides the best colour and texture match for facial and cervical skin. The advent of tissue expansion[100] has increased the role of cutaneous local flaps. This however is a multistaged prolonged procedure which necessitates opening up fresh tissue planes and is therefore not suitable for primary reconstruction. Tissue expansion however can be used to improve the final cosmetic results and enable excision of unmatched patches of skin inserted at the time of primary reconstruction.

Intra-orally, local mucosal flaps can sometimes be used to close small defects. Buccal flaps, for example, can be used effectively in the reconstruction of the lip and small defects in the retromolar trigone area. Tongue flaps can be used to recreate the vermillion margin of the lips and for closing palatal defects.

In the treatment of intra-oral malignancy there is a natural reluctance to use local mucosal flaps because of the fears of a field change and epithelial dysplasias. The limited amount of tissue available also restricts their use.

Pedicled flaps

Pedicled flaps, by definition, have to be situated within reach of the defect to be reconstructed. The donor sites are therefore confined to the upper trunk and head and neck regions. Several flaps have proved useful in reconstructing defects of the mouth and jaws.

Nasolabial flap

This is a cutaneous flap from the nasolabial fold which is raised at the level of the facial muscles. Based inferiorly it can be tunnelled through the cheek into the oral cavity. Bilateral nasolabial flaps are particularly useful for reconstructing small defects of the anterior floor of mouth. In this situation a two stage technique is employed with division of the bridge segment at 3 weeks.[101,102] This method can also be used as a single stage technique for reconstructing buccal mucosal defects by de-epithelialising the bridge segment (Fig. 7.6).

Deltopectoral flap

The deltopectoral flap is a cutaneous axial pattern flap based on perforating branches of the internal thoracic artery. It is usually raised based on the first three or four intercostal spaces. The flap is particularly useful for replacing cervical skin as a simple transposition flap or as a staged procedure for reconstructing external facial skin particularly

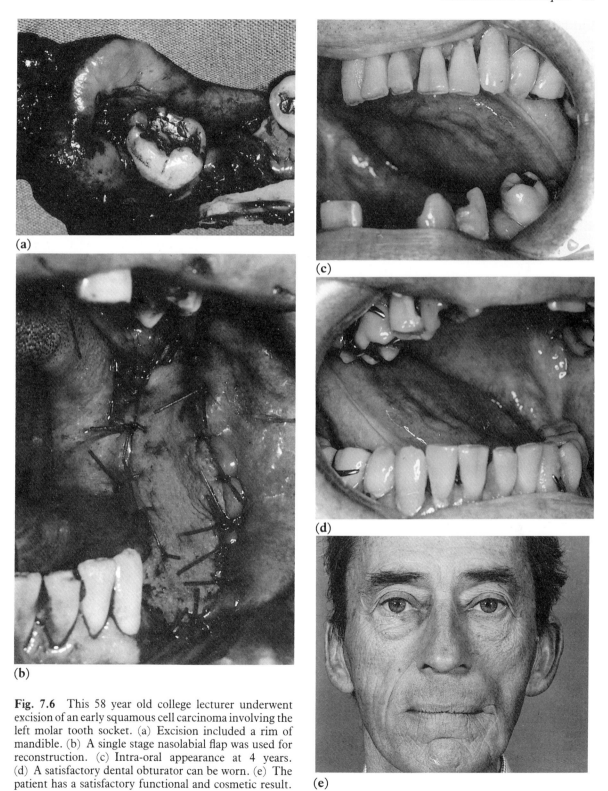

Fig. 7.6 This 58 year old college lecturer underwent excision of an early squamous cell carcinoma involving the left molar tooth socket. (a) Excision included a rim of mandible. (b) A single stage nasolabial flap was used for reconstruction. (c) Intra-oral appearance at 4 years. (d) A satisfactory dental obturator can be worn. (e) The patient has a satisfactory functional and cosmetic result.

in the parotid region. The skin gives a good thickness and texture match for both cervical and facial skin (Fig. 7.7).

Although the deltopectoral flap was originally described for replacement of mucosal lining[103] the authors no longer use this technique which has been superseded by more reliable single stage methods of reconstruction. The deltopectoral flap however does maintain a place for cutaneous reconstruction in the head and neck.

Pectoralis major flap

The pectoralis major is a myocutaneous flap and in many centres has become the work horse in head and neck reconstruction.[104,105] The vascular pedicle comprises the pectoral branch of the acromiothoracic axis as the arterial supply and vena commitantes as the venous drainage. A line drawn from the coracoid process to the xiphisternum gives the approximate axis of the vascular pedicle. An island of skin can be raised on a portion of muscle con-

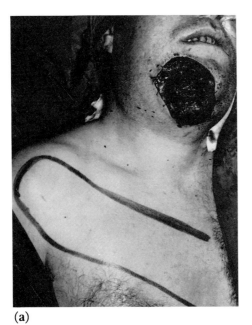

(a)

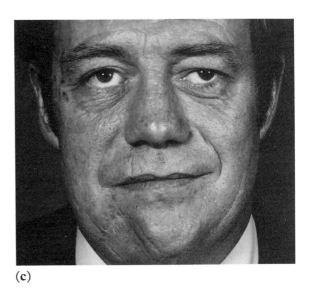

(c)

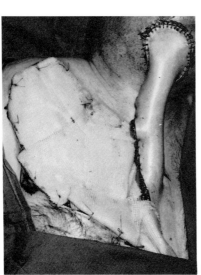

(b)

Fig. 7.7 (a) Deltopectoral flap outlined to reconstruct chin and submental defect. (b) Flap sutured in position. The flap was divided at 3 weeks and a revisionary procedure at 1 year. (c) The final appearance three years following surgery.

taining this vascular pedicle. The amount of skin and the amount of muscle can vary according to requirements. A composite flap including bone can be raised by incorporating a segment of the fifth rib which is said to receive a blood supply from the pectoralis major muscle.[106,107] Similarly a segment of sternum may be taken for osteocutaneous transfer relying on the origin of the pectoralis muscle from the sternum.[108] It is difficult to assess the vascularity in these bone grafts but they appear to survive most probably because they are surrounded by muscle that has a good blood supply.

The pectoralis major myocutaneous flap provides a single stage method of reconstruction that introduces a permanent blood supply to its new site (Fig. 7.8). The muscle can be used most effectively to protect the major vessels and structures in the neck and is particularly useful in previously irradiated cases. Some form of neck dissection or neck exposure is required to introduce this flap into the head and neck.

The cutaneous element of the flap can be used for intra-oral and pharyngeal reconstruction or for replacing skin in the cheek or neck. The flap is not without its problems and although total necrosis of the skin paddle is exceptionally rare, partial necrosis and wound dehiscence problems are not uncommon.[105,109] Other problems include excessive bulk, and a natural tendency to descend under the effects of gravity.

Our preference is to use the pectoralis major myocutaneous flap where bulk is required or where muscle is required to add additional protection. It is commonly used in palliative surgery where the bulk provides sufficient padding to cover inoperable tumour. The flap is most useful for reconstructing defects in the lower part of the face and neck but it has not proved reliable enough for routine reconstruction of defects that extend above the zygomatic arch.

There are other pedicled flaps that have very occasional use in reconstruction of defects following tumour excision. The temporalis muscle flap[110] and the masseter muscle crossover flap[111,112] are both useful local pedicled flaps that can be used to reconstruct posterior defects in the oral cavity. Both flaps are allowed to undergo spontaneous epithelialisation postoperatively. Although doubts have been raised regarding their dimensional stability, nevertheless they are a reliable method of closing such defects. The sternocleidomastoid flap[113,114] and the platysma flap[115,116] use cervical skin and require exploration of the neck. These are not favoured by the authors in primary reconstruction for head and neck tumours. The trapezius flap[117,118] has proved most effective in reconstructing posteriorly situated defects in the occipital and mastoid regions but is not used in our practice for reconstructing more anterior defects. The extensive dissection required to elevate and mobilise this flap together with its bulk detract from its use and the results that are achieved do not compare favourably in our hands with other techniques, notably free flaps.

Free flaps

The advent of microsurgery has opened up new horizons in reconstructive surgery in the head and neck. The surgeon is unrestricted in choosing elsewhere in the body to achieve whatever soft tissue and bone, in terms of quantity and quality, required for the reconstruction. Improvements in instrumentation and technique now mean that free tissue transfer is often more reliable than traditional techniques in head and neck reconstruction.[119,120] Free flaps offer a single stage method of reconstruction that provides well vascularised tissue and the introduction of a permanent new blood supply to the area. This has enabled combined modality treatment, either in the form of postoperative radiotherapy and/or postoperative chemotherapy, to be commenced at an early stage following the surgical procedure. The wide variety of tissues available for transfer have also resulted in improved results in reconstruction since the tissues can be more accurately replaced.

Free flaps have now become our first choice in reconstruction of many defects in the head and neck particularly those affecting the jaws. There are several free flaps that have proved consistently useful and reliable and are worthy of further consideration.

The radial forearm flap

The radial forearm flap is a fasciocutaneous flap based on the radial vessels. It provides thin pliable skin of variable dimensions and has a reliable vascular anatomy. The pedicle is easily dissected for a considerable length and its large size vessels simplify the microsurgical aspects of the procedure. The flap can be raised from the arm at the same time as excision in the head and neck using two surgical teams operating simultaneously.

The thin nature of the skin is suited for intra-oral reconstruction to replace oral lining particularly in areas where bulk is not required and a degree of

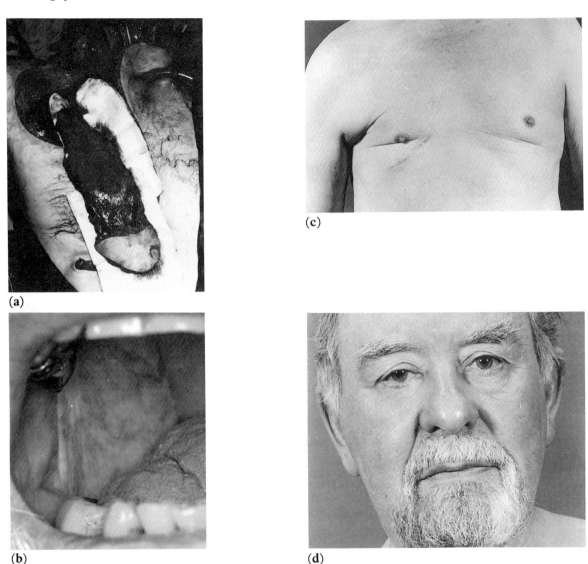

Fig. 7.8 (a) A right pectoralis major myocutaneous flap is raised and islanded on its vascular pedicle. (b) A similar islanded pectoralis major flap has been used to reconstruct a defect in the buccal mucosa retromolar trigone and tonsil region. (c) The donor defect was closed directly. (d) The appearance at 2 years is satisfactory but shows significant shoulder drop on the side of the right radical neck dissection.

mobility is to be maintained.[121,122] Thus, the most useful sites for this flap are the retromolar trigone, buccal mucosa and floor of the mouth extending onto the tongue, where tongue mobility is to be maintained. The flap can also be used to resurface the neck, chin and cheek skin and again provides a reasonable thickness and texture match at these sites. It also provides a better colour match than several other free flap donor sites but cannot of course compete favourably with local skin flaps as far as tissue matching is concerned.

It is also possible to raise a composite flap including a segment of radius.[123] Only 30 per cent of the circumference of the radius should be removed to avoid weakening this bone and the risk of fracture. The bone should be removed in a keel-shaped fashion[124] and approximately 11 cm in length can be achieved in a normal adult. The bone is very

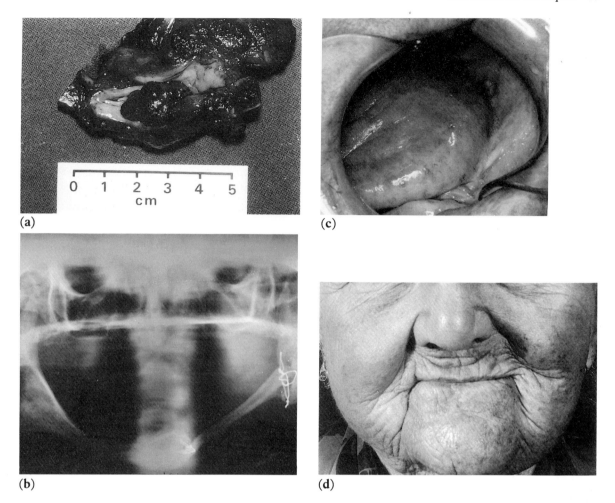

Fig. 7.9 (a) Segmental excision of a T4N0 squamous cell carcinoma of the left lower alveolus. (b) Composite osteocutaneous radial forearm flap was used for reconstruction incorporating a straight segment of radius. (c) Intra-oral appearance at 5 years. (d) This 79 year old patient continues to function well 8 years following surgery.

strong and is straight and therefore best suited for reconstructing lateral mandibular defects (Fig. 7.9). The cortical nature of the bone is ideally suited to rigid fixation using plates and screws and it is also possible to carry out osteotomies to alter the curvature of the radius where required (Fig. 7.10).

Care must be taken with the donor site to ensure that there is no loss of function in the hand or arm and to minimise any cosmetic deformity.[43] An Allen test should be performed pre-operatively to ensure the viability of the hand following division of the radial artery. A pre-operative X-ray of the arm is mandatory for all patients who are to undergo a composite flap including a segment of radius. This is required to assess the thickness of the bone and to exclude any pathology, such as previous fractures. With regard to harvesting bone, right angled osteotomy cuts should be avoided as they significantly weaken the radius and, as mentioned previously, the bone should be removed in a keel-shaped fashion.[124] Wherever possible we aim to close the donor defect completely and avoid the necessity of a skin graft on the arm. In intra-oral reconstruction, most commonly the flap is designed on the distal part of the arm closest to the wrist where the skin is thinnest and most pliable. A flap of up to 4 cm in width can be raised, the length varying between 5 and 7 cm. Such flaps are usually large enough for the majority of intra-oral defects not requiring

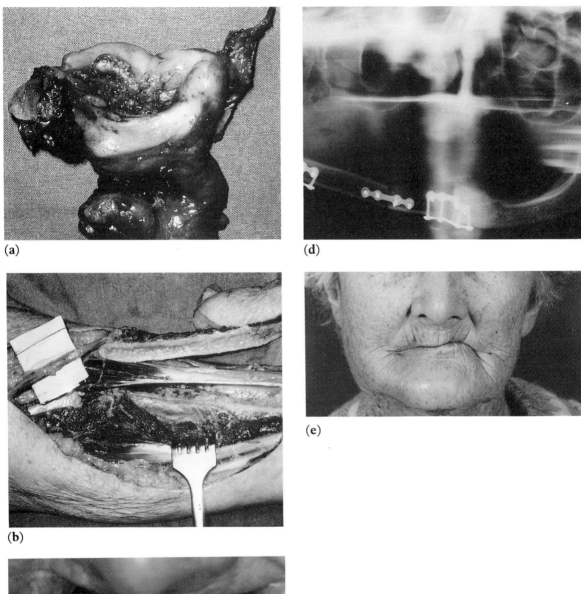

(a)

(b)

(c)

(d)

(e)

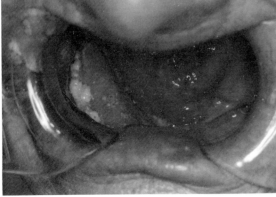

Fig. 7.10 This 77 year old female patient underwent segmental excision for a T4N0 squamous carcinoma of the right lower alveolus (a). (b) A composite radial osteocutaneous forearm flap was raised. (c) Intra-oral appearance at 3 weeks. (d) The orthopantomogram shows the extent of the mandible reconstruction with a single osteotomy to maintain chin prominence. (e) The patient is functionally stable and on full oral diet at 3 weeks.

bulk. Defects larger than this require both surface area and bulk and therefore the radial forearm flap is not usually suitable. It is now our practice to close the defect using an ulnar transposition flap[125] as this avoids the use of a skin graft and has contributed to improved primary wound healing and final cosmesis (Fig. 7.11).

In our experience the radial forearm flap has proved a very effective method, particularly in intra-oral reconstruction (Table 7.3). This reconstruction has consistently proved able to tolerate radical postoperative radiotherapy in the early postoperative period without wound breakdown or fistula formation or osteoradionecrosis.

Table 7.3 The radial forearm flap in intra-oral reconstruction

Total number of cases	175
Age (years)	35–85 (57)
Operating time (hours)	7.6
Postoperative mortality	5 (2.8%)
Flap survival	162 (92.5%)
Intra-oral healing (days)	6–30 (19)
Fistula	2 (1.2%)

Deep circumflex iliac artery groin flap
The deep circumflex iliac artery (DCIA) provides one of the best donor sites for vascularised bone.[126]

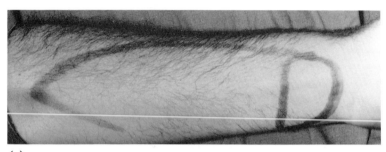

(a)

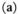

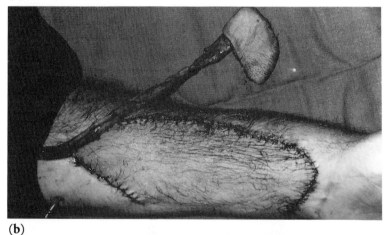

(b)

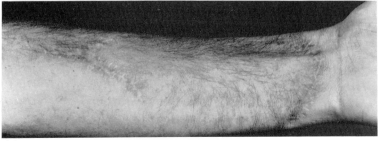

(c)

Fig. 7.11 (a) A distal radial forearm flap is designed together with the markings for an ulnar transposition flap. (b) The forearm flap is raised on its vascular pedicle comprising the radial artery and venae comitantes and the ulnar transposition flap used to close the defect. (c) Appearance at 1 year.

The vessel arises from the external iliac artery, passes laterally and divides into an ascending branch which enters the abdominal musculature and gives a supply particularly to the internal oblique muscle, before continuing on laterally in the curvature of the iliac bone to provide a blood supply to the bone. The natural curve of the iliac bone is well suited to mandibular replacement and particularly reconstruction of a hemimandible. (Fig. 7.12) The skin overlying the iliac crest however is less reliably supplied by the DCIA and as a composite flap the osteocutaneous flap has not proved to be uniformly successful. Furthermore the cutaneous segment can often be somewhat bulky, both for intra-oral or for facial reconstruction and groin skin is a poor match for cervicofacial skin.

To circumvent these problems an alternative is to take a segment of internal oblique muscle supplied by the ascending branch of the DCIA as the soft tissue component of a composite flap.[127] This muscle has a reliable vascular supply and can be draped over the bone and either left to re-epithelialise inside the mouth or be skin grafted.

Again consideration must be given to the donor

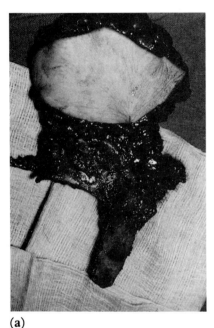

(a)

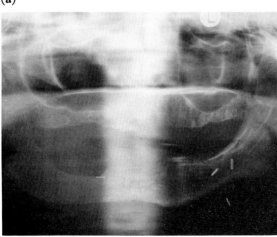

(b)

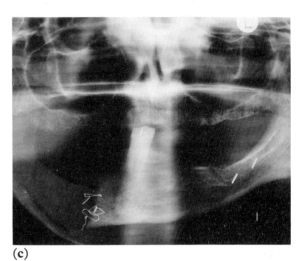

(c)

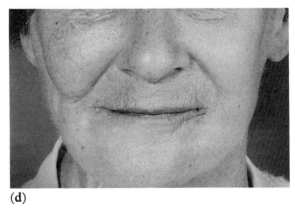

(d)

Fig. 7.12 (a) A composite deep circumflex iliac flap designed for reconstruction of the right hemimandible. (b) Orthopantomogram at 3 weeks shows the position of the vascularised bone. The bone was subsequently trimmed at 18 months and the X-ray appearance is shown at 3 years (c). (d) A satisfactory facial contour has been achieved.

site, and although the final scar is in the groin crease region there are often significant problems associated with removal of a segment of bone from the pelvis. Despite these criticisms the quality of bone and the accuracy with which the bone can be contoured for mandible reconstruction maintains its place in reconstruction of segmental defects[128–130] (Fig. 7.13). The bone also offers sufficient thickness and height to permit the subsequent use of osseo-integrated implants in dental rehabilitation.[42,128]

Scapula flap

The scapular and parascapular flaps were initially described as cutaneous flaps.[131,132] The reliable vascular anatomy with large size vessels and the long vascular pedicle often led to these cutaneous flaps being used in preference to traditional free groin flaps. The scapular flap however was often not a first choice in head and neck reconstruction at this time since it required the patient to be turned on the operating table and simultaneous operating was not possible. It was the introduction of the osteocutaneous scapular flap which included a segment of bone from the lateral border of the scapula that increased the role of this flap in head and neck reconstruction.[133,134] The osteocutaneous scapular flaps have the advantage of offering large amounts of skin that can be designed in a transverse or oblique fashion. A length of approximately 14 cm of bone, 3 cm wide, can be harvested from the lateral border of the scapula. The bone and the skin can therefore lie in a different axis and this differentiates this donor site from many other composite flaps where the skin has to lie in the same axis and direction as the bone. This gives the scapular flap a degree of manoeuverability in reconstructing complex and difficult defects.

The skin however is somewhat thick and the flap can be bulky but this can be used to good effect particularly in reconstructing the symphysis and anterior two thirds of tongue where a volume replacement is required (Fig. 7.14).

The donor site can usually be closed directly unless exceptionally large flaps are removed. The disadvantage of access which does not permit simultaneous operating and requires repositioning of the patient limits the usefulness of this technique. In addition, the skin is rather thick and does not provide a good colour match for cervico-facial reconstruction and is also somewhat rigid for intra-oral reconstruction. The bone is straight and requires careful manipulation with wedge osteotomies to change its shape. Harvesting the

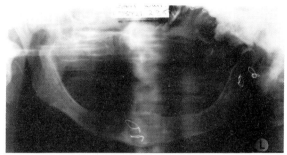

(a)

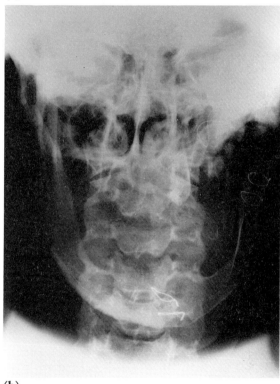

(b)

Fig. 7.13 Long term results of a vascularised deep circumflex iliac crest (DCIA) reconstruction of the left hemimandible. Revision of the bone was performed at 18 months and the X-rays show the final appearance at 8 years (a). There has been some remodelling as a result of functional muscle activity (b).

bone requires division of the teres musculature which should be re-attached to the scapula at the time of wound closure. In the author's experience an osteocutaneous scapula flap raised on the same side as a radical neck dissection which has denervated the trapezius leads to major shoulder dysfunction.

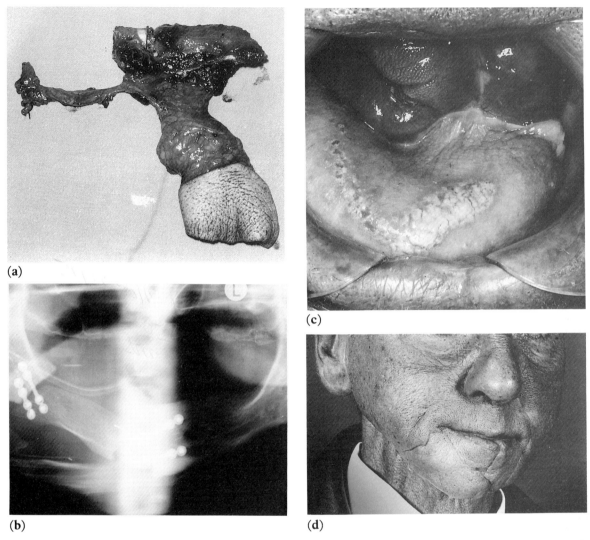

Fig. 7.14 (a) A composite osteocutaneous scapula flap demonstrating the mobility of the skin paddle in relation to the bone. (b) An orthopantomogram showing the extent of mandible reconstruction. (c) A skin paddle was used to reconstruct the floor of the mouth. (d) Appearance at 15 months following reconstruction.

Despite these problems the manoeuverability of skin and bone retain the place of this method of reconstruction in cases where it is difficult to orientate the bony and soft tissue reconstruction.

Fibula transfer

The fibula was first described as a donor site for vascularised bone.[135] The fibula is raised with the peroneal artery which supplies both a nutrient branch and, more importantly, a series of periosteal branches to the fibula. It was several years before the fibula was used in reconstruction of the jaw[136] and this followed the introduction of the osteocutaneous flap.[137] An elipse of skin overlying the fibula on the lateral border of the leg can be raised but the skin has to lie in the same axis and direction as the bone and there is very little degree of manoeuverability. The fibula however offers the surgeon the greatest length of bone and is therefore most suited for extensive defects of the mandible. In such defects, the straight bone has to be osteotomised into the required shape but with modern techniques of osteotomy and fixation satisfactory contouring of the bone can be achieved.[138] The authors find the fibula most useful for extensive symphyseal defects. Peroneal skin can be used effectively to reconstruct the floor of the mouth and maintain tongue mobility while the fibula reconstructs the bony prominence of the lower jaw (Fig. 7.15). The donor defect in the lower leg can also be closed directly unless a broad skin paddle is taken when closure necessitates the use of a skin graft. At least 5 cm of bone should be left intact distally to preserve the ankle mortise and prevent any subluxation or ankle deformity. Similarly the proximal few centimetres at the fibula head should be maintained intact to prevent damage to the peroneal nerve.

The fibula osteocutaneous flap is proving increasingly popular in major reconstruction of the lower jaw. It provides dense cortical bone ideally suited to rigid plate fixation and is similarly suitable for subsequent osseo-integrated implants at a later

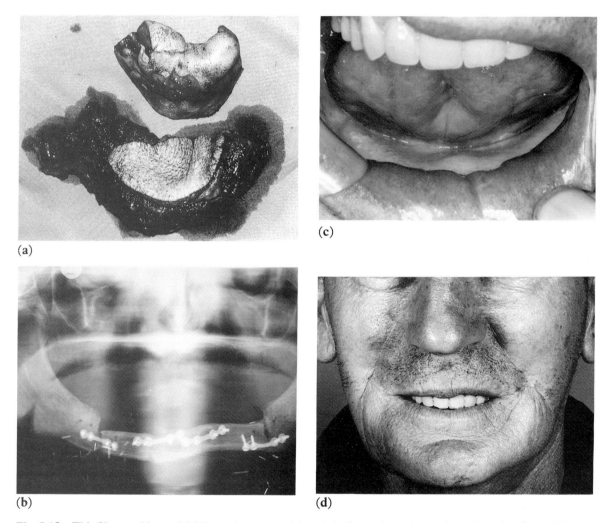

(a)

(b)

(c)

(d)

Fig. 7.15 This 52 year old man initially underwent excision of the floor of mouth together with a rim of mandible and reconstruction using nasolabial flaps. Histology showed a malignant salivary gland tumour extending into the bone. The whole area with the nasolabial flaps and the anterior symphysis of the mandible was excised and a composite fibula flap used for reconstruction. The excision specimen was used to form a template for the reconstruction (see Fig. 7.5, p. 79. (a) The excision specimen and the osteotomised fibular flap are shown together. (b) The orthopantomogram shows the extent of the symphyseal reconstruction. (c) The skin was used to line the floor of the mouth. (d) The patient underwent postoperative radiotherapy and remains disease free at 3 years.

date. One criticism of the fibula flap is that it can often have a short vascular pedicle which may necessitate the use of interpositional vein grafts in the neck. Provided a short length of fibula is maintained at the upper and lower ends to maintain knee and ankle joint stability, this flap has an acceptable donor defect.[139]

Rectus abdominis flap

The rectus abdominis flap based inferiorly on the deep inferior epigastric vascular pedicle has proved consistently reliable in terms of its vascular anatomy.[140] The present authors have found it particularly useful in reconstructing major defects in the head and neck where volume and bulk are required.[141] In addition, via the same incision in the lower abdomen, access can be gained to the iliac crest for a non-vascularised free bone graft. This combination of a free bone graft together with a microvascular free flap can be used effectively in reconstructing major defects following massive resections of upper jaw and maxillary sinus tumours. In such situations it is often difficult to orientate the bone and soft tissue aspects of the reconstruction and therefore traditional vascularised composite flaps are difficult to inset. The alternative is to use a free non-vascularised bone graft that can be shaped accurately to conform to the facial skeletal defect and to wrap this free bone graft in well vascularised muscle so that it will successfully revascularise and survive. The combination of iliac crest and rectus abdominis flap has proved very useful in such major upper jaw reconstructions (Fig. 7.16). Because the upper facial skeleton is not subject to major torsional forces or muscular attachments these grafts are well maintained. Furthermore, in our experience this technique can tolerate early postoperative radical radiotherapy without loss of bone grafts. There is some evidence of resorption unlike vascularised bone grafts but this does not occur to any significant extent or detract from the final result.

Elevation of the rectus abdominis flap can be carried out simultaneously with excision in the head and neck without necessitating any change in the patient's position. The vascular pedicle is long with good size vessels facilitating microvascular anastomosis. The major drawback of the rectus abdominis flap is that it tends to weaken the abdominal wall and it is often necessary to re-enforce closure using a marlex or prolene mesh to minimise weakness of the abdominal wall and reduce the risk of incisional hernia.

Latissimus dorsi flap

The latissimus dorsi free flap has become the work horse for major volume and bulk reconstructions at a wide variety of sites in the body.[142,143] Although it is possible to raise a rib with the latissimus dorsi, this rib is not well vascularised and the authors prefer to use a non-vascularised rib together with latissimus dorsi in a similar fashion to using rectus abdominus with free non-vascularised iliac crest. The rib together with latissimus dorsi has again proved useful in major upper jaw and maxillary reconstruction where there is a large volume defect requiring an abundance of tissue reconstruction and some bony skeletal support (Fig. 7.17).

It is not always necessary to change the position of the patient on the operating table to harvest a latissimus dorsi flap. By elevating the shoulder on a sand bag, small latissimus dorsi flaps can be raised with the patient lying on their back. The close proximity to the head and neck however does not allow simultaneous operating at both donor and recipient sites. Where larger flaps are to be harvested and ribs taken then it is often simpler to alter the position of the patient into a lateral decubitus position for harvesting the flap and closing the donor defect.

The donor defect can be closed directly unless massive amounts of skin are removed and acceptable cosmetic results are generally achieved.

There are now a wide variety of alternative donor sites available that are also of use in the head and neck.[144] The lateral arm flap for example has a similar role to the radial forearm flap but provides slightly more bulk should this be required. Patches of jejunum can be used to reconstruct intra-oral lining; we do not favour inflicting an abdominal wound with all its sequelae solely to obtain a patch for intra-oral lining but we do use free jejunal transfers for reconstructing circumferential defects of the pharynx and cervical oesophagus. Other free flaps such as the groin flap and dorsalis pedis flap are now no longer used in immediate reconstruction following tumour resection having been replaced by the more reliable techniques mentioned above.

Postoperative management

The majority of protocols adopted for postoperative care are aimed at preventing complications rather than treating them when established. As with any surgical procedure, there is a routine of postoperative care aimed at maintaining the general medical condition of the patient. Furthermore, there is the

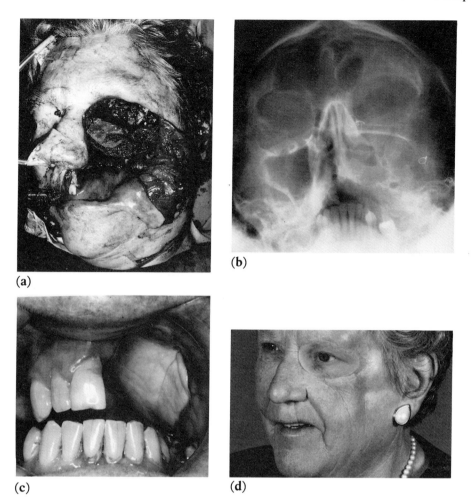

Fig. 7.16   This 65 year old patient underwent a left radical maxillectomy including exenteration of the orbit. (a) A free non-vascularised iliac crest bone graft was used to reconstruct the zygomatic/malar complex. The graft was revascularised by filling the soft tissue defect with a rectus abdominis free flap. The patient underwent postoperative radiotherapy and the appearance of the bone graft reconstruction is shown at 2 years (b). The skin paddle of rectus abdominis flap was used for intra-oral reconstruction, allowing a small upper dental obturator to be worn (c). (d) The patient remains disease free at 4 years.

management of the donor defect and particular problems associated with head and neck surgery.

General postoperative care

Throughout the operative procedure the patient will have been carefully monitored. Cardiac status, fluid balance, temperature and oxygen saturation will all have been regularly monitored as will the haemoglobin and urea, electrolytes and haematocrit as required. This careful monitoring must continue during the early postoperative period and requires either an intensive care unit or a high dependence nursing facility. The use of electrocardiogram (ECG) monitors, pulse oximeters and central venous pressure (CVP) lines can aid monitoring during this period. Hourly urine volume should be checked together with fluid and electrolyte balances. Particularly in major flap reconstructions, the haemodynamic status of the patient is exceptionally important and it is essential to maintain a good cardiac output in order to perfuse the reconstruction. Haemoglobin should also be maintained and should not be allowed to drop significantly

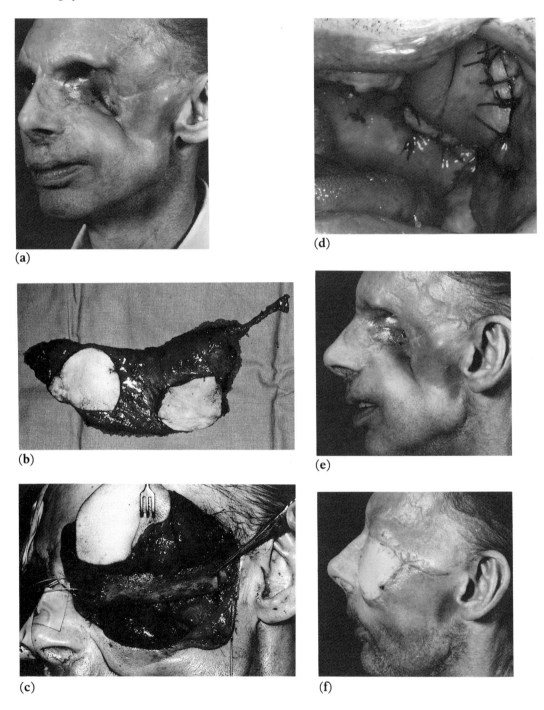

(a)

(b)

(c)

(d)

(e)

(f)

Fig. 7.17   (a) This patient presented with an extensive orocutaneous fistula and facial collapse some 8 years following a maxillectomy. A bipaddled latissimus dorsi flap was raised and free non-vascular rib grafts harvested (b). The rib grafts were used to reconstruct the zygoma/malar complex and lateral orbital wall (c). One skin paddle was used to reconstruct the oral cavity (d) and the other for external facial reconstruction. (e) The pre-operative appearance contrasts with the postoperative appearance at two months (f). The facial collapse has been corrected and the defect completely reconstructed forming the basis for subsequent dental and facial prosthetics.

below 10 grams since this will impair oxygenation. Similarly the patient should not be overtransfused since this might increase blood viscosity and hinder perfusion.

In our practice anticoagulation is not used as a routine even in microvascular free tissue transfers. However prophylaxis against deep venous thrombosis is routinely carried out. Any patient being temporarily immobilised by an operation or indeed having cancer is known to have an increased incidence of deep venous thrombosis and pulmonary thrombo-embolism. For these reasons we routinely use subcutaneous heparin (5000 units twice daily) commencing at the time of surgery and continuing until the patient is mobilised. Intra-operatively pneumatic leggings are used to prevent deep venous thrombosis while the patient is under anaesthetic.

Prophylactic antibiotics are used similarly. Routinely metronidizole is used together with a cephalosporin commencing at the time of surgery and continuing for a period of 5 days. Metronidizole in particular has proved effective in dealing with oral contamination.

Head and neck recipient site

There are particular complications that can arise in head and neck surgery and these require special consideration.

Management of the airway

In any patient undergoing major surgery to the jaws or oral cavity, there is likely to be a degree of postoperative intra-oral swelling. If there is any fear that the patient will become orally incompetent and unable to control their own secretions and saliva, then it is often safer to manage the patient with a tracheostomy. This will have been discussed previously in the presurgical planning and is performed at the beginning of the operation. We have found the morbidity of this procedure in adults is minimal and yet it can prevent fatal complications. Tracheostomy also provides easy access for the removal of bronchial secretions postoperatively and can be used to prevent aspiration until the patient regains co-ordination in swallowing. Postoperatively the tracheostomy tube requires regular toilet and changing.

Not every patient requires a tracheostomy. At the end of surgery an assessment has to be made. A nasal tube can be retained and the patient ventilated or allowed to breathe spontaneously until the patient is stable but this can only be carried out in an intensive care facility. As a general rule, if there is any doubt at the end of an operation as to whether the patient will manage with or without a tracheostomy then that in itself should serve as an indication to perform a tracheostomy rather than risk complications and necessitate an emergency tracheostomy.

Nutrition

Maintaining nutrition following major surgery is important to enable satisfactory wound healing. In major surgery of the mouth and jaws, nutritional deficiencies should be expected. It is our practice to pass a nasogastric tube peroperatively and to commence early enteral nutrition. Once the patient is able to swallow satisfactorily then the tube can be removed. Prolonged difficulties require a gastrostomy as discussed in Chapter 6.

Wound drainage

It is important to adequately drain wounds in the head and neck to prevent the accumulation of blood and haematoma, which might cause significant problems as a result of compression. It is our practice to use suction drainage in all neck wounds to allow the cervical skin to collapse and adhere to the deeper structures. Suction drains are often employed under major flap reconstructions, and where a microvascular free tissue transfer has been performed an additional simple corrugated drain is used to decompress the skin overlying the microvascular anastomosis.

Suction drains are maintained in position until drainage falls to approximately 15 ml/day. Prolonged drainage can occur in the neck, particularly when there is evidence of a lymphatic leak. Many lymphatic leaks resolve spontaneously with the altering of enteral nutrition to a non-fat diet. Where the lymphatic leak persists then parenteral nutrition may be required until the lymph leak ceases. Re-exploration of lymphatic leaks may be required but this is often technically difficult because of the friable nature of the tissues. Persistent leaks may require the import of muscle, usually local muscle flaps, to seal off and close the leak.

Donor defect

Some donor sites are particularly useful in head and neck surgery since they can be bandaged and to all intents and purposes ignored in the early postoperative phase. This particularly applies to the forearm flap, the lateral arm flap and the fibula flap. Other donor sites can cause significant problems, particularly intra-abdominal wounds which are painful and can often restrict breathing and postoperative respiratory recovery. The rectus abdominis and flaps based on the DCIA vessels similarly result in painful wounds in the early postoperative period and the management of pain in any postoperative recovery is very important. Large myocutaneous flaps are sometimes prone to prolonged wound drainage and are best treated with suction drains. This particularly applies to the latissimus dorsi and pectoralis major flaps.

Donor sites are subject to all the normal complications of surgery such as haematoma, infection, wound breakdown and dehiscence but careful surgical technique, wound drainage and the use of prophylactic antibiotics have significantly reduced these complications in major head and neck surgery. Despite simultaneous operating at two different sites cross infection between the head and neck and a donor site has not proved to be a problem and in our experience has been exceptionally rare.

Rehabilitation (See also Chapter 6)

Rehabilitation commences prior to the onset of surgery. This is essential if the patient is to be motivated towards achieving a good functional result. Pre-operatively high risk patients should be identified, as should those who are going to require additional support. Unfortunately all too often rehabilitation does not start until the patient is almost completely healed and the patient and therapist then have an uphill battle. To achieve the optimum functional and socio-economic results, we have found that excision, reconstruction and rehabilitation complement each other, the one affecting the other. It is a constant source of amazement that patients who undergo major resections of what appear to be vital structures in the head and neck can survive and function well in society.

This, in essence, is the aim of surgical treatment; to cure the disease, wherever possible, to reconstruct the patient and to provide a functional and cosmetic basis for rehabilitation so that the patient can return to society. It is likely that only minor advances will be made in excision and reconstructive techniques over the next decade. It is therefore to be hoped that further advances will be made in rehabilitation.

References

1 Bassett MR, Dobbie RA. Patterns of nutritional deficiency in head and neck cancer. *Archives of Otolaryngology – Head and Neck Surgery* 1982; **91**: 119.
2 Brookes GB. Nutritional status: a prognostic indicator in head and neck cancer. *Archives of Otolaryngology – Head and Neck Surgery* 1985; **93**: 69.
3 Tiwari RM, Gerritsen GJ, Balm AJM, Snow GB. Critical evaluation of the role of CT scanning in ethmoidal cancer. *Journal of Laryngology and Otology* 1986; **100**: 421.
4 Shaha AR. Preoperative evaluation of the mandible in patients with carcinoma of the floor of the mouth. *Head and Neck* 1991; **13**: 398.
5 Ahuja RB, Soutar DS, Moule B *et al*. Comparative study of technetium-99M bone scans and orthopantomography in determining mandible invasion in intraoral squamous cell carcinoma. *Head and Neck* 1990; **12**: 234.
6 Noyek AM. Diagnostic imaging in mandibular invasion by cancer. In: Fee WE, Goepfert H, Johns ME, Strong EW, Ward PH eds. *Head and Neck Cancer*, Volume II. Philadelphia, PA: BC Decker, 1990: 53–8.
7 Weisman RA, Kimmelman CP. Bone scanning in the assessment of mandibular invasion by oral cavity carcinomas. *Laryngoscope* 1982; **92**: 1–4.
8 Baker H, Krause CJ, Saxon KG. Evaluation of bone scan by scintigraphy to detect subclinical invasion of the mandible by squamous cell carcinoma of the oral cavity. *Otolaryngology – Head and Neck Surgery* 1982; **90**: 327–36.
9 Stevens MH, Harnsberger P, Mancuso AA *et al*. Computed tomography of cervical lymph nodes: staging and management of head and neck cancer. *Archives of Otolaryngology – Head and Neck Surgery* 1985; **111**: 735.
10 Feinmesser R, Freeman JL, Noyek *et al*. Metastatic neck disease: a clinical radiographic/pathological correlative study. *Archives of Otolaryngology – Head and Neck Surgery* 1987; **113**: 1307.
11 Stern WBP, Silver CE, Zeifer BA, Persky MS, Heller KS. Computed tomography of the clinically negative neck. *Head and Neck* 1990; **12**: 209–13.
12 Mafee MM, Kampos M, Raju S *et al*. Head and neck high field magnetic resonance imaging versus computed tomography. *Otolaryngological Clinics of North America* 1988; **21**: 513–46.

13 Kassel EE, Keller MA, Kucharzyk W. MRI of the floor of the mouth, tongue and oral pharynx. *Radiological Clinics of North America* 1989; **27**: 331–51.

14 Phillips CD, Gay SB, Newton RL, Levine PA. Gadolinium enhanced MRI of tumours of the head and neck. *Head and Neck* 1990; **12**: 308–15.

15 van de Brekel MWM, Castelijns JA, Stel HV *et al.* Occult metastatic disease detected with US and US guided fine needle aspiration cytology. *Radiology* 1991; **180**: 457.

16 Baatenburg de Jong RJ, Rongen RJ, Verwoerd CDA *et al.* Ultrasound guided fine needle aspiration of neck nodes. *Archives of Otolaryngology – Head and Neck Surgery* 1991; **117**: 402.

17 Hermanek P, Sobin LH eds. *International Union against Cancer TNM Classification of Malignant Tumours*, 4th edn. New York: Springer Verlag, 1987.

18 American Joint Committee on Cancer. *Manual for Staging of Cancer*, 3rd edn. Philadelphia, PA: JB Lippincott, 1987.

19 Eneroth CM, Franzen Z, Zajicek J. Cytological diagnosis on aspirate from 1,000 salivary gland tumours. *Acta Oto-Laryngologica Supplement* 1967; **244**: 168.

20 Abele JS, Miller TR. Fine needle aspiration of the thyroid nodule: clinical applications. In: Clark OH ed. *Endocrine Surgery of the Thyroid and Parathyroid Glands*. St Louis, MO: CV Mosby, 1985: 293.

21 Summers GW. Physiological problems following ablative surgery of head and neck cancer. *Otolaryngological Clinics of North America* 1974; **7**: 217.

22 Shedd DP. Rehabilitation problems of head and neck cancer patients. *Journal of Surgical Oncology* 1976; **8**: 11.

23 Dhillon RS, Palmer BV, Pittam MR, Shaw HJ. Rehabilitation after major head and neck surgery: the patient's view. *Clinical Otolaryngology* 1982; **7**: 319.

24 Freedlander E, Espie CA, Campsie LM, Soutar DS, Robertson AG. Functional complications of major surgery for intraoral cancer. *British Journal of Plastic Surgery* 1989; **42**: 266.

25 Finlay PM, Dawson F, Robertson AG, Soutar DS. An evaluation of functional outcome after surgery and radiotherapy for intraoral cancer. *British Journal of Oral and Maxillofacial Surgery* 1992; **30**: 14.

26 Teichgraeber J, Bowman J, Goepfert H. New test series for the functional evaluation of oral cavity cancer. *Head and Neck Surgery* 1985; **8**: 9.

27 List MA, Ritter-Sterr C, Lansky SB. A performance status scale for head and neck cancer patients. *Cancer* 1990; **60**: 564.

28 Shedd DP. Rehabilitation of head and neck cancer patients. In: McKenna PJ, Murphy GP eds. *Fundamentals of Surgical Oncology*. New York: Macmillan Publishing, 1986: 496.

29 Olson ML, Shedd DP. Disability and rehabilitation in head and neck cancer patients after treatment. *Head and Neck Surgery* 1978; **1**: 52.

30 David DJ, Barrett JA. Psychosocial aspects of head and neck cancer surgery. *Australia and New Zealand Journal of Surgery* 1977; **47**: 584.

31 Karnofsky DA, Burchenal JH. The clinical evaluation of chemotherapeutics in cancer. In: McLeod CM ed. *Evaluation of Chemotherapeutic Agents*. New York: Columbia Press, 1949: 191.

32 Jacobson MC. Intelligibility alterations in an oral cancer patient following primary surgery and two reconstructions: a case study. *South African Journal of Communication Disorders* 1983; **30**: 15.

33 Hufnagle J, Pullon P, Hufnagle K. Speech considerations in oral surgery. *Oral Surgery, Oral Medicine, Oral Pathology* 1978; **45**: 354.

34 Matloub HS, Larson DL, Kuhn JC, Yousif J, Sanger JP. Lateral arm free flap in oral cavity reconstruction: a functional evaluation. *Head and Neck* 1989; **11**: 205–11.

35 Mathog RH. Rehabilitation of head and neck cancer patients: consensus on recommendations from the International Conference on Rehabilitation of the Head and Neck Cancer Patient. *Head and Neck* 1991; **13**: 1–14.

36 Muz J, Mathog RH, Hamlet L, Davis LP, Kling GA. Objective assessment of swallowing function in head and neck cancer patients. *Head and Neck* 1991; **13**: 33–9.

37 Hamlet S, Jones L, Patterson R, Michou G, Cislo C. Swallowing recovery following anterior tongue and floor of mouth surgery. *Head and Neck* 1991; **13**: 334–9.

38 Barry WJ, Timmermann G. Mispronunciations and compensatory movements of tongue-operated patients. *British Journal of Disorders of Communication* 1985; **20**: 81–90.

39 Heller KS, Levy J, Speech CC, Sciuiba DMD. Speech patterns following partial glossectomy for small tumours of the tongue. *Head and Neck* 1991; **13**: 340–3.

40 McConnel FMS, Teichgraeber JF, Adler RK. A comparison of three methods of oral reconstruction. *Archives of Otolaryngology – Head and Neck Surgery* 1987; **113**: 496–500.

41 Branemark PI. Osseointegration and its experimental background. *Journal of Prosthetic Dentistry* 1983; **50**: 599.

42 Riediger D. Restoration of masticatory function by microsurgically revascularised iliac crest bone grafts using endosseous implants. *Plastic and Reconstructive Surgery* 1986; **77**: 530.

43 Bardsley AF, Soutar DS, Elliott D, Batchelor AG. Reducing morbidity in the radial forearm flap donor site. *Plastic and Reconstructive Surgery* 1990; **86**: 287–94.

44 Frank HA, Davidson TM. Ethical dilemmas in head and neck cancer. *Head and Neck* 1989; **11**: 22–6.

45 Morton RP, Davies DM, Baker J, Baker GA, Stell PM. Quality of life in treated head and neck cancer patients: a preliminary report. *Clinics of Otolaryngology* 1984; **9**: 181–5.

46 Aaronson NK, Beckman J eds. *The Quality of Life of Cancer Patients*. New York: Raven Press, 1987.

47 Schipper H, Clinch J, McMurray A, Levitt M. Measuring the quality of life of cancer patients: the functional living index-cancer: development and validation. *Journal of Clinical Oncology* 1984; **2**: 472–83.

48 Maguire P. Psychological and social consequences of cancer. In: Williams CJ, Whitehouse JWA eds. *Recent Advances in Clinical Oncology*. London: Churchill Livingstone, 1981.

49 Davies ADM, Davies C, Delco MC. Depression and anxiety in patients undergoing diagnostic investigations for head and neck cancer. *British Journal of Psychiatry* 1986; **114**: 491–3.

50 Espie CA, Freedlander E, Campsie LM, Soutar DS, Robertson AG. Psychological distress at follow up after major surgery for intraoral cancer. *Journal of Psychomatic Research* 1989; **33**: 441–8.

51 Zigmond AS, Snaith RP. The hospital anxiety depression scale. *Acta Psychiatrica Scandinavica* 1983; **67**: 361–70.

52 Platz H, Fries R, Hudec M. Retrospective DOSAK study of carcinoma of the oral cavity. Results and consequences. *Journal of Maxillofacial Surgery* 1985; **14**: 147–53.

53 Perez CA, Carmichael T, Venkata R *et al*. Carcinoma of the tonsillar fossa: a non randomised comparison of radiation alone or combined with surgery: long term results. *Head and Neck* 1991; **13**: 282–90.

54 Nathanson A, Agren K *et al*. Evaluation of some prognostic factors in small cell carcinoma of the mobile tongue: a multi-centre study in Sweden. *Head and Neck* 1989; **11**: 387–92.

55 Kramer S, Gelber RD, Snow JB *et al*. Combined radiation therapy and surgery in management of advanced head and neck cancer: final report of study 73–03 of the radiation oncology group. *Head and Neck* 1987; **10**: 19–30.

56 Mendelson BC, Hodgkinson DJ, Woods JE. Cancer of the oral cavity. *Surgical Clinics of North America* 1977; **57**: 585–96.

57 Cade S, Lee ES. Cancer of the tongue. A study based on 653 patients. *British Journal of Surgery* 1957; **44**: 433–6.

58 Spiro RH, Frazell EL. Evaluation of radical surgical treatment of advanced cancer of the mouth. *American Journal of Surgery* 1968; **116**: 571–7.

59 Ringe AH, Sako K, Rao U, Razack MS, Reese P. Immunologic pattern of regional lymph nodes in squamous cell carcinoma of the floor of the mouth. *American Journal of Surgery* 1985; **150**: 461–5.

60 Cunningham NJ, Johnston JT, Myers EM, Schramm VL, Thearle PB. Cervical lymph node metastasis after local excision of early squamous cell carcinoma of the oral cavity. *American Journal of Surgery* 1986; **152**: 361–5.

61 Spiro RH, Strong EW. Epidermoid carcinoma of the mobile tongue. Treatment by partial glossectomy alone. *American Journal of Surgery* 1971; **122**: 707–10.

62 Zelefsky MJ, Harrison LB, Fass EE *et al*. Postoperative radiotherapy of oral cavity cancers: impact of anatomic subsite on treatment outcome. *Head and Neck* 1990; **12**: 472–5.

63 Lefebvre JL, Coch-Dequeant B, Castelain B *et al*. Interstitial brachytherapy and early tongue squamous cell carcinoma management. *Head and Neck* 1990; **12**: 232–6.

64 Spiro RH, Huvos AG, Wong JY, Spiro JD, Gnecco CA, Strong EW. Predictive value of tumour thickness in squamous carcinoma confined to the tongue and floor of mouth. *American Journal of Surgery* 1986; **152**: 345–50.

65 Mohit-Tabatabai MA, Sobel HJ, Rush BF, Mashberg A. Relation of thickness of floor of mouth stage I and II cancers to regional metastasis. *American Journal of Surgery* 1986; **152**: 351–3.

66 MacComb WS, Fletcher GJ. Planned combination of surgery and radiation in treatment of advanced primary head and neck cancers. *American Journal of Roentology, Radium Therapy and Nuclear Medicine* 1957; **77**: 397–414.

67 Jesse RH, Lindberg RD. The efficacy of combining radiation therapy with a surgical procedure in patients with cervical metastasis from squamous cell carcinoma of the oropharynx and hypopharynx. *Cancer* 1975; **35**: 1163–6.

68 Vikram B, Strong EW, Shah J, Spiro EM. Elective postoperative radiation therapy in stage III and IV epidermoid carcinoma of the head and neck. *American Journal of Surgery* 1980; **140**: 580–4.

69 Robertson AG, McGregor IA, Flatman GE, Soutar DS, Boyle P. The role of radical surgery and postoperative radiotherapy in the management of intraoral carcinoma. *British Journal of Plastic Surgery* 1985; **38**: 314–20.

70 Robertson AG, McGregor IA, Soutar DS *et al*. Postoperative radiotherapy in the management of advanced intraoral cancers. *Clinical Radiology* 1986; **37**: 173–8.

71 Robertson AG, Rao GS, Al-Sammarie A, Soutar DS. The management of tumours arising in the maxillary antrum. *Clinical Oncology* 1992; **4**: 240–3.

72 Byers RM, Bland KI, Borlase B, Luna M. The prognostic and therapeutic value of frozen section determination in the surgical treatment of squamous carcinoma of the head and neck. *American Journal of Surgery* 1978; **136**: 525.

73 Looser KG, Shah JP, Strong EW. The significance of 'positive' margins in surgically resected epider-

moid carcinomas. *Head and Neck Surgery* 1978; **1:** 107.

74 Zieske LA, Johnson JT, Myers EN *et al.* Squamous cell carcinoma with positive margins. *Archives of Otolaryngology – Head and Neck Surgery* 1986; **112:** 863.

75 Byers RM, Newman R, Russell N. Results of treatment for squamous carcinoma of the lower gum. *Cancer* 1981; **47:** 2236–8.

76 Wald RM, Calcaterra TC. Lower alveolar carcinoma. *Archives of Otolaryngology* 1983; **109:** 578–82.

77 Bartelbort SW, Bahn SL, Ariyan S. Rim mandibulectomy for cancer of the oral cavity. *American Journal of Surgery* 1987; **154:** 423.

78 Fleming WB. Marginal resection of the mandible in the treatment of cancer of the floor of the mouth. *Australian and New Zealand Journal of Surgery* 1987; **57:** 521.

79 Totsuka Y, Usui Y, Tei K *et al.* Results of surgical treatment for squamous carcinoma of the lower alveolus: segmental versus marginal resection. *Head and Neck Surgery* 1991; **13:** 114–20.

80 Skolnik EM, Tenta LT, Wineiger DM *et al.* Preservation of XI cranial nerve in neck dissection. *Laryngoscope* 1967; **77:** 1304.

81 Bocca E, Pignataro O. A conservation technique in radical neck dissection. *Annals of Otology, Rhinology and Laryngology* 1967; **76:** 975.

82 Jesse RH, Ballantyne AJ, Larson A. Radical or modified neck dissection: a therapeutic dilemma. *American Journal of Surgery* 1978; **136:** 516.

83 Leemans CR, Tiwari RM, van der Waal I *et al.* The efficacy of comprehensive neck dissection with or without postoperative radiotherapy in nodal metastasis of squamous cell carcinoma of the upper respiratory and digestive tracts. *Laryngoscope* 1990; **100:** 1194.

84 Ariyan S, Chicarilli ZN. Cancer of the oral cavity. In: Ariyan S ed. *Cancer of the Head and Neck.* St Louis, MO: CV Mosby, 1987.

85 Riley RW, Fee WE, Goffinet D *et al.* Squamous cell carcinoma of the base of the tongue. *Otolaryngology – Head and Neck Surgery* 1983; **91:** 143.

86 Vikram B, Strong EW, Shah JP, Spiro R. Failure at the primary site following multi-modality treatment in advanced head and neck cancer. *Head and Neck* 1984; **6:** 720–3.

87 Henry AK. *Extensile Exposure*, 2nd edn. Edinburgh: E & S Livingstone, 1966.

88 Osborne JE, Clayton M, Fenwick JD. The Leeds modified Weber Fergusson incision. *Journal of Laryngology and Otology* 1987; **101:** 465–6.

89 Hernandez Altimar F. Transfacial access to the retromaxillary area. *Journal of Maxillofacial Surgery* 1986; **14:** 165.

90 Brown AMS, Lavery KM, Millar BG. The transfacial approach to the post nasal space and retro-

maxillary structures. *British Journal of Oral and Maxillofacial Surgery* 1991; **29:** 230.

91 Spiro RH, Gerold FP, Strong EW. Mandibular swing approach for oral and oropharyngeal tumours. *Head and Neck Surgery* 1981; **3:** 371–8.

92 McGregor IA, McDonald DG. Mandibular osteotomy in the surgical approach to the oral cavity. *Head and Neck Surgery* 1983; **5:** 457–62.

93 Clayman GL, Adams GL. Modifications of the mandibular swing for preservation of occlusion and function. *Head and Neck* 1991; **13:** 102–6.

94 Dubner S, Spiro RH. Median mandibulotomy; a critical assessment. *Head and Neck* 1991; **13:** 389–93.

95 Lindberg R. Distribution of cervical lymph node metastases from squamous cell carcinoma of the upper respiratory and digestive tracts. *Cancer* 1972; **29:** 1446.

96 Skolnik EM, Yee KF, Friedman M, Goldon TA. The posterior triangle in radical neck surgery. *Archives of Otolaryngology* 1976; **102:** 1–4.

97 Sharpe DT. The pattern of lymph node metastases in intraoral squamous cell carcinoma. *British Journal of Plastic Surgery* 1981; **34:** 97–101.

98 Robbins T, Medicina JE, Wolfe GT *et al.* Standardising neck dissection terminology. *Archives of Otolaryngology – Head and Neck Surgery* 1991; **117:** 601–5.

99 Freedlander E, Schecker LR. The longterm results of intraoral split skin grafting. *British Journal of Plastic Surgery* 1982; **35:** 376–83.

100 Argenta LC. Controlled tissue expansion in reconstructive surgery. *British Journal of Plastic Surgery* 1984; **37:** 520.

101 Zarem HA. Current concepts in reconstructive surgery in patients with cancer of the head and neck. *Surgical Clinics of North America* 1971; **55:** 1.

102 Soutar DS, McGregor IA. Nasolabial flaps to anterior floor of mouth. In: Strauch B, Vasconez LO, Hall-Findlay EJ eds. *Encyclopaedia of Flaps*, Volume I. Boston: Little Brown & Co., 1990: 352.

103 Bakamjian VY. A two stage method for pharyngoesophageal reconstruction with a primary pectoral skin flap. *Plastic and Reconstructive Surgery* 1965; **36:** 173.

104 Ariyan S. The pectoralis major myocutaneous flap: a versatile flap for reconstruction in the head and neck. *Plastic and Reconstructive Surgery* 1979; **63:** 73–81.

105 Baek S, Lawson W, Biller H. An analysis of 133 pectoralis major myocutaneous flaps. *Plastic and Reconstructive Surgery* 1982; **69:** 460–7.

106 Cuono CB, Ariyan S. Immediate reconstruction of a composite mandibular defect with a regional osteomusculo cutaneous flap. *Plastic and Reconstructive Surgery* 1980; **65:** 477–83.

107 Reid C, Taylor GI. The vascular territory of the

thoraco–acromial axis. *British Journal of Plastic Surgery* 1984; **37**: 194–212.

108 Green MF, Gibson JR, Bryson JR, Thomson E. A one stage correction of mandibular defects using a split sternum pectoralis major osteomusculo cutaneous transfer. *British Journal of Plastic Surgery* 1981; **34**: 11–16.

109 Ossoff RA, Wurster CF, Berktold RE *et al*. Complications after major myocutaneous flap reconstruction of head and neck defects. *Archives of Otolaryngology* 1983; **109**: 812–14.

110 Bradley P, Brockbank J. The temporalis muscle flap in oral reconstruction. *Journal of Maxillofacial Surgery* 1981; **9**: 139.

111 Tiwari R. Masseter muscle cross-over flap in primary closure of oro-pharyngeal defects. *Journal of Laryngology and Otology* 1987; **101**: 172–217.

112 Langdon JD. The masseter muscle cross-over flap – a versatile flap for reconstruction in the oral cavity. *British Journal of Oral and Maxillofacial Surgery* 1989; **27**: 124–31.

113 Ariyan S. One stage reconstruction for defects of the mouth using a sternocleidomastoid myocutaneous flap. *Plastic and Reconstructive Surgery* 1979; **63**: 618.

114 Larson DL, Goepfert H. Limitations of the sternocleidomastoid musculocutaneous flap in head and neck cancer reconstruction. *Plastic and Reconstructive Surgery* 1982; **70**: 328.

115 Coleman JJ, Jurkiewicz MJ, Nahai F, Mathes SJ. The platysma musculocutaneous flap: experience with 24 cases. *Plastic and Reconstructive Surgery* 1983; **72**: 315–321.

116 Hurwitz DJ, Rabson JA, Futrell JW. The anatomic basis for the platysma skin flap. *Plastic and Reconstructive Surgery* 1983; **72**: 302–312.

117 Demergasso F, Piazza M. Trapezius myocutaneous flap in reconstructive surgery for head and neck cancer: an original technique. *American Journal of Surgery* 1979; **128**: 533.

118 Guillamondegui OM, Larson DL. The lateral trapezius musculocutaneous flap: its use in head and neck reconstruction. *Plastic and Reconstructive Surgery* 1981; **67**: 143.

119 Percival NJ, Sykes PJ, Early MJ. Free flap surgery. The Welsh Regional Unit experience. *British Journal of Plastic Surgery* 1989; **42**: 435.

120 Shaw WW, Converse JM. A survey of 2680 free flaps: survival, donor site and applications amongst experienced microvascular surgeons. *Plastic Surgery Forum* 1987; **4**: 93.

121 Soutar DS, Schecker LR, Tanner NSB, McGregor IA. The radial forearm flap: a versatile method for intraoral reconstruction. *British Journal of Plastic Surgery* 1983; **36**: 1–8.

122 Soutar DS, McGregor IA. The radial forearm flap in intraoral reconstruction: the experience of 60 consecutive cases. *Plastic and Reconstructive Surgery* 1986; **78**: 1.

123 Soutar DS, Widdowson WP. Immediate reconstruction of the mandible using a vascularised segment of radius. *Head and Neck Surgery* 1986; **8**: 232.

124 Soutar DS, Ray AK. The radial forearm flap in head and neck reconstruction. In: Jackson IT, Sommerland B eds. *Recent Advances in Plastic Surgery 4*. London: Churchill Livingstone, 1992.

125 Elliot D, Bardsley AF, Batchelor AG, Soutar DS. Direct closure of the radial forearm flap donor defect. *British Journal of Plastic Surgery* 1988; **41**: 358.

126 Taylor GI, Townsend P, Corlett R. Superiority of the deep circumflex iliac vessels as a supply for free groin flaps: clinical work. *Plastic and Reconstructive Surgery* 1979; **64**: 595.

127 Ramasastry SS, Tucker JB, Swartz WM, Hurwitz DJ. The internal oblique muscle flap: an anatomic and clinical study. *Plastic and Reconstructive Surgery* 1984; **73**: 721.

128 Sanger JR, Matloub HS, Yousif NJ, Larson DL. Enhancement of rehabilitation by the use of implantable adjuncts with vascularised bone grafts for mandible reconstruction. *American Journal of Surgery* 1988; **15**: 243.

129 Rosen IB, Manktelow RB, Zuker RM, Boyd JB. Application of microvascular free osteocutaneous flaps in the management of postradiation recurrent oral cancers. *American Journal of Surgery* 1985; **150**: 474.

130 Boyd JB. Reconstruction of the mandible. In: Soutar DS ed. *Microvascular Surgery and Free Tissue Transfer*. London: Edward Arnold, 1992.

131 Hamilton SGL, Morrison WA. The scapular free flap. *British Journal of Plastic Surgery* 1982; **35**: 2.

132 Nassif TM, Vidal L, Bover JL, Baudet J. The parascapular flap: a new cutaneous microsurgical free flap. *Plastic and Reconstructive Surgery* 1982; **69**: 591.

133 Swartz WM, Banis JC, Newton ED *et al*. The osteocutaneous scapular flap for mandibular and maxillary reconstruction. *Plastic and Reconstructive Surgery* 1987; **77**: 530.

134 Baker SR, Solivan M. The osteocutaneous scapular flap for one stage reconstruction of the mandible. *Archives of Otolaryngology* 1988; **114**: 267.

135 Taylor GI, Miller G, Ham F. The free vascularised bone graft. *Plastic and Reconstructive Surgery* 1975; **55**: 533.

136 Hidalgo DA. Fibular free flap: a new method of mandibular reconstruction. *Plastic and Reconstructive Surgery* 1989; **84**: 71.

137 Zhong-Wei Chen, Wang Yan. The study and clinical application of the osteocutaneous flap of the fibula. *Microsurgery* 1983; **4**: 11.

138 Hidalgo DA. Aesthetic improvements in free flap

mandible reconstruction. *Plastic and Reconstructive Surgery* 1991; **88**: 574.

139 Goodacre TEE, Walker CJ, Jawad AS *et al.* Donor site morbidity following osteocutaneous free fibular transfer. *British Journal of Plastic Surgery* 1990; **43**: 410.

140 Taylor GI, Corlett RJ, Boyd JB. The versatile deep inferior epigastric (inferior rectus abdominus) flap. *British Journal of Plastic Surgery* 1984; **37**: 330.

141 Harii K. Inferior rectus abdominus flaps. In: Baker SR ed. *Microsurgical Reconstruction of the Head and Neck*. New York: Churchill Livingstone, 1989.

142 Maxwell GP, Manson PN, Hoopes JE. Experience with 13 latissimus dorsi myocutaneous free flaps. *Plastic and Reconstructive Surgery* 1979; **64**: 1.

143 Quillen CG. Latissimus dorsi myocutaneous flaps in head and neck reconstruction. *Plastic and Reconstructive Surgery* 1979; **63**: 664.

144 Webster MHC, Soutar DS. *Practical Guide to Free Tissue Transfer*. London: Butterworths, 1986.

8 Radiotherapy

JM Henk and JD Langdon

Physical nature of radiation

Radiotherapy means treatment using ionising radiation, i.e. radiation that interacts with fluids to produce free ions. The type of radiation most commonly used is electromagnetic in the energy range 60 KeV – 25 MeV. The source of the electromagnetic radiation may be from a machine, e.g. a deep X-ray set or a linear accelerator, or from decay of a radioactive isotope, especially 60-Cobalt. Occasionally particulate radiation, i.e. electrons, neutrons or protons, is used.

Radiotherapy dosage is expressed in terms of absorbed dose. This is the quantity of ionising radiation energy absorbed per unit mass of tissue, and is therefore a concentration of radiation effect, not a quantity of energy. The SI unit of absorbed dose is the gray (Gy), defined as an energy absorption of 1 joule/kg. All doses in this chapter are expressed in gray, although in many cases the old unit, the rad, was used in the original publications quoted (100 rads = 1 Gy).

Biological action

In cells exposed to ionising radiation, free radicals are formed in the intracellular water. Adjacent large molecules may be denatured by the action of these free radicals. Most of the changes produced have no observable effect on cell function, unless a strand of DNA is broken in such a way that the cell is unable to go through a subsequent mitosis. Cell death will ensue if the cell attempts to divide, which it may do at an interval after radiotherapy that may be as short as a few minutes or as long as several years. This phenomenon of 'mitotic death' is responsible for nearly all the observed effects of radiotherapy on tumours and normal tissues.

Tumour effects

Irradiated tumour cells undergo mitotic death. The interval between irradiation and cell death depends on the rate of cell proliferation in the tumour. In the case of a rapidly proliferating tumour, e.g. squamous cell carcinoma, cell death and lysis is often seen within a few days. On the other hand, a very slowly proliferating tumour, e.g. a pleomorphic adenoma, may not manifest radiation changes for many months or even years.

The chance of a given dose of radiation sterilising all tumour cells depends on three factors:

Radiosensitivity is an inherent biological property of a cell type; it is determined by biochemical factors such as the ability of the cell to repair DNA damage.

Oxygenation influences the probability of cells killed. The greater the concentration of oxygen present in the cell at the instant of radiation, the more likely is a free radical to cause a lethal event.

Tumour size, the number of tumour cells initially present, is of critical importance.

Radiotherapy is rather like shooting randomly with a machine gun, so that the dose–response relation can be described by an exponential function (Fig. 8.1). A constant increment of dose kills a constant fraction of cells; therefore the fewer the cells present initially the greater the probability of killing them all.

If a tumour is relatively radioresistant, e.g. an adenocarcinoma of the mucus or salivary glands, radiotherapy can usually effect a cure only if there is a very small population of tumour cells present, such as immediately after near-total surgical removal. With more radiosensitive tumours, e.g. squamous cell carcinoma, there is a fair chance of success which diminishes with increasing tumour

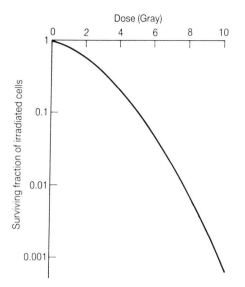

Fig. 8.1 Survival curve of mammalian cells exposed to radiation in tissue culture.

size. However, there is a wide variation in radiocurability between squamous carcinomas that appear clinically and histologically identical, because of differences in oxygenation, proliferation kinetics and intrinsic radiosensitivity.

Normal tissue effects

Mitotic death of normal cells accounts for the side effects of radiotherapy. Rapidly proliferating tissues manifest radiation changes quickly; mucosa after about 12 days and the skin after about 21 days following the start of a course of radiotherapy. These effects are known as acute reactions; they normally heal completely.

Mitotic death of vascular endothelial cells accounts for most of the delayed normal tissue effects. Endothelial cells have a turnover time of several months. Consequently, devascularisation of irradiated tissues does not begin until at least 3 months after radiotherapy and tends to progress for several years with little or no recovery. Tissue changes occurring as a result of devascularisation are known as 'late damage' and are irreversible.

Some normal cells do not normally undergo mitosis unless stimulated to do so. An example is the osteoblast, which may be stimulated to divide in order to remodel bone after trauma. Bone is largely unaffected by radiotherapy, unless trauma such as dental extraction provides a mitotic stimulus, in which case osteoblasts undergo mitotic death so that bone necrosis may ensue.

Normal tissue tolerance

The concept of normal tissue tolerance to radiotherapy has developed from many years of observation of late normal tissue effects. The tolerance dose is defined as the maximum dose of irradiation that can be given to the volume of tissue being treated without producing an unacceptable incidence of late damage.

The tolerance dose depends on the type of tissue; for example, it is low in the case of the lens of the eye and the spinal cord, and high in the case of skin and muscle. It also depends on the volume of tissue being irradiated; the larger the volume the lower the tolerance dose.

Principles of radiotherapy

There are two fundamentally different methods of administering radiotherapy. *Teletherapy*, or external beam irradiation, uses a machine to deliver beams of irradiation directed at the tumour from outside the patient. In *brachytherapy* the source of radiation is placed within, or in close proximity to, the tumour.

In oral cancer radiotherapy may be used as the sole treatment, or in combination with other modalities of treatment. Irradiation which aims at cure is termed radical radiotherapy. Here the object is local control, i.e. the complete destruction of the irradiated tumour, which requires the killing of all those tumour cells with unlimited capacity for cell division, while keeping dosage within normal tissue tolerance levels. The chance of achieving local control will vary according to the radiosensitivity, size, oxygenation and site of the tumour.

External beam therapy

Teletherapy is the form of radiotherapy most widely used in treatment. The absorption properties of radiation in tissue depend on the energy of the photons, which is inversely proportional to wavelength.

In the early days of radiotherapy (until the 1950s), the only sources of teletherapy available were X-ray machines operating in the orthovoltage range, i.e. up to 300 kV. The X-rays emitted by these machines were of relatively low penetration and delivered their maximum dose to the skin surface, which inevitably caused severe skin reactions. They had the additional disadvantage of very high absorption in materials with high atomic numbers, such as calcium in bone, so that their use to treat lesions in the mouth carried a high risk of osteoradionecrosis of the mandible. In the past 40 years sources of higher energy radiations have become available, such as telecobalt machines emitting gamma rays of energy just over 1 MeV and linear accelerators emitting X-rays of 4 MeV and higher. These supervoltage radiations are more penetrating than orthovoltage X-rays and deliver their maximum energy at a depth of several millimetres below the skin surface, so that severe skin reactions are no longer a problem. Their absorption in matter is less dependent on atomic number, so that bone absorbs very little more energy than does soft tissue; osteoradionecrosis is therefore less likely to occur. It is usual to employ two or more beams of supervoltage radiation converging on the tumour volume, so that the latter is irradiated homogeneously to the required dose while the neighbouring tissues through which the beam passes receive a lower dose (Fig. 8.2).

A course of external beam radiotherapy is *fractionated*, i.e. the total dose is divided into a number of smaller doses delivered over a period of several weeks. The larger the number of fractions, the greater the total dose required to produce the same effect (e.g. 50 Gy in 15 treatments over 3 weeks is roughly equivalent to 65 Gy in 30 treatments over 6 weeks).

The aim of fractionation is to increase the differ-

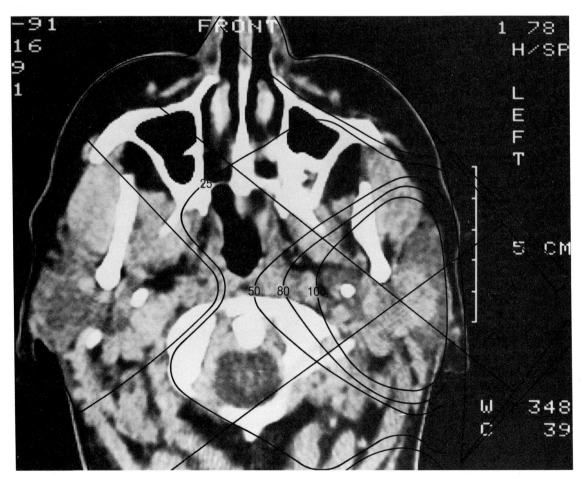

Fig. 8.2 Treatment plan for external radiation to a parotid tumour. The isodose lines indicate radiation dosage expressed as a percentage of that delivered to the centre of the tumour.

ential effect of the radiation on the tumour compared with the normal tissues. There are several mechanisms contributing to the beneficial effects of fractionation. Normal cells have a higher capacity than tumour cells to repair damage to DNA after exposure to small doses of radiation. The tumour response is enhanced by re-oxygenation of hypoxic cells as the tumour regresses, and there is the opportunity to irradiate tumour cells as they pass through more sensitive phases of the cell cycle.

The optimum treatment time and number of fractions remains the subject of controversy. In the early days of radiotherapy many different fractionation schemes were tried over a wide range, from one to 60 fractions, with treatment times of up to 12 weeks. Coutard,[1] working mainly with carcinomas of the larynx, eventually decided that the optimum was treatment once daily over a period of 5 or 6 weeks. This remains the most widely used fractionation scheme in current clinical practice, although both shorter and longer treatment times are also extensively used. A 6 week course of treatment is inevitably taxing on a patient and on the resources of a hospital department. Accordingly, there has been a tendency to give longer treatments to the fitter patients with the better prognoses, and to give shorter treatments to the older or less fit patients with more advanced tumours and poorer prognoses. As a result, almost all retrospective analyses show better results from longer treatment times.

An exception is the large study by Paterson of results at the Christie Hospital, Manchester.[2] Wartime conditions compelled this centre to reduce their treatment times from the previously standard 5 weeks to 3 weeks, and then to 8 days. It was found that the patients treated over 8 days did less well, but the results of the 3 week treatment were identical to those of 5 weeks in terms of local control and survival, with no significant differences in morbidity. Some radiotherapists have accepted Paterson's evidence and routinely use a 3 week treatment time, while others still maintain that 6 week treatment gives a better therapeutic ratio. Unfortunately, there is no evidence from prospective controlled trials to support either point of view; in most trials carried out the numbers of patients were too small to draw meaningful conclusions, but no evidence of the superiority of the longer treatment time emerged. The weight of evidence from all published series suggests that the 3 and 6 week treatment times give similar local control rates and late effects on normal tissues if a total dose appro-

priate to the fractionation scheme is chosen. There is some difference for morbidity, more qualitative than quantitative. Compared with 6 week treatments, 3 week treatments give brisker but shorter mucosal reactions and milder skin reactions.

We believe that for treating oral and salivary gland cancer with small treatment volumes of 300 cm^3 or less, there is no proven advantage in protracting treatment beyond 4 weeks, and so we give 55 Gy in 20 fractions over 4 weeks for radical treatments of this type. When the treatment volume is larger, the less severe mucositis resulting from a longer treatment time may be an advantage by making it easier for the patient to maintain adequate nutrition during treatment, so we give daily fractions of 2 Gy to a total dose of 66 Gy. The latter scheme is also used where central nervous system tissue, such as the spinal cord or optic nerve, is within or close to the irradiated volume, as there is a more profound effect of fraction size on the radiovulnerability of these tissues.

So-called 'altered' or 'unconventional' schedules using more than one fraction of radiotherapy per day are now under investigation (see below).

Results of external beam therapy
The results of external beam irradiation as a sole treatment of oral cancer are not entirely satisfactory. As stated previously, the probability of local control of a tumour depends on its size, and to a lesser degree on its morphology. Typical local control rates of external radiotherapy range from as high as 90 per cent for T1 tumours to as low as 10 per cent for T4, with intermediate figures for T2 and T3 of about 70 per cent and 40 per cent respectively. It is never possible to predict the outcome of any form of treatment in an individual cancer patient, and this is particularly true of external radiotherapy. Occasionally a very small carcinoma will completely fail to respond to radiotherapy, and sometimes an enormous tumour where the prognosis seems virtually hopeless will unexpectedly disappear and not recur.

Methods of improving results of external beam therapy
Better results from radiotherapy can be achieved only by increasing the differential effect of the radiation on the tumour compared with the normal tissues. Radiotherapists are therefore looking for exploitable differences between tumour cells and normal cells which are responsible for the dose-limiting late radiation effects. Two possible exploit-

able differences between tumour cells and normal cells are the oxygen effect and cell proliferation kinetics.

The presence of viable hypoxic cells in tumours but not in normal tissues is believed to be one of the major causes of radiotherapy failure, thus many of the efforts to improve the results of radiotherapy in the past 25 years have been directed towards overcoming this so-called 'oxygen effect'. The relative importance of the oxygen effect in clinical radiotherapy, however, remains controversial. As a course of fractionated radiotherapy proceeds, re-oxygenation of tumour cells occurs; therefore, some radiotherapists believe that hypoxia is a relatively insignificant factor in clinical radiotherapeutic practice. Nevertheless, many experimental animal tumours have been shown not to re-oxygenate adequately, and clinical studies with high pressure oxygen and chemical sensitisers of hypoxic cells are strongly suggestive that the same is true of many human cancers. Several methods of overcoming the oxygen effect have been tried in oral cancer, especially hyperbaric oxygen, neutron therapy and hypoxic cell radiosensitising drugs.

Hyperbaric oxygen

The most obvious approach to the problem of the radioresistant hypoxic tumour cell is to provide it directly with more oxygen. In order to bring about a large reduction in the proportion of hypoxic cells, oxygen must be inhaled at raised pressure. In pure oxygen at a pressure of 3 atmospheres absolute, the maximum the human brain can tolerate without general anaesthesia, it has been calculated that only 0.1 per cent of tumour cells are likely to remain hypoxic.[3] This calculation, however, assumes normal blood flow rate in capillaries. Unfortunately, high pressure oxygen induces vasoconstriction, so that in practice it may be less effective. The oxygen must be present at the instant of irradiation so the radiotherapy is delivered while the patient is in a hyperbaric oxygen chamber (Fig. 8.3). This technique has been used in the past with some success in oral cancer.

Churchill-Davidson[4] reported encouraging results in a group of 25 patients, and subsequently reported a 62 per cent local control rate of lymph node metastases. Prospective controlled trials under the aegis of the Medical Research Council showed a significant benefit in terms of both survival and local control from the use of hyperbaric oxygen in a variety of head and neck sites.[5,6] In these trials, statistical significance was reached only when the results from all head and neck sites were added together, but the results in oral cavity carcinomas followed the general trend (Table 8.1). These trials showed that the effectiveness of hyperbaric oxygen diminishes as the tumour increases in size; the significant benefit was demonstrated in lesions, both primary and nodal, of 2–5 cm diam-

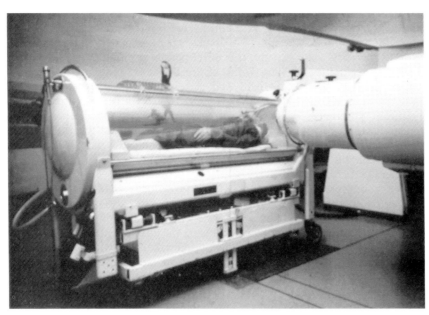

Fig. 8.3 Hyperbaric chamber for use in radiotherapy.

Table 8.1 Results of Cardiff hyperbaric oxygen trial in patients with oral cavity carcinomas, 1966–71

	Hyperbaric oxygen	Air
No. treated	24	25
5 year survival	38%	27%
2 year local control	45%	15% ($P<0.05$)

eter. The lack of benefit in the case of large tumours is presumably because the oxygen failed to penetrate into larger masses.

Hyperbaric oxygen has largely been abandoned, mainly because of its complexity and hazards, which make radiotherapists and technicians unwilling to use it. Also, a high proportion of patients with head and neck cancer in the UK are unfit for the procedure. Nevertheless, the results of the controlled trials are important because they show that almost certainly the oxygen effect is real, and not totally overcome by fractionation alone.

Hypoxic cell sensitising agents
The property of oxygen that is responsible for its radiosensitising action is its electron affinity. There has been much interest in developing electron-affinitive compounds that have the same radiobiological properties as oxygen, and that are non-toxic and freely diffusible so that they can be administered systemically and reach hypoxic tumour cells. Several electron-affinitive compounds have been tried in head and neck cancer, all belonging to the nitro-imidazole family. Unfortunately, these substances are neurotoxic, and in general it has been found that the doses which can safely be given are insufficient to improve significantly the results of radiotherapy.[7,8] A possible exception is nimorazole, which showed a benefit in a control trial of radiotherapy in oropharyngeal carcinoma conducted in Denmark.[9]

Neutron therapy
Another approach to the problem of the oxygen effect is the use of types of radiation that are less dependent on the presence of oxygen for their cell killing effect. Fast neutrons have been used in radiotherapy because of this property. They have a major disadvantage, however, because late responding normal tissues accumulate more radiation damage than in the case of electromagnetic irradiation. Consequently, there is a greater risk of late normal tissue complications, such as fibrosis and necrosis.

There have been several trials of neutron therapy in oral cancer with no evidence of benefit, and the method has been largely abandoned because of severe complications.[10–12] A benefit is still claimed for inoperable salivary gland carcinoma by some radiotherapists (see Chapter 15).

A multicentre randomised trial in 32 patients showed a significantly higher tumour control rate 2 years after treatment,[13] but more evidence on late morbidity is required before neutron treatment can be recommended for routine use in the treatment of salivary tumours.

Altered fractionation
There is some evidence that the effect of radiotherapy on late reacting normal tissues can be reduced relative to tumour effect by the use of small fraction sizes. Hence, a higher total dose can be given safely if fraction sizes are reduced below the conventional 2 Gy. Inevitably, the total number of fractions must be increased. This increase in number and reduction in size of fractions is known as *hyperfractionation*. This approach is gaining in popularity, with several authors claiming improved results.[14,15] A controlled trial conducted by the European Organisation for Research on Treatment of Cancer (EORTC) compared standard 2 Gy fractions once per day to a total dose of 70 Gy over 7 weeks with a hyperfractionated regime consisting of fractions of 1.15 Gy twice daily to a total dose of 80.5 Gy over 7 weeks in carcinoma of the oropharynx; local control in the hyperfractionation arm of the study was significantly better.[16]

Many human tumours, especially squamous cell carcinoma, contain malignant cells that are capable of rapid proliferation. The rate of cell turnover in a tumour may be expressed as the potential doubling time (T_{pot}), which is the time the tumour would take to double in volume if all cells survived and none were shed, died or differentiated. T_{pot} can be estimated in human tumours by biopsy after injection of bromodeoxyuridine, which labels cells in the synthetic phase of the cell cycle. Typical values of T_{pot} for squamous carcinomas have been found to be between 3 and 5 days.[17] The significance of this rapid proliferation is that tumour cells surviving the early part of a course of radiotherapy can repopulate the tumour, so that effectively there are more cells to be killed, so the chance of cure is reduced. There is evidence that the rate of repopulation actually increases during a course of radiotherapy.[18] Hence, it is to be expected that shorter treatment times should be more effective. Several retrospective reviews have indeed shown that prolonging treatment time militates against cure.[19,20] Shortening of treatment time to overcome the effect of repopulation is known as *acceleration*. Acceleration must be combined with an element of hyperfractionation, otherwise the fraction size will be too large. Several accelerated hyperfraction regimes are now the subject of multicentre controlled trials. An example is the 'CHART' (Continuous Hyperfractionated Accelerated Radiation Therapy) regime introduced by Dische and Saunders,[21] in which radiotherapy is given to a dose of 54 Gy in 36 fractions of 1.5 Gy, administered three times a day over 12 consecutive days. This regime showed better control rates and lower late morbidity compared with historical controls.

Concomitant cytotoxic agents
Numerous studies have been performed in which cytotoxic drugs have been administered at the same time as radiotherapy. Some have shown a significant improvement in local tumour control, but usually with an increase in morbidity. It is not clear to what extent cytotoxic drugs can enhance the relative effect of radiotherapy on tumours compared with normal tissues, and it may be that in most instances the effect is merely additive. The subject is discussed in Chapter 9.

Brachytherapy

Brachytherapy is a general term applied to radiotherapy delivered from a source of radiation placed very close to the tumour. There are two methods; surface moulds and interstitial implants. The former now have little part to play in the treatment of mouth cancer, but the latter are widely used.

Principle
The principle of brachytherapy depends on the law of inverse squares, which states that the intensity of dosage of radiation at a point is inversely proportional to the square of the distance of that point from the source of the radiation. In interstitial treatment, solid sources of radiation are implanted directly into the tumour, producing a high intensity of radiation in the immediate vicinity of the sources, while the dose to surrounding normal tissues is low because of rapid fall-off.

For interstitial treatment to be successful the whole visible and palpable tumour plus a margin of safety of at least 1 cm must receive an adequate dose of radiation delivered as homogeneously as possible, avoiding underdosed areas where disease may survive and overdosed areas where necrosis may ensue. In practice this usually means that the radiation sources must encompass the whole lesion; therefore interstitial irradiation is generally applicable only to tumours confined to the soft tissue. Sources cannot be inserted into bone, so tumours involving or fixed to bone are unsuitable for interstitial irradiation.

Radiation sources
Radioactive material used for brachytherapy may be either permanently implanted or removed. Permanent implants use short lived radioactive isotopes that rapidly decay to a negligible activity, so they can be safely left in the tumour site permanently. Gold-198, in the form of seeds introduced with a specially designed 'gun', is occasionally used. It is difficult to distribute gold seeds accurately and ensure a uniform dose distribution is obtained, and so the technique is now rarely used. It may still have a place as a method of boosting the dose in awkward sites, such as the soft palate, where it is difficult to use removable sources.

Nowadays nearly all brachytherapy is carried out using removable radiation sources. In the early days of radiotherapy radium was the only radioactive material available. It was enclosed in platinum needles 2.5 mm in diameter and 1.5–6 cm in length. Radium has now been superseded by artificially produced isotopes which are safer to handle.

Caesium-137 is available in needles of the same dimensions and activity as the old radium needles. Insertion of needles involves radiation exposure to the operator and other operating theatre personnel. The thick needles are traumatic and uncomfortable for the patient.

The most popular radioactive material for interstitial irradiation of oral cancer is now iridium-192. This is produced in the form of fine wire which is inserted into the tissues using either slotted guide needles or plastic tubing.[22]

The slotted guide needle technique is used for intra-oral insertion of 'hairpins' or single pins of iridium wire of 0.6 mm diameter (Fig. 8.4). This method is applicable to smaller tumours of the tongue, floor of the mouth and buccal mucosa where the introducers can be inserted intra-orally, i.e. the same types of lesions which were previously treated by radium needles. In this method, the positioning of sources does not involve handling of a radioactive material. The operator does not feel obliged to hurry and can take great care to ensure

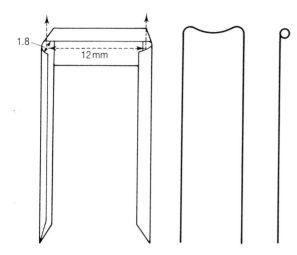

1.8

12 mm

Fig. 8.4 Slotted guide needle and iridium-192 sources for intra-oral brachytherapy.

that the introducers are correctly positioned to give the desired dose and distribution of radiation. The position of the guide needles can be checked by X-rays on the operating table before they are loaded with radioactive material (Fig. 8.5). The only radiation exposure to the operating theatre staff occurs during the last few minutes of the procedure when the iridium is inserted into the guide needles and the latter removed. The flexible and thinner wires cause less discomfort to the patient than the thick rigid caesium or radium needles. They permit easier feeding and oral hygiene. The change from radium or caesium needles to iridium hairpins was reported to bring about improved results in the treatment of tongue and floor of mouth cancer.[23,24] This is probably because it is possible to take more time over the procedure and check the position of the sources when using iridium.

Another technique using iridium-192 involves the introduction of finer iridium wire of diameter 0.3 mm via plastic tubing (Fig. 8.6). The tubing is inserted in loops via straight hollow guide needles which must be inserted through the skin into the oral cavity. With this technique, there is true after-loading, i.e. the tubes are positioned under general anaesthesia but not loaded with radioactive wire until the patient is returned to the ward. In this way radiation exposure to the operator and operating theatre staff is completely eliminated. This technique is useful for the cheek, and also for the posterior third of the tongue where the needles can be inserted between the mandible and the hyoid bone.

It can also be used in the neck as an adjuvant to salvage neck dissection (see Chapter 13).

Dosage
If an oral cancer is treated by brachytherapy alone, a dose of 65–70 Gy is given over a time ranging between 5.5 and 8 days at a dose rate of 0.3–0.5 Gy per hour. It is believed that shorter times at a higher dose rate increase the risk of necrosis without improving the chances of tumour control.[25]

External radiotherapy and brachytherapy can be used in combination, in which case the external beam is usually given first to a dose of 40 Gy over 4 weeks, followed by an implant as soon as possible giving a further 35–40 Gy, using the same dose rate as above. It is important that the total treatment time should not exceed 6 weeks because of the risk of failure due to tumour cell repopulation.[26]

Results of brachytherapy
The value of interstitial irradiation in the treatment of oral cancer is well established. It was used extensively between 1930 and 1950. During this period mouth cancer was particularly common in western countries, so that radiotherapists gained plenty of experience and became skilled at the quick and accurate positioning of radium needles. During the same period the only external beam sources available were in the orthovoltage range with their high associated morbidity and poor efficacy. From about 1950 onwards there was a fairly rapid swing away from interstitial therapy towards external irradiation, because of the greater awareness of the hazards to staff of handling radioactive materials, and the advent of supervoltage external beam radiotherapy. A third factor in the UK was the declining incidence of the disease. As a result the younger radiotherapists were not able to obtain adequate experience in radium needle implants, were concerned about radiation exposure to themselves and other hospital staff, and preferred to use the newer supervoltage external radiation which, it was believed, would be equally effective. It is possible that this swing away from interstitial therapy was a significant factor in the failure to improve survival rates in oral cancer over recent years. In the past 15 years there has been something of a renaissance of interstitial therapy, with the advent of the newer techniques, especially those using iridium wire, involving much less radiation exposure to hospital staff, and with the realisation that results of supervoltage external radiotherapy were not as good as at first hoped.

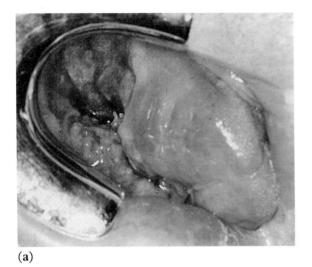

(a)

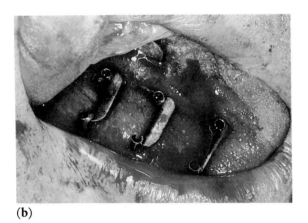

(b)

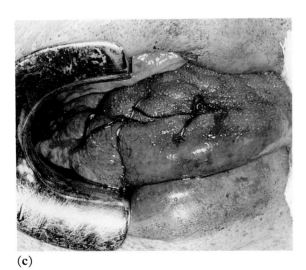

(c)

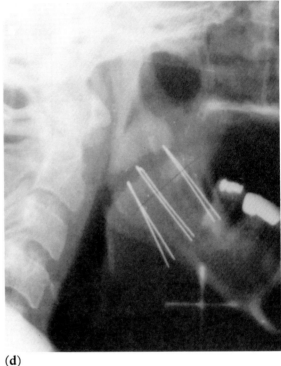

(d)

Fig. 8.5 (a) Carcinoma of the tongue to be treated by brachytherapy. (b) Slotted guide needles in position. (c) Iridium-192 hairpins inserted and slotted guides removed. (d) X-ray to check position of sources.

It is now well recognised that the results of interstitial irradiation are superior to those of external irradiation. This is partly because the smaller earlier lesions are usually selected for implant, whereas the very advanced disease can only be treated by external beam. However, there are published results of the treatment of earlier tumours by both methods that show appreciable superiority for interstitial irradiation.[27] The Patterns of Care Study conducted by the American College of Radiology in 96 institutions in the USA[28] revealed that, overall, the local recurrence rate in carcinoma of the tongue and floor of mouth was 41 per cent when treatment was by external beam alone, and 26 per cent when brachytherapy was used for all or part of the treatment. From single institutions specialising in brachytherapy, local recurrence rates for T1 and T2 oral cancer of between 5 and 15 per cent are typical.[29] The reasons for the greater efficacy of brachytherapy compared with external

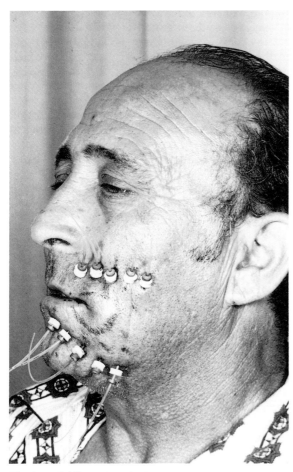

Fig. 8.6 Iridium-192 wire inserted via plastic tubing for treatment of carcinoma of the buccal mucosa adjacent to the angle of the mouth.

beam are the subject of some controversy. The short treatment time preventing the effect of tumour cell repopulation is undoubtedly one factor. There is some evidence for a lower oxygen effect with low dose rate continuous irradiation, but this effect seems slight and it is uncertain whether it is important clinically. The most important factor is probably the localised concentration of the radiation dose, which enables a higher effective dose to be delivered to the tumour without excessive normal tissue effect.[30]

Palliative radiotherapy

The aim of palliative radiotherapy is to relieve the symptoms of the disease, without attempting to cure the patient or causing new symptoms from acute normal tissue reaction. Palliative radiotherapy is only appropriate for patients with incurable disease and a short life expectancy. It is useful for relieving bleeding or pressure symptoms caused by the bulk of the tumour, such as pain or obstruction.

A moderate dose of radiation is administered over a short time; for example, 20 Gy over 5 days. This dose is sufficient to kill a substantial proportion of the malignant cells, but not to effect a cure. As a result the tumour regresses considerably and symptoms are relieved.

This approach is useful for palliation of metastases, especially in bone, brain or skin. With advanced primary disease or nodal metastases not a great deal can be achieved, as a brief period of regression of the tumour and amelioration of symptoms is followed by regrowth and a return of symptoms before the death of the patient. In head and neck cancer in general nothing short of complete control of the local disease can provide really worthwhile palliation, so palliative radiotherapy is not often advisable.

Combined radiotherapy and surgery

Salvage surgery

Where radical radiotherapy fails and there is residual or recurrent tumour, surgical cure may yet be possible. Surgery performed after failure of radical radiotherapy is termed 'salvage' surgery. After radical radiotherapy the heavily irradiated tissues tend to have an impaired blood supply and poor healing properties. Consequently, salvage surgery carries a higher risk than elective surgery of complications such as delayed wound healing, fistula formation, wound breakdown and carotid artery rupture. The hazards of salvage surgery tend to increase with time after irradiation, as delayed radiation changes progress in the vasculoconnective tissues, as described above. The complication rate is lowest when surgery is performed within 3 months of completion of radiotherapy. Unfortunately it is not often possible to know whether or not radiotherapy has been successful within that period. Some tumours regress slowly after radiotherapy although completely sterilised, especially those with a low rate of cell turnover, such as many types of salivary gland tumours. In such cases postradiotherapy induration, and recognisable tumour cells on biopsy, may persist for several weeks after completion of the radiotherapy. Sobel and Rubin[31] found from their own experience, and after reviewing the literature, that an accurate clinical and histological assessment of tumour persistence after radical radiotherapy could not be made until 90 days had elapsed from the date of starting the treatment. Consequently clinicians must beware of being too hasty in diagnosing residual tumour and proceeding to salvage surgery.

The same considerations apply to attempts to predict the radiation response during a course of radiotherapy. A policy sometimes adopted consists of assessing the response of the tumour two-thirds of the way through a course of radical radiotherapy, usually after 40 Gy has been given over 4 weeks. If the tumour seems to be regressing well it is regarded as radioresponsive and further radiotherapy is given to a full radical dose. If there is little or no regression surgery is performed. This policy has little to recommend it, as the rate of tumour shrinkage depends on the cell turnover rate and the rate at which dead tumour cells lyse or can be removed by phagocytic activity, and does not necessarily indicate ultimate radiocurability. Suit et al.[32] showed that there was a poor correlation between regression rate and ultimate prognosis. It is therefore not logical or justifiable to abandon a course of radiotherapy two-thirds of the way through because of apparent poor response, except perhaps in the very rare instance where the tumour continues to grow during radiotherapy.

Pre-operative radiotherapy

This term should be reserved for radiotherapy given to a patient for whom a decision to treat by elective surgery has been made. The aim of pre-operative radiotherapy is to increase the chance of surgical cure, based on the assumption that local recurrence or metastases result from dissemination at operation of cells derived from the actively growing periphery of the tumour. These cells have a good blood supply, are well oxygenated, and are therefore radiosensitive. A moderate dose of radiotherapy insufficient to cause severe acute reaction or to delay wound healing can eliminate the majority of these well oxygenated peripheral cells. The more radioresistant poorly oxygenated cells, which can be sterilised only by much larger doses of irradiation, are situated towards the centre of the

tumour and are therefore most likely to be removed at operation without risk of dissemination.

Pre-operative radiotherapy became very popular in the 1960s following animal experiments which demonstrated its effectiveness. In most experimental animal tumours tested, e.g. those of Powers and Palmer,[33] a low dose of radiation administered immediately before excision significantly increased survival rates. As a result a large number of clinical trials of pre-operative radiotherapy were set up. These were based on two different concepts; the low dose and the high dose.

The low dose technique consists of giving a relatively small dose of radiation in a few largish fractions over a few days, and operating immediately before any vasodilatation from acute radiation reaction occurs. Radiotherapy given in this way makes little or no difference to the difficulty of the operation or the postoperative morbidity; on the other hand, there is no regression of the tumour to make the operation easier. Two randomised controlled trials in the USA demonstrated a significant reduction in local recurrence but with no improvement in survival.[34,35]

The high dose approach consists of treatment with more conventionally sized daily fractions over 4 or 5 weeks, administering 70–80 per cent of a radical tumour dose, i.e. 40–50 Gy. This dosage results in some acute normal tissue reaction and hyperaemia, so surgery must be delayed for a further 3 to 4 weeks after the end of the course of radiotherapy to allow the reaction to subside. Advocates of this approach consider that the larger the number of cells that can be killed by radiation, the greater the chance of cure, and that tumour regression prior to surgery leads to an improvement in the patient's general condition and makes the operation easier and safer. This method has been more popular than the low dose method, but its value in oral cancer has never been demonstrated by prospective controlled clinical trials. It is fraught with practical difficulties. Problems may particularly be encountered in the patient whose tumour regresses considerably after the irradiation. The question then arises: 'Should the surgery proceed as originally planned, or will a lesser excision now suffice?' It is generally accepted that the surgery should remove all tissue initially involved by tumour, to give the patient the best chance of avoiding local recurrence. To this end, preradiotherapy photographs and tattooing of the mucosa at the edges of the lesion are valuable aids to the surgeon at the time of operation, indicating how extensive the resection should be. The situation is occasionally encountered where either the patient or the surgeon may be so impressed by the response that one or the other refuses the operation, so that the radiotherapist is then left with the problem of converting the pre-operative treatment into a radical treatment after an interval of several weeks, with the consequent reduced chances of a radiotherapy cure.

Postoperative radiotherapy

The rationale of postoperative radiotherapy is that a small number of malignant cells may be left behind after a radical operation, either implanted into the operative field or left at the deep margin of an excision, and postoperative recurrences subsequently develop from such cells left behind. Immediately after operation the residual cells should be few in number and therefore likely to be eliminated by a dose of radiation which would not have been sufficient to cure the original tumour.

Postoperative radiotherapy might be expected to be less effective than pre-operative radiotherapy. It can be expected to prevent only local recurrence, whereas pre-operative radiotherapy may also serve to sterilise cells disseminated into the blood at the time of operation, and therefore reduce the incidence of distant metastases. Cells left behind in an operation field are likely to be poorly vascularised and therefore relatively radioresistant. In experimental animal tumours pre-operative radiotherapy was shown to be more effective in increasing survival rates than postoperative radiotherapy.[36] Clinical studies nevertheless suggest that in head and neck cancer generally postoperative radiotherapy can prevent local recurrence in a proportion of patients with definite or probable microscopic residual disease after surgery.[37] In a retrospective review from the Memorial Sloan-Kettering Cancer Centre,[38] patients receiving postoperative radiotherapy had a much lower rate of local recurrence, both at the primary site and in the neck, compared with historical controls who received no radiotherapy. The largest effect was at the primary site where surgical margins were considered unsatisfactory; the local recurrence rate was reported as 73 per cent without postoperative radiotherapy, and 10.5 per cent with postoperative radiotherapy.[38] It is thought that radiotherapy is best commenced within 6 weeks of the end of surgery, in which case 50 Gy in 25 treatments is an adequate dose. If radiotherapy is delayed for more than 6 weeks for any reason, a dose of 60 Gy in 30 treatments is necessary.[39]

A multicentre prospective randomised controlled trial in the USA compared 50 Gy pre-operatively with 60 Gy postoperatively. All head and neck sites were included; the largest group was hypopharyngeal cancer, but only 15 per cent of the patients had oral cancer. The number of patients included in the trial was 277. Local regional control was significantly better in the postoperative radiotherapy group (70 per cent, $P = 0.04$). However, there was no significant difference in survival.[40]

There now seems little doubt that despite the theoretical considerations and animal experiments favouring pre-operative radiotherapy, postoperative radiotherapy is preferable in clinical practice. Postoperative radiotherapy is indicated whenever there is a histological appearance of aggressive disease, close or involved surgical margins, or lymph node involvement (see Chapter 13).

Side-effects of radiotherapy

Acute effects

Mucositis
The acute mucosal reaction to radiotherapy results from mitotic death of cells in the epithelium lining the oral cavity and pharynx. The cell cycle time of the basal epithelial cells is about 4 days, and the epithelium is 3 or 4 cells thick. Hence radiation changes begin to appear at about 12 days after the start of irradiation. The time of onset is almost independent of the dose, fractionation or radiation technique. Initially there is erythema of the mucosa followed after a few days by the appearance of a patchy fibrinous exudate. If a high dose of radiation is given over a short time, ulceration may supervene with a thick fibrinous membrane covering the denuded surface.

Mucositis is painful and interferes with nutrition. It should be treated conservatively, to avoid damaging the few remaining cells from which the epithelium will regenerate. The patient should be advised to take a soft bland diet, avoiding irritants such as smoking, spirits or spicy foods. The mouth should be kept clean using saline mouthwashes. Bacterial infection plays no part in the pathogenesis of mucositis, so there is no need for local antiseptics which tend to increase discomfort in the mouth. Anti-inflammatory agents such as aspirin used as a mouthwash, or sucralfate, help to ease the pain.

Surviving epithelial cells respond to radiation damage by dividing more rapidly, so that complete healing is the rule. The length of time mucositis takes to heal depends on the dose intensity of the radiotherapy, but is usually complete within 3 weeks after the end of treatment. Cytotoxic drugs which have a selective action on cells in the mitotic cycle kill regenerating epithelial cells, so that the simultaneous use of chemotherapy and radiotherapy results in more severe and prolonged mucosal toxicity.

Skin reaction

The cell turnover in the skin is a little slower than in the mucosa, so skin changes take longer to appear. Erythema usually appears during the third week of treatment and may progress to a dry and then a moist desquamation according to the dose delivered. Most radiotherapy for oral cancer is given using supervoltage beams which have a surface-sparing effect, so that skin changes are usually mild. Healing is normally complete within 3 weeks of finishing treatment.

Epilation

Hair loss occurs with quite small doses of radiation, so in the treatment of oral cancer it is seen at both the entrance and the exit of radiation beams. Skin close to the tumour being treated usually receives a dose sufficient to cause permanent epilation, but elsewhere the hair regrows after a few months.

Loss of the taste sensation

Patients receiving radiotherapy to the mouth invariably experience some disturbance or loss of taste sensation, the mechanism of which has not been elucidated. The taste receptor cells are relatively radioresistant; a dose of 60 Gy causes only a 10 per cent loss of taste cells.[41] There is a loss of microvilli on the surface of the taste receptors, which is also seen in conditions resulting in a diminished salivary flow in the absence of radiation, e.g. Sjøgren's syndrome. Disturbance of taste is frequently seen after irradiation of the parotid glands, suggesting that change in the volume and composition of saliva is one of the mechanisms underlying radiotherapy-induced taste loss. Taste loss can be a distressing symptom, and contributes to poor nutrition in patients receiving radiotherapy. Taste function usually recovers slowly within a few months after the end of radiotherapy, but in some patients the changes are permanent. No reliable method of improving taste sensation in these patients has been found; there is a suggestion that taste thresholds may be lowered by oral administration of zinc sulphate.[42]

Xerostomia

Salivary and mucous glands are especially vulnerable to radiation damage. Loss of secretory cells occurs as an acute effect, but the acini are incapable of regenerating and recovering their function. The vulnerability of salivary tissue is both age and dose dependent; as little as 20 Gy in adults can cause permanent cessation of salivary flow, so that glands in both the entry and exit path of radiation beams are at risk.

Salivary flow diminishes within a few days of the start of radiotherapy. After 5 weeks, the flow from irradiated salivary glands falls to zero and never recovers.[43] However, in most patients the sensation of dryness of the mouth tends to diminish after a few months. This may be partly subjective as they adjust to their diminished salivary flow, but also results from compensatory hypertrophy of unirradiated glandular tissue. Radiotherapy fields used in the treatment of oral cancer normally avoid at least part of the parotid glands, so that xerostomia tends not to be a severe problem. In contrast, radiotherapy to the nasopharynx destroys both parotid glands and causes a severe permanent xerostomia. When a salivary tumour is irradiated, it should be possible to avoid the contralateral gland and not cause xerostomia.

Dryness of the mouth is a distressing symptom, and carries an increased risk of dental decay. Oral administration of pilocarpine may help to stimulate residual salivary tissue, but is rarely very successful. Many patients find a saliva substitute solution helpful.[44] Several proprietary 'artificial salivas' are now available.

Infection

Acute bacterial infection during radiotherapy is uncommon. However, as a course of treatment progresses with increasing mucositis and xerostomia secondary superinfection with *Candida* sp. often occurs. This may present as increased pain and widespread fiery erythema of the mucosa or as discrete white plaques of 'thrush'. In order to prevent this, some clinicians advocate the routine use of chlorhexidine mouthwash throughout the radiotherapy and until the mucositis has resolved. However, the 0.2 per cent commercial preparation is irritant in this situation and should be diluted with warm water to a concentration of 0.01 per cent. We do not advocate the routine use of chlorhexidine for this purpose as our patients find it unpleasant to use. Preferably, candidal infections are treated as and when they occur using specific antifungal agents. In practice, miconazole gel, 10 ml used four times daily, is effective and well tolerated. Severe infections require systemic treatment with fluconazole.

Late effects

Ischaemia and fibrosis
Vascular endothelial cells are slow replicating, with a turnover time of several months. Poststenotic dilatation of venules also occurs, which appears on skin and mucosal surfaces as telangiectasia. This process begins several months after irradiation and may progress for several years. The extent of devascularisation depends on the dose of radiation administered and the volume of tissue irradiated. After excessive doses of radiation, tissue necrosis may supervene.

Cell death in connective tissues attracts migrating fibroblasts, leading to excess deposition of collagen which appears clinically as fibrosis.

Soft tissue necrosis
Acute mucositis normally heals within a few weeks of the end of radiotherapy. Over a period beginning within a few months and extending to several years, vascular changes in the submucosa lead to varying degrees of atrophy, telangiectasia, dryness and fragility of the mucosa. The mucosa can then be damaged by quite minor trauma, leading to ulceration that is slow to heal because of the impaired blood supply. The higher the radiation dose and the larger the volume irradiated, the more marked are the mucosal changes and the greater the risk of ulceration. Brachytherapy gives a higher but more localised mucosal dose, and tends to carry a higher risk of radionecrotic ulceration compared with external beam, although necrosis from the latter is more difficult to treat because of the larger area of devascularised mucosa.

A radionecrotic ulcer is typically flat with little surrounding induration. In some cases there may be associated fibrosis, giving the ulcer a leathery feel. Occasionally, when there is thickening at the edges of the ulcer, it is difficult to distinguish from recurrent carcinoma. A clinical diagnosis should be made if possible, trying to avoid biopsy which may make the radionecrosis worse. A useful distinguishing feature is the character of pain. A deep boring pain, especially if referred to the ear, is suggestive of carcinoma. The pain of radionecrosis is usually more superficial, often with local tenderness. Treatment consists of scrupulous oral hygiene, irrigation of the ulcer to keep it free of food debris and a course of antibiotics. Most radionecrotic ulcers, especially those following brachytherapy, heal with conservative treatment. If there is no improvement after 2 weeks of treatment, recurrent carcinoma must be suspected and a biopsy performed.

A small minority of radionecrotic ulcers fail to heal and require surgery. Local diathermy excision is usually adequate. It is very rare for a major excision and repair procedure to be required.

Bone necrosis
The radiovulnerable cells in bone are the vascular endothelium and the osteocytes. There is relatively little mitotic activity in the latter in the adult, so bone necrosis normally occurs only when there has been a high dose of radiation and a mitotic stimulus such as trauma (see below).

Osteoradionecrosis

Definition
Osteoradionecrosis literally means death of irradiated bone. In clinical practice, the term is normally used to define the condition in which dead bone in an irradiated volume loses its mucosal covering, so becoming exposed.

Aetiology

Biological basis
In normal healthy adult bone, most cells are in the resting phase of the mitotic cycle. However, there is a slow but constant cell turnover accompanied by remodelling of the bone structure. Osteoclasts proliferate, resorb bone and disappear; osteoblasts proliferate to reconstruct the bone. This process continues throughout life. Trauma stimulates proliferation of osteoblasts mainly from the periosteum to repair the damage to the bone.

Irradiation lethally damages some osteoclasts and osteoblasts, which continue to survive and perform their vegetative functions until they attempt to divide, when mitotic death occurs and they disintegrate. An individual bone cell may undergo mitotic death at an interval of months or years after irradiation, or it may never in fact divide unless stimulated by trauma. There is therefore a slow loss of bone cells over a long period after radiotherapy with a consequent slowing down of the remodelling process, which may eventually lead to thinning and reduced strength of the bone. There is also diminished vascularity of the periosteum as a late effect of radiation on endothelial cells, which may also contribute to bone damage. The direct effect on the bone cells is probably the more important, as histological changes in bone after irradiation have been observed in the absence of any visible changes in the vasculature.

The mandible is affected much more commonly than the maxilla. The mandible consists of more compact bone with a higher density and therefore greater radiation absorption. Its blood supply in the age group who develop cancer is poor, being almost entirely via the periosteum. The maxilla with its lower density and rich vasculature is rarely the site of osteoradionecrosis.

Radiation dose

The very high absorbed dose from orthovoltage radiation was associated with a high incidence of bone necrosis. Watson and Scarborough[45] reported an incidence of 13 per cent in a series of 1819 patients with oral cancer treated by irradiation. With modern supervoltage radiation, the incidence is lower and markedly dose dependent. Bedwinek et al.[46] reported the incidence of necrosis of the healthy, uninvolved mandible at varying dose levels of supervoltage irradiation using daily fractions of 2 Gy. No cases of osteoradionecrosis were recorded with doses below 60 Gy, up to 70 Gy the incidence was 1.8 per cent, and above 70 Gy was 9 per cent.

Dental factors

Murray et al.[47] found that the incidence of osteoradionecrosis was three times higher in dentate than in edentulous patients as a result of infection from periodontal disease and trauma from tooth extraction. An extraction increases the demand on the remodelling process. If dental extraction is performed at an interval after radiotherapy when there is devascularisation in addition to lethal damage to osteoblasts, there is a particularly high risk of bone necrosis. The risk of necrosis is less if dental extraction is performed before radiotherapy, but is still present as a consequence of the enhanced re-

modelling of bone which proceeds for some months after the extraction. Hinds[48] reported that at the MD Anderson Hospital the highest incidence of mandibular necrosis occurred in those patients having dental extractions immediately prior to radiotherapy. Improvements in dental management of patients receiving radiotherapy is now tending to reduce the difference in incidence of necrosis between dentate and edentulous patients.

Infection

Infection can gain entry to the bone via traumatic injuries, tooth extractions, pulpal infection or periodontal infection. It acts as a mitotic stimulus and thereby precipitates necrosis. The infection can then spread diffusely through the bone. Radionecrotic ulceration of the overlying mucosa allows entry of infection to the bone. Bragg et al.[49] stated that clinical radiation necrosis of the mandible was associated with open mucosal wounds in most cases. In some cases the mucosal necrosis is the precipitating factor, and in others the mucosal necrosis is secondary to necrosis of the underlying bone.

Tumour involvement of bone

Invading tumour suppresses osteoblastic remodelling,[50] but if the malignant cells are killed by treatment the bone will attempt to regenerate so that mitotic death of osteoblasts occurs. Consequently, successful treatment by radiotherapy of a carcinoma invading the bone is almost inevitably followed by osteoradionecrosis.

General condition of the patient

Many patients with mouth cancer are alcoholic and in poor general condition. In these patients poor nutritional status and lack of oral hygiene make them particularly prone to mucosal ulceration and consequent osteoradionecrosis.

Diagnosis

If a segment of mandible undergoes necrosis, the process starts on the alveolar margin and is accompanied by ulceration of the alveolar mucosa. This gives a characteristic appearance of a flat ulcer with the brownish-looking dead bone at its base. Pain is not normally a feature of osteoradionecrosis *per se*, and even a pathological fracture due to this cause may be completely painless. However, the necrosis is often complicated by secondary infection, in which case there may be severe pain with trismus,

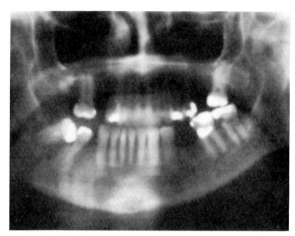

Fig. 8.7 Osteoradionecrosis of the right side of the mandible, 3 years after high dose external radiotherapy to an adenoid cystic carcinoma of the submandibular salivary gland. A painless pathological fracture has occurred at the site of the necrosis.

foetor and general ill health. The characteristic X-ray appearances are shown in Fig. 8.7. As in the case of soft tissue necrosis, bone necrosis must be distinguished from tumour recurrence.

Treatment

A conservative approach should be adopted. Meticulous oral hygiene is essential, including the use of 0.01 per cent chlorhexidine mouthwash after every meal. Loss of the mucosa usually results in a cavity in the gum over the necrotic bone; this cavity should be regularly irrigated to dislodge any food debris and necrotic tissue. The patient should be instructed to do this himself or herself wherever possible. It is unimportant what solution is used for irrigation as it is the mechanical removal of debris that is important; possibly hydrogen peroxide or chlorhexidine solution may help to destroy anaerobic organisms.

Sequestra should be allowed to separate spontaneously. Any surgical interference only encourages extension of the necrotic process. When a sequestrum becomes loose, it should be removed gently and any sharp edges or spicules of bone smoothed off with bone rongeurs to prevent irritation of the tongue. Osteoblastic activity and re-absorption of non-vital bone may take many months or even years, because of the relatively avascular nature of irradiated bone. Therefore, great patience is required to resist the temptation to intervene surgically, even when a pathological fracture occurs.

Pain, when present, usually indicates secondary infection. Attempts should be made to control the infection by the local measures outlined above and administration of systemic antibiotics. Antibiotics are not very effective because of the avascularity of the tissues, so prolonged treatment is necessary. The tetracyclines are the most useful antibiotics because of their selective bone uptake; a dosage of 250 mg four times a day for 10 days is recommended, followed by 250 mg twice daily continued for several months. Metronidazole, 200 mg three times a day, should be added in cases of severe infection in an attempt to combat anaerobic organisms. There are advocates of long term low dose tetracycline for all cases of osteoradionecrosis, but the value of this is difficult to assess because healing is always slow with or without treatment and no controlled study has been done.

Hyperbaric oxygen therapy has been shown to promote healing. Ketchum *et al.*[51] showed in animal studies that hyperbaric oxygen promoted rapid revascularisation and increased both osteoblastic and osteoclastic activity. Hart and Mainous[52] reported a series of 46 patients with osteoradionecrosis of the mandible treated with hyperbaric oxygen. They put their patients into a hyperbaric chamber at 2 atmospheres pressure for 2 hours per day for 60 days, i.e. a total of 120 hours in the chamber. Daily irrigation and long term tetracycline were also employed. Of the 46 patients 37 became symptom free after one course of treatment, with complete soft tissue healing intra-orally. A further five healed after a second course. The remaing four patients required bone grafts to restore mandibular continuity – all were successful. This method of treatment is undoubtedly effective, but is cumbersome and time-consuming for both patients and hospital staff, and there are risks in subjecting patients with cardiovascular or respiratory disease to raised pressures. Consequently, hyperbaric oxygen cannot be recommended for routine use, but may have a place for the younger, fitter patient treated in a centre where the resources are available.

A simpler method which has been claimed to promote cell growth is ultrasound. Harris[53] recommends therapeutic ultrasound at a frequency of 3 mHz pulsed one in four at an intensity of 1 W/cm^2 applied to the mandible for 10 mins daily for 50 days.

Spontaneous healing occurs in about 50 per cent

of cases using the conservative measures described. Failure of healing may be due to excessive radiation dosage, uncontrollable infection or the presence of persistent tumour. In those cases where there is no improvement after a few months of conservative therapy, surgical treatment must be undertaken.

Surgical treatment

The key to successful surgical management is the introduction of new vascularised soft tissue to cover the irradiated bone. The problem arises in deciding how much of the necrotic bone to resect. When surgery becomes inevitable, i.e. for persistent severe pain in an area of osteoradionecrosis which has failed to respond to other measures, the necrotic bone must be trimmed back until all obviously infected tissue is removed. The overlying soft tissue is then resected until viable non-friable margins are seen. A muscle flap is then raised and brought into the area to cover all exposed bone. Temporalis, trapezius, pectoralis major and latissimus dorsi flaps are all suitable, the choice being based on the size of the defect and any previous surgical intervention. Theoretically, all bone within the high dose irradiated volume should be resected so that the bone margins are well vascularised. However, in some cases this would lead to massive defects, and in practice may not be necessary.

In most circumstances, it is better to avoid bone grafting even when a pathological fracture is present. If bone reconstruction is essential, then conventional bone grafting techniques combined with a course of hyperbaric oxygen pre- and postoperatively give the most reliable results.[54] Vascularised free flaps are rarely indicated in these circumstances as suitable recipient vessels are not usually available in the heavily irradiated patient.

Dental care of patients receiving radiotherapy

The teeth of a patient treated by radiotherapy for oral cancer are at risk both from the direct effect of radiation and from the secondary effects of xerostomia. Teeth receiving a high dose of radiation suffer killing of odontoblasts and atrophy of the pulp, but these changes in themselves are unlikely to contribute to decay. Salivary changes as described above are a more potent factor provoking caries. The reduction in volume and increased viscosity of the saliva after radiotherapy encourages bacterial growth. Frank *et al.*[55] showed that in patients receiving irradiation for carcinoma of the oral cavity, only those in whom the salivary glands had been irradiated developed rampant caries. The caries developed whether or not the teeth had also been within the fields of irradiation.

Taste loss and difficulty with mastication lead many patients to turn to a semi solid high carbohydrate diet. There is consequent food stagnation and accumulation of dental plaque. A further factor may be the reduction in pH of the saliva; this encourages enzymatic action by bacteria producing pyruvic and lactic acids from carbohydrate, which are active in destruction of enamel. The caries rate after irradiation is far more rapid than that of ordinary caries in the unirradiated mouth, and the entire dentition may be destroyed within 1 or 2 years unless special care is taken of the teeth. The radiation caries are characteristically marginal in type (Fig. 8.8).

To prevent radiation caries in patients who have had radiotherapy to the oral cavity or salivary glands, meticulous dental hygiene and dental supervision are essential.

Teeth not in irradiated volume

Teeth outside the radiation fields are at risk of caries, secondary to xerostomia. The following measures help to minimise the risk of caries formation.

Mouthwashes

A dilute solution of chlorhexidine gluconate used as a mouthwash is an effective antibacterial agent which inhibits the formation of dental plaque, an essential precursor of both caries and gingival inflammation. It is available commercially as a 0.2 w/v solution, which requires dilution as at this concentration it is quite irritant. The patient should be instructed to rinse the mouth for 1 min, timed by a watch, with 5 ml of the solution in 100 ml of water after every meal and before retiring at night. This regimen should be continued indefinitely following radiotherapy.

Topical fluoride applications

Local application of a fluoride reduces the incidence of caries. For example, in children, a sodium fluoride mouthwash was shown by Brandt *et al.*[56] to reduce caries by 37 per cent. In the postirradiation patient, fluoride must be applied to the whole surface of all teeth to have a protective effect. In order to apply fluoride to the teeth, custom built carriers

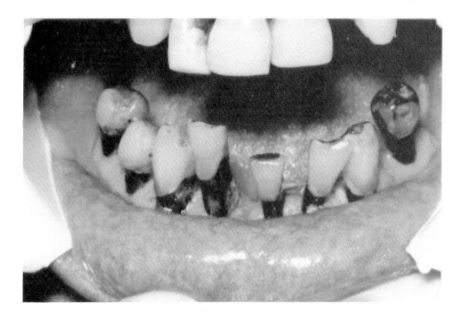

Fig. 8.8 Postradiotherapy caries.

are made for each patient. The patient is provided with a viscose gel containing 1 per cent sodium fluoride in a squeezy bottle and is instructed to put 10 drops of gel into the carriers and apply to the teeth for 5 mins per day, as described by Daly.[57] A controlled trial of this method was reported by Daly *et al.*[58] Patients were randomised to receive topical applications of fluoride. Caries developed in 47 out of 69 control patients, but in only 20 of 65 patients given fluoride, a highly significant difference. Possibly, a daily fluoride mouthwash can give similar protection, but no controlled studies have been done.

Acrylic splints

Coffin[59] advocated covering the teeth with acrylic splints during radiotherapy and for 2 years afterwards, thereby protecting the teeth from the unfavourable intra-oral environment. This appears to be an effective method of preventing radiation caries, but no controlled studies have been carried out; it is probably no more effective than fluoride application, but is considerably more inconvenient.

Saliva substitute

Saliva substitutes as described above help to keep the mouth moist, raise the pH and also protect the teeth. Shannon *et al.*[60] found that their saliva substitute would produce remineralisation of enamel in extracted teeth *in vitro* provided calcium phosphate and fluoride were present in the solution.

Teeth within irradiated volume

Care of teeth that have received a high dose of irradiation is aimed at prevention of osteoradionecrosis. Formerly, it was standard practice to extract all teeth which were likely to be within the high dose irradiated volume prior to starting radiotherapy, because it was thought that such teeth would inevitably decay and that extraction subsequent to radiotherapy was more likely to precipitate necrosis than extraction prior to radiotherapy. This policy was advocated by many authors,[61,62] but others have indicated the risk of irradiating a mandible shortly after extraction.[63,64]

It is now generally accepted that loss of teeth in the high dose irradiation volume is by no means inevitable, and that the incidence of bone necrosis is lowest if extraction can be avoided altogether. The only teeth that need to be extracted before radiotherapy are any that are not vital, needing root filling or elaborate restorative techniques, or which are associated with active periodontal disease. Extractions of these teeth should be performed atraumatically and the gums sutured to promote rapid healing. All other teeth should be cleaned and restored before radiotherapy begins.

Subsequent to radiotherapy, the teeth should be cared for as described above. If extractions of teeth in the high dose irradiated volume become necessary, these should be performed atraumatically under general anaesthesia with antibiotic cover. The authors prescribe tetracycline 250 mg four times daily for 10 days prior to extraction. At the time of extraction, metronidazole is added and both antibiotics are continued until the socket is epithelialised.

References

1 Coutard J. Roentgen therapy of epitheliomas of the tonsillar region, hypopharynx and larynx from 1926. *American Journal of Roentgenology* 1932; **25**: 313–18.
2 Paterson R. Studies in optimum dosage. *British Journal of Radiology* 1952; **25**: 505–16.
3 Thomlinson RH. Oxygen therapy – biological considerations. In: Deeley TJ ed. *Modern Trends in Radiotherapy*. London: Butterworths, 1967.
4 Churchill-Davidson, I. Oxygen therapy – clinical experiences. In: Deeley TJ ed. *Modern Trends in Radiotherapy*. London: Butterworths, 1967.
5 Henk JM, Smith CW. Radiotherapy and hyperbaric oxygen in head and neck cancer. Interim report of the second clinical trial. *Lancet* 1977; **ii**: 104–5.
6 Berry GH, Dixon B, Ward AJ. The Leeds results for radiotherapy in HBO for carcinoma of the head and neck. *Clinical Radiology* 1979; **30**: 591–2.
7 Fazekas J, Pajak TF, Wasserman T *et al*. Failure of misonidazole-sensitized radiotherapy to impact upon outcome among stage III–IV squamous carcinoma of the head and neck. *International Journal of Radiation Oncology, Biology, Physics* 1987; **13**: 1155–60.
8 MRC Working Party on Misonidazole in Head and Neck Cancer. A study of the effect of misonidazole in conjunction with radiotherapy for the treatment of head and neck cancer. *British Journal of Radiology* 1984; **57**: 585–95.
9 Overgaard J, Sand Hansen H, Lindelor B *et al*. Nimorazole as a hypoxic radiosensitizer in the treatment of supraglottic larynx and pharnyx carcinoma. *Radiotherapy and Oncology* 1991; **suppl. 20**: 143–9.
10 Cohen L. Absence of a demonstrable gain factor for neutron beam therapy of epidermoid carcinoma of the head and neck. *International Journal of Radiation Oncology, Biology, Physics* 1982; **8**: 2173–6.
11 MacDougall RH, Orr JA, Kerr GR, Duncan W. Fast neutron treatment for squamous cell carcinoma of the head and neck: final report of Edinburgh Randomised Trial. *British Medical Journal* 1990; **301**: 1241–2.
12 Wells G, Koh W, Pelton J *et al*. Fast neutron teletherapy in advanced epidermoid head and neck cancer: a review. *American Journal of Clinical Oncology* 1989; **12**: 293–300.
13 Griffin TW, Pajak TF, Laramore GE *et al*. Neutron vs photon irradiation of inoperable salivary gland tumours. *International Journal of Radiation Oncology, Biology, Physics* 1989; **15**: 1085–90.
14 Parsons JT, Mendenhall WM, Cassisi NJ *et al*. Hy-
perfractionation for head and neck cancer. *International Journal of Radiation Oncology, Biology, Physics* 1988; **14**: 649–58.
15 Wang CC, Blitzer PH, Suit HD. Twice-a-day radiation therapy for cancer of the head and neck. *Cancer* 1985; **55**: 2100–4.
16 Horiot JC, le Fur T, N'Guyen C *et al*. Hyperfractionation compared with conventional radiotherapy in oropharyngeal carcinoma. *European Journal of Cancer* 1990; **26**: 779–80.
17 Wilson GD, McNally NJ, Dische S *et al*. Measurement of cell kinetics in human tumours *in vivo* using bromodeoxyuridine incorporation and flow cytometry. *British Journal of Cancer* 1988; **58**: 423–31.
18 Withers HR, Taylor JMG, Maciejewski B. The hazard of accelerated tumour clonogen repopulation during radiotherapy. *Acta Oncologica* 1988; **27**: 131–46.
19 Barton MB, Keane TJ, Gadalla T, Marks E. The effect of treatment time and treatment interruption on tumour control in the radical radiotherapy of laryngeal cancer. *Radiotherapy and Oncology* 1992; **23**: 137–43.
20 Maciejewski B, Withers HR, Taylor JMG *et al*. Dose fractionation and regeneration in radiotherapy for cancer of the oral cavity and oropharynx; tumour dose-response and repopulation. *International Journal of Radiation Oncology, Biology, Physics* 1989; **16**: 831–43.
21 Dische S, Saunders MI. The rationale for continuous hyperfractionated accelerated radiation therapy. *International Journal of Radiation Oncology, Biology, Physics* 1990; **14**: 649–58.
22 Paine CH. Modern after-loading methods for interstitial radiotherapy. *Clinical Radiology* 1972; **23**: 262–73.
23 Pierquin B, Chassagne D, Cachin Y, Baillet F, Fournell le Bois F. Carcinomes epidermoides de la langue mobile et du plancher buccal. *Acta Radiologica* 1970; **9**: 465–80.
24 Dearnaley DP, Dardoufas C, A'Hern RP, Henk JM. Interstitial irradiation for carcinoma of the tongue and floor of mouth; Royal Marsden experience (1970–1986). *Radiotherapy and Oncology* 1991; **21**: 183–92.
25 Mazeron JJ, Simm JM, Le Pechoux C *et al*. Effect of dose rate on local control and complications in definitive irradiation of T1–2. Squamous cell carcinoma of mobile tongue and floor of mouth with interstitial iridium-192. *Radiotherapy and Oncology* 1991; **21**: 39–47.
26 Mendenhall WM, van Gise WS, Bova FJ, Million RR. Analysis of time-dose factors in squamous cell carcinoma of the oral tongue and floor of mouth treated with radiation therapy alone. *International Journal of Radiation Oncology, Biology, Physics* 1981; **7**: 1005–11.
27 Chu A, Fletcher GH. Incidence and causes of failures

to control by irradiation the primary lesions in squamous cell carcinomas of the anterior two-thirds of the tongue and floor of mouth. *American Journal of Roentgenology* 1973; **117**: 502–8.

28 Wallner PE, Hanks GE, Kramer S, McLean CT. Patterns of care study: analysis of outcome survey data – anterior two-thirds of tongue and floor of mouth. *American Journal of Clinical Oncology* 1986; **9**: 50–7.

29 Pierquin B, Chassagne D, Baillet F, Castro JR. The place of implantation in tongue and floor of mouth cancer. *Journal of the American Medical Association* 1971; **215**: 961–3.

30 Hall EJ, Lam YM. Renaissance of interstitial brachytherapy. In: Vaeth JM ed. *Frontiers of Radiation Therapy and Oncology*, Volume 12. Basel: Karger, 1978.

31 Sobel S, Rubin P. Tumour persistence as a predictor of outcome after radiation therapy of head and neck cancers. *International Journal of Radiation Oncology, Biology, Physics* 1976; **1**: 873–7.

32 Suit HD, Lindberg R, Fletcher GH. Prognostic significance of extent of tumour regression at completion of radiation therapy. *Radiology* 1965; **84**: 1100–7.

33 Powers WE, Palmer LA. Biologic basis of preoperative radiation treatment. *American Journal of Roentgenology* 1968; **102**: 176–92.

34 Terz JM, King ER, Lawrence W. Pre-operative irradiation for head and neck cancer: results of a prospective study. *Surgery* 1981; **89**: 449–53.

35 Strong EW. Pre-operative radiation and radical neck dissection. *Surgical Clinics of North America* 1969; **49**: 271–6.

36 Perez CA, Olsen J. Preoperative vs. postoperative irradiation comparison in an experimental animal tumour system. *American Journal of Roentgenology* 1970; **108**: 396–404.

37 Cachin Y, Eschwege F. Combination of radiotherapy and surgery in the treatment of head and neck cancers. *Cancer Treatment Reviews* 1975; **2**: 177–91.

38 Vikram B, Strong EW, Shah J, Spiro RH. Elective post-operative radiation therapy in stages III and IV epidermoid carcinoma of the head and neck. *American Journal of Surgery* 1980; **140**: 580–4.

39 Vikram B. Post-operative irradiation for squamous cell carcinoma of the head and neck. *International Journal of Radiation Oncology, Biology, Physics* 1990; **18**: 267.

40 Tupchong L, Scott CB, Blitzer PH *et al.* Randomized study of pre-operative vs. post-operative radiation therapy in advanced head and neck carcinoma: long term follow-up of RTOG study 73–03. *International Journal of Radiation Oncology, Biology, Physics* 1990; **20**: 21–8.

41 Conger AD. Loss and recovery of taste acuity in patients irradiated to the oral cavity. *Radiation Research* 1973; **53**: 338–47.

42 Mossman KL, Henkin RI. Radiation-induced changes in taste acuity in cancer patients. *International Journal of Radiation Oncology, Biology, Physics* 1978; **4**: 663–70.

43 Mira JG, Westcott WB, Starcke EN, Shannon IL. Some factors influencing salivary function when treating with radiotherapy. *International Journal of Radiation Oncology, Biology, Physics* 1981; **7**: 535–41.

44 Shannon IL, McGrary BR, Starcke EN. A saliva substitute for use by xerostomic patients undergoing radiotherapy to the head and neck. *Oral Surgery* 1977; **44**: 656–61.

45 Watson WL, Scarborough JE. Osteoradionecrosis in intra oral cancer. *American Journal of Roentgenology* 1938; **40**: 524–8.

46 Bedwinek JM, Shukovsky LJ, Fletcher GH, Daly TE. Osteonecrosis in patients treated with definitive radiotherapy for squamous cell carcinomas of the oral cavity and naso and oropharynx. *Radiology* 1976; **119**: 665–7.

47 Murray CG, Herson J, Daly TE, Zimmerman S. Radiation necrosis of the mandible: a 10-year study. Part 1, factors influencing the onset of necrosis. *International Journal of Radiation Oncology, Biology, Physics* 1980; **6**: 543–8.

48 Hinds EC. Dental care and oral hygiene before and after treatment. *Journal of the American Medical Association* 1971; **215**: 964–6.

49 Bragg DG, Shidnia H, Chu F, Higinbotham NL. Clinical and radiographic aspects of radiation osteitis. *Radiology* 1970; **97**: 103–11.

50 Carter RL, Pitnam MR. Squamous carcinoma of the head and neck: some patterns of spread. *Journal of the Royal Society of Medicine* 1980; **73**: 420–7.

51 Ketchum SA, Thomas AM, Hall AD. Angiographic studies of the effect of hyperbaric oxygen on burn wound vascularization. In: Wada J, Ina T eds. *Proceedings of the 4th International Congress on Hyperbaric Medicine*. Baltimore, MD: Williams & Wilkins, 1970: 388.

52 Hart GB, Mainous EG. The treatment of radiation necrosis with hyperbaric oxygen. *Cancer* 1976; **37**: 2580–5.

53 Harris M. The conservative management of osteoradionecrosis of the mandible with ultrasound therapy. *British Journal of Oral and Maxillofacial Surgery* 1992; **30**: 313–18.

54 Marx RE, Ames JR. The use of hyperbaric oxygen therapy in bony reconstruction of the irradiated and tissue-deficient patient. *Journal of Oral and Maxillofacial Surgery* 1982; **40**: 412–20.

55 Frank RM, Herdley J, Philippe E. Acquired dental defects and salivary gland lesions after irradiation for carcinoma. *Journal of the American Dental Association* 1965; **70**: 868–83.

56 Brandt RS, Slack GL, Walter DF. The effect of sodium fluoride mouthwash on caries incidence in British school children – a two year study. *Proceedings of the British Paediatric Society* 1972; **2**: 23.

57 Daly TE. Dental care in the irradiated patient. In: Fletcher GH ed. *Textbook of Radiotherapy*. Philadelphia, PA; Lea and Febiger, 1980: 299.

58 Daly TE, Drane JB, MacComb WS. Management of problems of the teeth and jaws in patients undergoing irradiation. *American Journal of Surgery* 1972; **124:** 539–42.

59 Coffin F. The control of radiation caries. *British Journal of Radiology* 1973; **46:** 365–8.

60 Shannon IL, Trodahl JN, Starcke EN. Remineralisation of enamel by a saliva substitute designed for use by irradiated patients. *Cancer* 1978; **41:** 1746–50.

61 Moss WT. *Therapeutic Radiology*. St Louis, MO: CV Mosby, 1959.

62 Vermund H, Rappaport I, Nethery W. Role of radiotherapy in the treatment of oral cancer. *Journal of Oral Surgery* 1974; **32:** 690–5.

63 Wildermuth O, Cantril ST. Radiation necrosis of the mandible. *Radiology* 1953; **61:** 771–85.

64 Carl W, Schaaf N, Sako K. Oral surgery and the patient who has radiation therapy for head and neck cancer. *Oral Surgery* 1973; **36:** 651–9.

9 Medical treatment of malignant tumours of the mouth, jaw and salivary glands

AL Jones and ME Gore

Cytotoxic chemotherapy

Over the last decade the potential role of chemotherapy in head and neck malignancy has been extensively investigated. Initially studies focused on patients with locally advanced or metastatic disease to establish which cytotoxic drugs had activity. Few, if any, of these patients were cured by chemotherapy, and there is now increasing interest in the use of chemotherapy as adjuvant therapy to eradicate micrometastatic disease and as induction or 'neo-adjuvant' therapy before surgery to achieve maximum tumour shrinkage thus allowing organ preservation, and to facilitate local treatment with surgery and radiotherapy in an attempt to improve disease-free survival.

In this chapter we have reviewed randomised trials of chemotherapy in patients with squamous cell carcinomas of the head and neck region and where possible comment specifically on the implications for tumours arising in the oral cavity, jaw and salivary glands. Unrandomised Phase II trials are only discussed in the context of developing new regimens that warrant evaluation in comparative studies.

Chemotherapy in advanced disease

Approximately 20 per cent of patients with squamous cell carcinoma of the head and neck develop metastatic disease. Less than 10 per cent of these patients are alive 2 years after development of metastases and there is no evidence that chemotherapy improves survival. Indeed, response rates average 25–40 per cent with median response duration of 4–6 months and median survival of 6–10 months. The main aim of chemotherapy in patients with recurrent or metastatic squamous cell carcinoma of the oral cavity therefore is the palliation of disease-related symptoms. Fit patients with advanced disease may be eligible for Phase II trials of new cytotoxic drugs which, if active and with a response rate ≥ 20 per cent, could warrant further evaluation in combination regimens.

Single agent chemotherapy

A number of drugs have single agent activity in squamous cell carcinoma of the head and neck. These include methotrexate, cisplatin, 5-fluorouracil (5-FU) and vincristine. The response rates to these drugs alone or in combination regimens in randomised trials is shown in Table 9.1. There is wide variation in the doses and scheduling of most drugs, but overall responses are usually partial and of short duration (4–6 months). Complete responses are rare and there are no cures in advanced disease.[5] In most patients with advanced disease response is defined by clinical and radiological assessment but it is uncommon for investigators to assess true histological response although cancers of the oral cavity are often accessible for repeat biopsy. This may be of interest in a research setting but would have little relevance outside clinical trials. The achievement of a partial response (≥ 50 per cent reduction in tumour volume) is of little consequence in terms of survival but is important to identify active drugs that may be associated with useful palliation. Even patients who have a minor reduction (< 50 per cent) in tumour volume which does not amount to a partial response may have relief of disease-related symptoms such as pain and dysphagia.[7] Once maximum response has been reached chemotherapy should be discontinued as there is no evidence that maintenance treatment

Table 9.1 Chemotherapy for advanced/recurrent squamous carcinoma of the head and neck

Treatment	No. of points	Response (%) CR (PR)		Reference
Methotrexate	21	6 (28)	No	Hong and
Cisplatin	23	6 (26)	significant difference	Bromer[1]
Methotrexate	50	8 (16)	No	Grose et al.[2]
Cisplatin	50	4 (12)	significant difference	
Methotrexate (high dose) (leucovorin)	19	6 (29)	No significant	Taylor et al.[3]
Methotrexate (low dose)	18	4 (32)	difference	
Cisplatin (high dose)	31	5 (16)	No	Veronesi et al.[4]
Cisplatin (low dose)	28	5 (18)	significant difference	
Cisplatin Bleomycin Cisplatin + Bleomycin Symptomatic care only				Morton and Stell[5]
Cisplatin + Methotrexate + Bleomycin + Vincristine		(50)	$P = 0.003$	Clavel et al.[6]
Methotrexate + Bleomycin + Vincristine		(28)		
Methotrexate	83	29 (35)		Vogl et al.[7]
Cisplatin + Bleomycin + Methotrexate	80	38 (48)	$P < 0.05$	
Cisplatin + 5-FU (infusion)	18	13 (72)	$P < 0.05$	Kish et al.[8]
Cisplatin + 5-FU (bolus)	20	4 (20)		
Cisplatin	50	14 (28)	No	Liverpool
Methotrexate	50	6 (12)	significant	Head and
Cisplatin + 5-FU	50	12 (24)	difference	Neck
Cisplatin + Methotrexate	50	11 (22)		Oncology Group[9]
Cisplatin + 5-FU	87	28 (32)	$P < 0.01$ (vs Methotrexate)	Forestiere et al.[10]
Carboplatin + 5-FU	86	18 (21)	$P = 0.05$ (vs Methotrexate)	
Methotrexate	88	9 (10)		

5-FU, 5-Fluorouracil.

will prolong remission and indeed patients may experience cumulative toxicity. In practice most patients receive 3–4 cycles of chemotherapy and it is rare to exceed 6 cycles.

Methotrexate is the most commonly used drug and can be safely administered by weekly intravenous injection at doses of 40–60 mg/m^2 in the outpatient setting.[11,12] The response rates with methotrexate varied between 8 per cent and 50 per cent in different series and average approximately 30 per cent. Methotrexate is used as the 'gold standard' against which the efficacy of other drugs used as single agents can be assessed. Dose escalations of methotrexate have not been associated with any consistent increase in response rates and may result in increased mucosal toxicity.[3,13] This complication can be a major problem in this patient population because of previous treatment, e.g. radiotherapy to the oral cavity, and the use of folinic acid rescue 24 hours after methotrexate may not completely avoid mucosal toxicity. In one comparative study the response rate for standard dose methotrexate with folinic acid was 17 per cent compared with 37 per cent for methotrexate + placebo, but there was a significant increase in toxicity in those patients receiving methotrexate without folinic acid.[14]

Cisplatin, 80–120 mg/m^2, also achieved response rates of approximately 30 per cent in Phase II trials.[15,16] In one controlled trial there was superior survival for those patients treated with cisplatin compared with an untreated control group who received symptomatic care.[17] It is important to note that 30 per cent of patients were not fit enough for treatment in this trial and this would bias the results in favour of cisplatin. In randomised trials cisplatin has similar response rates and duration of response as methotrexate; however, toxicity is higher with cisplatin.[1,2] In a four arm randomised study comparing single agent methotrexate, single agent cisplatin, cisplatin–methotrexate combinations and cisplatin–fluorouracil combinations, the response rates were similar for cisplatin (14 per cent), cisplatin + methotrexate (11 per cent) and methotrexate (6 per cent) but there was a survival benefit for cisplatin-containing chemotherapy at 6 months (52 per cent) compared with single agent methotrexate (31 per cent).[9] Non-comparative studies have suggested a dose–response relation for cisplatin but this has not been confirmed in randomised trials and cisplatin should be given in standard doses of 60–120 mg/m^2.[4] Carboplatin, which has a better side effect profile than cisplatin with reduced incidence of emesis and neuropathy, has been evaluated in a Phase II trial with a response rate of 24 per cent[18] but direct comparisons of cisplatin and carboplatin have not yet been reported either as single agents or as part of combination regimens.

The activity of 5-FU appears to be schedule dependent rather than dose dependent. The response rates are low with bolus administration but significant activity has been obtained using infusion.[19]

When used in combination with cisplatin a 4 day infusion of 1000 mg/m^2 5-FU gave a higher response rate (72 per cent; complete response (CR), 22 per cent) than bolus 600 mg/m^2 5-FU (20 per cent; CR, 10 per cent) on days 1 and 8.[8]

Combination chemotherapy

The aim of combination chemotherapy using two or three cytotoxic drugs is to develop regimens with a higher complete response rate which in turn may affect survival. There have been many small non-comparative studies in single institutions suggesting that a higher overall response rate is achieved with combination chemotherapy, but the number of randomised studies is limited. The response rates to combination chemotherapy regimens in advanced trials is shown in Table 9.1.

Several comparative studies have shown higher response rates with combination chemotherapy compared with single agent treatment, in particular for cisplatin-containing regimens compared with non-cisplatin based chemotherapy.[6,7,17,20,21] In these studies the complete response rate was also higher in those patients receiving a cisplatin-containing regimen. This apparent improvement in response rate has not resulted in improved duration of response or median survival and there may be some increase in toxicity.

Results of a Phase II study of cisplatin with a 96 hour infusion of 5-FU were reported in 1984.[22] There was an overall response rate of 70 per cent, with a complete response rate of 27 per cent in patients with recurrent and/or metastatic disease. The importance of infusional 5-FU in this regimen was confirmed in a randomised trial in which cisplatin + 5-FU infusion had a higher response rate (72 per cent; CR, 22 per cent) than cisplatin + 5-FU bolus (20 per cent; CR, 10 per cent).[8] Since then this combination has been extensively investigated in non-randomised studies: overall response rates have varied between 11 per cent and 79 per cent with 0 per cent to 27 per cent of patients achieving CR.[23] The difference in response rates may reflect different pretreatment prognostic factors, variations in drug scheduling and the inclusion of patients with locally advanced disease receiving neo-adjuvant chemotherapy. This emphasises the need for controlled trials. Many now consider the combination of cisplatin and 5-FU as the standard treatment for squamous cell carcinoma of the head and neck.

The combination of cisplatin and 5-FU has been shown to have a higher response rate than single agent methotrexate in two trials.[9,10] The combination has also been compared with single agent cisplatin and 5-FU separately.[24] In this study cisplatin + 5-FU had a higher overall response rate (32 per cent) than cisplatin alone (17 per cent) or 5-FU alone (13 per cent) ($P = 0.035$). Toxicity was higher with combination treatment and the median time to progression was similar for all three groups (range, 1.7–2.4 months), although this small difference does represent a statistically significant improvement in response duration for patients receiving combination treatment. There was no overall survival difference between the three treatment groups in this trial. The Southwest Oncology Group[10] compared cisplatin + 5-FU, carboplatin + 5-FU and single agent methotrexate; there was an increased response rate for each of the combination regimens (cisplatin + 5-FU, 32 per cent; carboplatin + 5-FU, 21 per cent) compared with methotrexate. There was no improvement in overall survival and there was increased toxicity for the combination arms. The trial was not designed for direct comparison between cisplatin + 5-FU and carboplatin + 5-FU but as two randomised Phase II trials with a shared control arm (methotrexate). The sample size was not sufficient to detect any differences between the platinum containing arms.

Outside the research setting single agent methotrexate, cisplatin or infusional 5-FU, or the combination of cisplatin + infusional 5-FU, all provide a reasonable chance of palliation and can be regarded as standard treatment. Only combination chemotherapy has reproducibly produced complete responses and is probably the treatment of choice for fit patients whose performance status suggests they can tolerate the higher level of toxicity. Unfortunately only approximately 10 per cent of patients with squamous cell carcinomas of the head and neck are currently entered into clinical trials,[25] and further advances in the management of these cancers will only occur if participation in randomised trials is increased so that questions of response, survival and quality of life can be properly addressed.

Factors affecting response to chemotherapy

It is still questionable whether the choice of chemotherapy regimen has any effect on survival in squamous cell carcinoma of the head and neck. However there are a number of patient- and dis-

Table 9.2 Prognostic factors affecting response to chemotherapy in recurrent/metastatic disease

Favourable	*Unfavourable*
Performance status 0–2	Performance status 3–4
Small volume disease	Bulky disease
Local disease	Metastatic spread
No bone erosion	Bone erosion
Long disease-free interval	Short disease-free interval
Previous complete response to chemotherapy	Poor response to chemotherapy
Previous complete response to radiotherapy	Poor response to radiotherapy

ease-related factors that may influence response to chemotherapy both in patients with recurrent disease and in the neo-adjuvant setting (Table 9.2).

The majority of patients with malignancy of the oral cavity are aged greater than 50 years and may have concurrent medical problems such as ischaemic heart disease, liver disease and obstructive airway disease, conditions themselves related to alcohol and tobacco abuse which are major aetiological factors for oral cavity cancer.[26] Patients may therefore have a poor pretreatment performance status which is an important determinant in response to chemotherapy and survival.[24,27]

Many tumour-related factors used to predict response to chemotherapy have been derived empirically from clinical observations in patients undergoing radiotherapy and surgery.

Patients with bulky disease and/or distant metastases have an inferior response rate to patients with small volume disease.[28] Bone and skin involvement are features associated with particularly poor response rates and short overall survival. In the adjuvant or neo-adjuvant setting the presence of involved regional lymph nodes is an adverse prognostic factor. For patients with advanced or metastatic disease there is no evidence that oral cavity carcinoma has any different chance of response to chemotherapy from other primary sites within the head and neck region. The influence of previous treatment such as radiotherapy is important in assessment of toxicity, as patients with oral cavity malignancy are more likely to have mucositis, dysphagia and xerostomia if the salivary glands have been irradiated. Patients who fail chemotherapy are extremely unlikely to respond to a second line regimen, hence drugs that are expected to have clinical activity in squamous cell carcinoma on the basis of preclinical data and Phase I trials should be evaluated in Phase II trials.

Although these clinical observations may have some relevance in predicting response there is marked variation in response rates and survival for a given tumour stage and a more rigorous definition of prognostic subgroups may be useful to design trials and compare treatment results.[29] Some investigators have reported that patients with poorly differentiated tumours have a higher response rate.[24] The histological grade of malignancy, DNA ploidy and nuclear DNA index predict for relapse and disease-free survival, with a poorer response rate in aneuploid compared with diploid tumours. The importance of immunological factors in the prediction of response to chemotherapy is also being investigated.

Chemotherapy combined with radical local treatment

Chemotherapy maybe used in conjunction with radical local treatment by surgery with or without radiotherapy, in an attempt to improve local control rates, decrease metastases, and thereby improve survival.

Chemotherapy may be combined with radical local treatment in one of three ways:

(1) *Adjuvant* chemotherapy, i.e. chemotherapy given after the local treatment. The aim of adjuvant chemotherapy is to sterilise a possible small population of residual cancer cells at the primary site or in the neck, and also to eliminate micrometastases. Autopsy studies indicate that micrometastatic dissemination, especially in lung and liver, is much higher than the 20 per cent incidence of overt metastases.[30]

(2) *Neo-adjuvant* or *induction* chemotherapy is given before local treatment. The aim is to reduce the bulk of the disease, thereby either increasing the chance of radiotherapy success or facilitating surgery.

(3) *Concomitant* or *simultaneous* chemotherapy is given at the same time as radiotherapy with the objective of increasing the chance of a radiotherapy cure.

Many studies of combined treatment involving chemotherapy have been reported, but have many drawbacks. They mostly involve patients with very advanced disease and a poor prognosis; however, patients are able to tolerate chemotherapy better at an early stage of the disease, so a benefit may be more easily demonstrated in less advanced stage disease. In most studies the number of patients is insufficient to detect any statistically significant benefit. In an overview of 23 trials, Stell and Rawson[31] concluded that the numbers of patients in individual trials might at best detect a median increase in survival of 25 per cent (range, 11–51 per cent) but were not large enough to detect the 5 per cent improvement in survival that might be expected with chemotherapy. Moreover, selection criteria for the entry of patients into trials was not clearly defined and the toxicity of chemotherapy was rarely reported according to accepted criteria. In many studies patients were unable to tolerate the prescribed treatment, so compliance with protocols was low, resulting in a rather low actual dose intensity of drugs delivered.

Adjuvant chemotherapy

The largest controlled trial of adjuvant chemotherapy was the Head and Neck Intergroup Study. Four hundred and forty-six patients were randomised to surgery and radiotherapy or to surgery followed by adjuvant chemotherapy (cisplatin + 5-FU) and radiotherapy. There was a significant reduction in distant metastases in the patients receiving chemotherapy (15 per cent) compared with the no chemotherapy group (23 per cent; $P = 0.03$).[32] There was no significant difference in disease-free survival (46 versus 38 per cent) or 4 year actuarial survival.

Other randomised studies have also suggested that adjuvant therapy may reduce locoregional recurrence in patients at high risk of local relapse, e.g. patients with extracapsular lymph node spread. Some of these trials were conducted in patients who had already responded to neo-adjuvant therapy or were in a selected 'chemosensitive' group and there was not always a control group who did not receive chemotherapy at some time during primary treatment. In the study by Ervin *et al.*[33] patients were treated with two cycles of induction chemotherapy with cisplatin, bleomycin and midcycle methotrexate before radical local treatment; responders were randomised to further chemotherapy or observation only. Only 46 of 144 patients consented to the adjuvant study and of the 26 randomised to chemotherapy only 10 received all three cycles of adjuvant treatment. The apparent superior disease-free survival in the patients receiving adjuvant treatment (88 versus 55 per cent) is based on relatively small numbers and may reflect biological differences, with patients fit enough to tolerate chemotherapy having an intrinsically better prognosis.

Other trials have confirmed a decrease in the occurrence of distant metastases but have not demonstrated any consistent effect on survival.[34,35] These trials also reinforce the problems of delivering adjuvant therapy; for example, in the Head and Neck Contracts Programme only 15 per cent of patients received the prescribed course of adjuvant therapy with 4-weekly single agent cisplatin for 6 months.[36]

Subset analyses have shown statistical differences in disease-free, and in some cases overall, survival for smaller tumours (T1 or T2) and certain anatomical sites. In the report by Jacobs and Makuch,[34] there were 192 patients with oral cavity cancer; those patients who received induction chemotherapy with cisplatin and bleomycin followed by surgery and adjuvant chemotherapy with cisplatin had superior 3 year disease-free survival (67 per cent) compared with the standard arm who received no chemotherapy (49 per cent) or patients receiving induction chemotherapy without subsequent adjuvant chemotherapy (44 per cent). This analysis does have the problems inherent in retrospective subset analysis and any differences in survival with adjuvant chemotherapy would require prospective evaluation to detect modest benefits which may be important. Other studies examining adjuvant therapy have not shown any impact of tumour site on outcome.[37]

Rao *et al.*[38] carried out a study investigating the use of 'peri-operative' adjuvant chemotherapy with methotrexate 50 mg/m^2 on days 3, 10 and 17 postoperatively compared with untreated controls in 135 patients who had undergone curative resection for alveolobuccal cancer. There was a significant advantage in terms of disease-free survival at 12 months with 71 per cent disease-free survival in the treated arm compared with 45 per cent in the control arm. This is a simple approach which warrants further study.

Adjuvant chemotherapy has not fulfilled the main stated aim of improving survival in squamous cell carcinoma of the head and neck, although there may be a reduction in the development of distant metastases. It is possible that patients with primary cancers at certain sites such as the oral cavity may benefit although this could only be proven in large stratified trials using effective regimens at the prescribed dose intensity.

Neo-adjuvant (induction) chemotherapy

There have been many small pilot trials of induction chemotherapy, with overall response rates ranging from 37–100 per cent and complete response rates of 0–54 per cent.[39,40] These response rates are higher than predicted from similar regimens in metastatic disease and may reflect either the fact that patients are better able to tolerate chemotherapy early in their disease and can receive a higher dose intensity, or the inherent differences in chemosensitivity between early and advanced disease. Single agent chemotherapy achieves complete response rates of only 0–5 per cent and combination regimens are preferred. The complete response rate might be expected to have an impact on organ preservation and possibly survival following surgical resection. In general those patients who have a complete response to chemotherapy have a better prognosis than patients who do not respond, but this may reflect biological differences between 'responders' and 'non-responders' which influence survival rather than an actual benefit of chemotherapy. Patients who respond well to chemotherapy have a higher response rate to subsequent radiotherapy.[41,42] There is a reduction in distant metastases as would be anticipated from the adjuvant data. A number of factors have been evaluated to determine their influence on response to induction chemotherapy (Table 9.3). Carcinoma arising in the oral cavity may have a higher response rate than at other primary sites (with the exception of nasopharyngeal cancer) but again this requires confirmation in a prospective trial stratified by site.

Table 9.3 Prognostic factors affecting response to induction chemotherapy

Factor	Favourable prognosis
Primary site	Oral cavity
T status	T1 and T2
N status	N1
Histology	No definite effect
Performance status	0–2
Drug	Combination regimen

In a randomised study by the Southwest Oncology Group[43] 158 patients with advanced, but resectable, head and neck cancer were enrolled. Treatment was either standard surgery and radiotherapy or induction chemotherapy using cisplatin, methotrexate, bleomycin and vincristine for 3 months followed by standard treatment. The overall response rate to induction chemotherapy was approximately 70 per cent but there was no survival difference between the two treatment arms.

With the recognition of the activity of cisplatin and infusional 5-FU in metastatic disease this regimen was tested as induction chemotherapy. Phase II trials demonstrated high response rates in excess of 90 per cent with a high clinical complete response rate of >50 per cent and histological complete responses in 75 per cent of patients at surgery.[44-46] Despite this high response rate, controlled clinical trials have failed to demonstrate a survival benefit from the use of this regimen as neo-aduvant treatment.[47-49]

In general, in randomised trials comparing chemotherapy followed by radical local treatment or with local treatment without chemotherapy, there has been no evidence to support a survival advantage for the use of induction chemotherapy.[50] These trials show a trend towards a reduction in distant metastases and also confirm that the use of induction chemotherapy does not compromise subsequent local treatment.[34,35,43] Locoregional control, however, remains a major problem, and may possibly even be reduced by induction chemotherapy in non-responders.[49]

There are a number of problems interpreting the results of these trials. In some studies chemotherapy was used at suboptimal doses, i.e. lower than those associated with the high response rates reported in Phase II trials.[50] This was either due to trial design or, in most cases, related to dose reduction and delays because of toxicity resulting in reduction in planned dose intensity. There were often insufficient patient numbers to detect any differences in survival rates, while imbalances in patient characteristics and subsequent treatment could bias the outcome. In some trials induction chemotherapy was given for two or three courses and only responders received adjuvant therapy.[33,34] This results in a higher dose intensity in responders to neo-adjuvant treatment and may influence survival figures. Induction chemotherapy has mainly been investigated in patients with Stage III/IV tumours and unresectable tumours and it is perhaps not surprising that survival rates have not improved. There may be a case for induction chemotherapy in patients with less advanced disease.

Concomitant chemotherapy and radiotherapy

Despite the use of induction and adjuvant chemo-

therapy most patients with squamous cell carcinoma of the head and neck die as a result of local recurrence. The use of simultaneous chemotherapy and radiotherapy has been proposed to maximise both local and systemic control. Chemotherapy may potentiate cytotoxicity of radiotherapy by a number of mechanisms. Drugs may kill specifically cells in the S phase of the mitotic cycle (methotrexate, hydroxyurea) at which phase the cells are at their most radioresistant, or drugs may be more toxic to hypoxic than fully oxygenated cells (mitomycin C). There may be inhibition of the DNA repair enzymes that enable cells to recover from radiation damage. The effect of cytotoxic drugs on non-dividing cells is thought to be minimal, so chemotherapy may have a greater potentiating effect of radiotherapy on tumours than on the critical dose-limiting late responding normal tissues (see Chapter 8). The details of mechanisms of interaction between cytotoxic drugs and radiation is beyond the scope of this book; there are comprehensive reviews by Steel,[51] Tannock[25] and Vokes and Weichselbaum.[52]

Clinical studies have explored simultaneous treatment with chemotherapy and radiotherapy using a variety of radiotherapy fractionation schedules and alternating chemotherapy with radiotherapy.

A number of cytotoxic drugs have been evaluated either because of their presumed effects on radiosensitisation or because of activity in squamous cell carcinoma of the head and neck. S phase specific agents tested include hydroxyurea and methotrexate. Hydroxyurea inhibits ribonucleotide reductase and may inhibit enzymes involved in DNA repair after radiation;[53] in the study by Richards and Chambers[54] it was found that hydroxyurea increased the local toxicity of radiotherapy without any improvement in locoregional control. In a controlled trial involving oral and oropharyngeal carcinoma treated with a 3 week course of radiotherapy, methotrexate 100 mg/m^2 on days 1 and 15 of radiotherapy gave superior relapse-free ($P<0.016$) and overall ($P<0.07$) survival compared with radiotherapy alone; however there was significant increase in acute mucositis in the patients receiving methotrexate ($P<0.02$).[55] This increase in acute normal tissue toxicity from the use of concomitant chemoradiotherapy has been seen with most drugs, including fluorouracil[56] and bleomycin.[57,58] Both these later drugs appear also to enhance late radiation toxicity.[59,60] In one study mitomycin C significantly increased locoregional control without any observed increase in radiation morbidity.[61]

The data for improvement in survival with single agent chemotherapy are not conclusive.[62] The reason for the lack of impact on overall survival is possibly that in many studies the doses of the drugs used are suboptimal, because they are often tested as radiosensitisers rather than being exploited as cytotoxic agents in their own right.

Combination chemotherapy regimens have also been used concomitantly with radiotherapy. The response rate with cisplatin + fluorouracil regimens is high, with a complete response rate in excess of 50 per cent.[63] This approach has been compared with induction chemotherapy in several randomised trials, all of which showed a higher disease-free survival for the concomitant group, but no significant advantage in overall survival and significantly more severe acute mucositis and weight loss in the simultaneous group.[64–66]

The increase in acute toxicity seen with concomitant chemotherapy and radiotherapy may lead to interruptions in radiotherapy or reduction in dose of radiotherapy, which may have an adverse effect on local control. A strategy designed to overcome this is the planned use of alternating chemotherapy with divided courses of radiotherapy. Some of these trials use accelerated fractionation or hyperfractionation schedules to try to deliver the planned radiation dose within a sufficiently short time. In the trial reported by Merlano *et al.*[67] four courses of chemotherapy using methotrexate, bleomycin and vinblastine were given either alternating with radiotherapy or followed by radiotherapy. Only advanced cases were admitted to the study and both disease-free survival and overall survival were very low, although there was a significant advantage to the alternating arm ($P<0.02$) but at the expense of a very significant increase in mucositis ($P<0.00004$). A later study by the same group compared chemotherapy using cisplatin + infusional fluorouracil, alternating with radiotherapy 20 Gy per course with radiotherapy alone up to 70 Gy.[68] The number of patients enrolled was 157 although 13 did not start treatment. There was a significantly higher response rate and median survival in the patients receiving the rapidly alternating schedule (complete response, 42 per cent; median survival, 16.5 months), compared with the radiotherapy only group (complete response, 22 per cent; median survival, 11.7 months). Acute mucositis was similar in the two arms of the trial; the lack of enhanced acute toxicity in the concomitant group was attributed to not using methotrexate. However, haematological toxicity was higher in the combination group. The combined therapy group had a greater number of patients who subsequently were able to undergo salvage surgery, probably because the enhanced response was more likely to render a previously inoperable tumour operable.

The overall trend in trials of concomitant radiotherapy and chemotherapy is for chemotherapy to improve locoregional control rates at the expense of increased acute toxicity, but clear cut evidence of a survival benefit has not yet been established. Also there is insufficient data on late radiation morbidity, so it is not clear whether the addition of concomitant chemotherapy has any greater effect on tumour control than higher doses of radiotherapy or more rapid fractionation.

Regional chemotherapy

The earliest studies of chemotherapy in head and neck cancer used intra-arterial infusion in an attempt to concentrate the effects of the drugs in the tumour-bearing areas. Sullivan *et al.*[69] pioneered the technique of infusing methotrexate into the external carotid artery while protecting the patient from systemic effects of methotrexate using folinic acid. A number of studies were performed in the 1960s using a variety of single agents intra-arterially (mainly methotrexate, fluorouracil, bleomycin and ethoglucid). However it became apparent that the technique of intra-arterial infusion was complicated and hazardous, and had the additional disadvantage of not being applicable to treatment of cervical lymph node metastases. In the belief that systemic chemotherapy could be at least equally as effective, intra-arterial chemotherapy became less popular. Some studies suggested a benefit from intra-arterial chemotherapy pre-operatively,[70,71] and interest in the method has been maintained in some centres. Newer drugs including cisplatin have been tried intra-arterially.[72,73]

A randomised study of pre-operative intra-arterial vincristine and bleomycin involving 222 patients and stratified into floor of mouth and posterior oral cavity was reported by Richard *et al.*[74] The overall response rate to the chemotherapy in the two groups was 48 per cent and 41 per cent respectively. In the floor of mouth group there was a significant improvement in local control and a small survival benefit.

There have been no randomised trials comparing intra-arterial chemotherapy with systemic chemotherapy and the actual benefit of this mode of administration over intravenous delivery needs further evaluation, which can only be achieved by randomised trials.

Salivary gland tumours

Salivary gland tumours of high grade malignancy (squamous cell carcinoma and high grade muco-epidermoid carcinoma) are managed according to the general principles governing head and neck cancer and there may be a place for chemotherapy although the development of chemotherapy regimens has been limited by the heterogeneity of the disease and the relatively small numbers of patients who develop recurrence. It is likely that cisplatin-based regimens would be effective although randomised trials would be necessary to see whether these tumours have similar chemosensitivity as squamous cell carcinoma of the head and neck.[75]

For further discussion of the role of chemotherapy in salivary gland tumours see Chapter 15.

Conclusion

The oral cavity may represent an anatomical site where tumours have a more favourable response to chemotherapy than at other head and neck sites,[31] but despite the high response rates there is no convincing survival benefit from the addition of chemotherapy to radical local treatment and most patients who die have locoregional relapse. The impact of concomitant chemoradiotherapy on reduction in local recurrence may prove important, but the optional drug combinations and scheduling require further investigation.

Biological therapy

Interferon-α has been used to modulate 5-FU in experimental systems and in patients with colorectal cancer.[76] The mechanism underlying the interaction is not fully understood but may involve intracellular biochemical modulation of 5-FU. Similarly interferon has also been used to modulate cisplatin in non-small cell lung cancer including tumours with squamous cell histology.[77] A preliminary report of a Phase I trial of interferon-α in combination with cisplatin and 5-FU in patients with advanced head and neck cancer suggested a high response rate with 20 of the 20 evaluable patients responding and a 70 per cent complete re-

sponse rate.[52] The toxicity normally attributed to cisplatin or 5-FU (mucositis and renal impairment) was higher than expected. There is an ongoing comparative Phase III trial to evaluate the role of interferon in squamous cell carcinoma of the head and neck.

Interleukin-2 (Il-2) administered intravenously has activity against a variety of human tumours.[78] Its main site of action is probably at a local level and locoregional administration might allow concentration of tumouricidal lymphocytes with less systemic toxicity. Phase I and II trials using peri-lymphatic bolus injection or continuous intra-arterial infusion of IL-2 have been reported.[79,80] These studies suggest a lower incidence of systemic toxicity but response rates are variable. Cancers of the head and neck region offer an opportunity to study the effects of biological agents because of the relative ease of performing repeat biopsies. Further studies to investigate dose and scheduling should be performed with careful biological monitoring and may provide useful information for future work on targeted gene therapy.

Chemoprevention

The most effective methods of preventing oral cancer are avoidance of the major aetiological factors, tobacco and alcohol. However patients with premalignant conditions in the mouth have a high risk of developing carcinoma (see Chapter 3), and patients successfully treated for oral cancer have a high risk of developing second primary neoplasms. Accordingly there is now a considerable interest in measures to prevent the development of cancer in this high risk group, including the use of chemical agents.

Retinoids

Vitamin A and related compounds have several properties which suggest that they may be useful as chemopreventive agents in oral squamous cell carcinoma. They are modulators of epithelial cell differentiation, both *in vitro* and *in vivo*. They probably act by regulating gene expression. Cell nuclei contain retinoic acid receptors that mediate the biological effects of retinoids. The ligand for these receptors is probably all-trans-retinoic acid, to which retinoids must be metabolised to exert their biological effect.[81] In experimental animals vitamin A deficiency causes squamous metaplasia similar to that induced by chemical carcinogens. It has been found that vitamin A and related retinoids can reverse the metaplasia in vitamin A deficient animals. They have also been shown to inhibit the growth of squamous carcinoma cell lines *in vitro*.[82,83]

There have been several studies of treatment of oral dysplastic leukoplakia by retinoids. Hong *et al*.[84] used isotretinoin in a dose of 1–2 mg/kg per day for 3 months in a placebo-controlled trial involving 44 patients. The drug produced major clinical responses in 67 per cent of patients compared with 10 per cent who received placebo ($P = 0.0002$) and reversed the dysplastic change in 56 per cent. At this dosage isotretinoin has appreciable toxicity, with peeling of the skin, cheilitis, facial erythema and hypertriglyceridaemia in about 75 per cent of patients. Headaches and dyspepsia also occasionally occur. The leukoplakic changes recurred after stopping treatment. However a subsequent study demonstrated that low dose maintenance treatment (0.5 mg/kg) after the end of the 3 months of high dose therapy was well tolerated and prevented recurrences.[85]

Vitamin A in high dosage was shown to reverse premalignant changes in Indian betel chewers.[86] Vitamin A is generally less toxic than isotretinoin, but effective dose levels, i.e. 300 000 IU per day, produce similar if less severe side effects. In both of the above studies β-carotene was also tested as maintenance treatment because of its lower toxicity, but was significantly less effective than either vitamin A or isotretinoin, probably because it is less easily metabolised to the active ligand.

Experience with isotretinoin in the treatment of leukoplakia has led to its being tested as adjuvant treatment in patients with oral and laryngeal carcinoma who were disease-free after primary treatment.[87] There was no influence on recurrence rates of the original tumours, but there was a significant reduction in the incidence of second primary tumours. This experience led to the setting up of larger multicentre chemopreventive trials in cured head and neck cancer patients, for example the Euroscan trial using vitamin A.[88]

Antioxidants

Agents with antioxidant properties can inhibit the effects of many toxins including carcinogens. *N*-acetylcysteine, a precursor of intracellular glutathione, inhibits the mutagenic effect of carcinogens such as benzpyrene *in vitro*,[89] and reduces the incidence of chemically induced tumours in experimental animals. It has no major side effects and is therefore under investigation as a chemoprotective

agent in oral cancer. It is being compared with vitamin A in the Euroscan trial.

References

1 Hong WK, Bromer R. Chemotherapy in head and neck cancer. *New England Journal of Medicine* 1983; **308**: 75–9.

2 Grose W, Lehane DE, Dixon DO, Fletcher WS, Stuckey WJ. Comparison of methotrexate and cisplatin for patients with advanced squamous cell carcinoma of the head and neck region: a Southwest Oncology Group study. *Cancer Treatment Report* 1985; **69**: 577–81.

3 Taylor SG, McGuire WP, Hauck WW, Showel JL, Lad TE. A randomised comparison of high dose infusion methotrexate verses standard dose weekly therapy in head and neck squamous cancer. *Journal of Clinical Oncology* 1984; **2**: 1006–11.

4 Veronesi A, Zagonel V, Tirelli V *et al*. High-dose versus low-dose cisplatin in advanced head and neck squamous carcinoma: a randomized study. *Journal of Clinical Oncology* 1985; **8**: 1105–8.

5 Morton RP, Stell PM. Cytotoxic chemotherapy for patients with terminal squamous cell carcinoma – does it influence survival? *Clinical Otolaryngology* 1984; **9**: 175–80.

6 Clavel M, Cognetti F, Dodion P *et al*. Combination chemotherapy with methotrexate, bleomycin, and vincristine with or without cisplatin in advanced squamous cell carcinoma of the head and neck. *Cancer* 1987; **60**: 1173–7.

7 Vogl SE, Schoenfield D. Is partial response of value in the chemotherapy of head and neck cancer? In: Chretien PB, Johns ME, Shedd DP, Strong EW, Ward PH eds. *Head and Neck Cancer*, Volume 1. Philadelphia PA: BD Decker Inc. 1985: 404–6.

8 Kish JA, Ensley JF, Jacobs J, Weever A, Comings G, Al-Sarraf M. A randomised trial of cisplatin (CACP) plus 5-fluorouracil (5-FU) infusion and CACP plus 5-FU bolus for recurrent and advanced squamous cell carcinoma of the head and neck. *Cancer* 1985; **56**: 2842–4.

9 The Liverpool Head and Neck Oncology Group. A stage III randomised trial of cisplatiun, methotrexate, cisplatinum and methotrexate and cisplatinum and 5-FU in end stage squamous carcinoma of the head and neck. *British Journal of Cancer* 1990; **61**: 311–15.

10 Forestiere AA, Metch B, Schuller DE *et al*. Randomised comparison of cisplatin plus fluorouracil and carboplatin plus fluorouracil versus methotrexate in advanced squamous-cell carcinoma of the head and neck: a Southwest Oncology Group study. *Journal of Clinical Oncology* 1992; **10**: 1245–51.

11 Lane M, More JE, Levin H, Smith SE. Methotrexate

therapy for squamous cell carcinoma of the head and neck. *Journal of the American Medical Association* 1968; **204**: 561–4.

12 Leone LA, Albala MM, Rege VB. Treatment of carcinoma of the head and neck with intravenous methotrexate. *Cancer* 1968; **21**: 828–37.

13 Woods RL, Fox RM, Tattersall MHN. Methotrexate treatment of squamous cell head and neck cancers: dose response evaluation. *British Medical Journal* 1981; **282**: 600–2.

14 Browman GP, Goodyear MDE, Levin MM, Russel R, Archibald SD, Young JEM. Modulation of the antitumour effect of methotrexate by low dose leucovorin in squamous cell head and neck cancer: a randomised placebo-controlled clinical trial. *Journal of Clinical Oncology* 1990; **8**: 203–8.

15 Jacobs C, Bertino JR, Goffinet DR, Fee WE, Goode RL. 24 hour infusion of cisplatinum in head and neck cancer. *Cancer* 1978; **42**: 2135–40.

16 Pinto HA, Jacobs C. Chemotherapy for recurrent and metastatic head and neck cancer. *Hematological Oncological Clinics of North America* 1991; **5**: 667–86.

17 Morton RP, Rugman F, Dorman EB *et al*. Cisplatinum and bleomycin for advanced or recurrent squamous cell carcinoma of the head and neck: a randomised factorial phase III controlled trial. *Cancer Chemotherapy Pharmacology* 1985; **15**: 283–9.

18 Al-Sarraf M, Metch B, Kish J *et al*. Platinum analogs in recurrent and advanced head and neck cancer: a Southwest Oncology Group and Wayne State University study. *Cancer Treatment Reports* 1987; **71**: 723–6.

19 Tapazoglou E, Kish J, Ensley J, Al-Sarraf M. The activity of single agent 5-fluorouracil infusion in advanced and recurrent head and neck cancer. *Cancer* 1986; **57**: 1105–9.

20 Jacobs C, Meyers F, Hendrickson C, Kahler M, Carter S. A randomised phase III study of cisplatin with or without methotrexate for recurrent squamous cell carcinoma of the head and neck. *Cancer* 1983; **52**: 1563–9.

21 Chauvergne J, Cappelaere P, Fargeot P *et al*. Randomised study with cisplatin alone or in combination for palliative chemotherapy in head and neck carcinoma of 209 patients. *Bulletin du Cancer* 1988; **75**: 9–22.

22 Kish JA, Weaver A, Jacobs J *et al*. Cisplatin and 5-fluorouracil infusion in patients with recurrent and disseminated epidermoid cancer. *Cancer* 1984; **53**: 1819–24.

23 Urba EG, Forestiere AA. Systemic therapy of head and neck cancer: most effective agents, areas of promise. *Oncology* 1989; **3**: 79–88.

24 Jacobs C, Lyman G, Velez Garcia E *et al*. A phase III randomised study comparing cisplatin and 5-fluorouracil as single agents and in combination for advanced squamous cell carcinoma of the head and neck. *Journal of Clinical Oncology* 1992; **10**: 257–63.

25 Tannock IF. Combined modality treatment with radiotherapy and chemotherapy. *Radiotherapy and Oncology* 1989; **16**: 83–101.

26 Johnson NW. *Risk Markers for Oral Diseases. Volume 2. Detection of Patients and Lesions at Risk*. Cambridge: Cambridge University Press, 1991.

27 Fountzilas G, Kosmidis P, Beer M, Sridhar KS, Banis K, Vritsios A, Daniilidis J. Factors influencing complete response and survival in patients with head and neck cancer treated with platinum-based induction chemotherapy. A Hellenic Co-operative Oncology Group study. *Annals of Oncology* 1992; **3**: 553–8.

28 Cognetti F, Pinnaro P, Ruggeri EM *et al*. Prognostic factors for chemotherapy response and survival using combination chemotherapy as initial treatment of advanced head and neck squamous cell cancer. *Journal of Clinical Oncology* 1989; **7**: 829–37.

29 Recondo G, Cvikonic E, Azli N *et al*. Neoadjuvant chemotherapy consisting of cisplatin and continuous infusions of bleomycin and 5-fluorouracil for advanced head and neck cancer. The need for a new stratification for stage IV (M0) disease. *Cancer* 1991; **68**: 2109–19.

30 Zharan P, Lehmann W. Frequency and sites of distant metastases in head and neck squamous cell carcinoma. *Archives of Otolaryngology – Head and Neck Surgery* 1987; **113**: 762–4.

31 Stell PM, Rawson NSB. Adjuvant chemotherapy in head and neck cancer. *British Journal of Cancer* 1990; **61**: 779.

32 Hong WK. Adjuvant chemotherapy for resectable squamous carcinoma of the head and neck: report on Intergroup Study 0034. *International Journal of Radiation Oncology, Biology, Physics* 1992; **23**: 885–6.

33 Ervin TJ, Clarke JR, Weichselbaum RR *et al*. An analysis of induction and adjuvant chemotherapy in the multi-disciplinary treatment of squamous cell carcinoma of the head and neck. *Journal of Clinical Oncology* 1987; **5**: 10–20.

34 Jacobs C, Makuch R. Efficacy of adjuvant chemotherapy for patients with resectable head and neck cancer; a subset analysis of the Head and Neck Contracts Programme. *Journal of Clinical Oncology* 1990; **8**: 838–47.

35 Laramore GE, Scott CB, Al-Sarraf M *et al*. Adjuvant chemotherapy for resectable squamous cell carcinoma of the head and neck. *International Journal of Radiation Oncology, Biology, Physics* 1992; **23**: 705–13.

36 Anonymous. Adjuvant chemotherapy for advanced head and neck squamous carcinoma. Final report of the Head and Neck Contracts Programme. *Cancer* 1987; **60**: 301–11.

37 Taylor SG, Applebaum E, Showel JL *et al*. A randomised trial of adjuvant chemotherapy in head and neck cancer. *Journal of Clinical Oncology* 1985; **3**: 672–9.

38 Rao RS, Parikh DM, Parikh HK, Bhansali MB, Fakih AR. Perioperative chemotherapy in oral

cancer. *Journal of Surgical Oncology* 1991; **47**: 21–6.

39 Al-Sarraf M. Head and neck cancer: chemotherapy concepts. *Seminars in Oncology* 1988; **15**: 70–85.

40 Choksi AJ, Dimery IW, Hong WK. Adjuvant chemotherapy of head and neck cancer: the past, the present, and the future. *Seminars in Oncology* 1988; **15**: 45–9.

41 Tannock IF, Browman G. Lack of evidence for a role of chemotherapy in the routine management of locally advanced head and neck cancer. *Journal of Clinical Oncology* 1986; **4**: 1121–6.

42 Ensley JF, Jacobs JR, Weaver A *et al*. Correlation between response to cisplatinum-combination chemotherapy and subsequent radiotherapy in previously untreated patients with advanced squamous cell cancers of the head and neck. *Cancer* 1984; **54**: 811–14.

43 Schuller DE, Metch B, Mattox D, McCracken JD. Preoperative chemotherapy in advanced resectable head and neck cancer: final report of the Southwest Oncology Group. *Laryngoscope* 1988; **98**: 1205–11.

44 Rooney M, Kish J, Jacobs J *et al*. Improved complete response rate and survival in advanced head and neck cancer after three-course induction therapy with 120 hour 5-FU infusion and cisplatin. *Cancer* 1985; **55**: 1123–8.

45 Vokes EE, Weischelbaum RR, Ratain MJ *et al*. PFL with escalating doses of interferon-alpha-2B (IFN) as neoadjuvant chemotherapy for stage IV head and neck cancer (HNC): A clinical and pharmacokinetic analysis. *Proceedings of the American Society of Clinical Otolaryngologists* 1991 (abstract).

46 Al Kourainy K, Kish J, Ensley J *et al*. Achievement of superior survival for histologically negative versus histologically positive clinically complete responders to cisplatin combination chemotherapy in patients with locally advanced head and neck cancer. *Cancer* 1987; **59**: 233–8.

47 Toohill RJ, Anderson T, Byhardt RW *et al*. Cisplatin and fluorouracil as neo-adjuvant therapy in head and neck cancer. *Archives of Otolaryngology – Head and Neck Surgery* 1987; **113**: 758–61.

48 Martin N, Hazan A, Verngnes L *et al*. Randomised study of 5-fluorouracil and cisplatin as neoadjuvant therapy in head and neck cancer: a preliminary report. *International Journal of Radiation Oncology, Biology, Physics* 1990; 973–5.

49 Jaulerry C, Rodriguez J, Brunin F *et al*. Induction chemotherapy in advanced head and neck tumours; results of two randomized trials. *International Journal of Radiation Oncology, Biology, Physics* 1992; **23**: 483–9.

50 Forestiere AA. Randomised trials of induction chemotherapy. *Haematological and Oncological Clinics of North America* 1991; **54**: 811–14.

51 Steel GG. The search for therapeutic gain in the combination of radiotherapy and chemotherapy. *Radiotherapy and Oncology* 1988; **11**: 31–53.

52 Vokes EE, Weichselbaum RR. Concomitant chemotherapy: rationale and clinical experience in patients with solid tumours. *Journal of Clinical Oncology* 1990; **8**: 911–34.

53 Phillips RA, Tolmach LJ. Repair of potentially lethal damage in x-irradiated He La cells. *Radiation Research* 1966; **29**: 413–32.

54 Richards GJ, Chambers RG. Hydroxyurea in the treatment of neoplasms of the head and neck. A resurvey. *American Journal of Surgery* 1973; **128**: 513–18.

55 Gupta NK, Pointon RCS, Wilkinson PM. A randomised clinical trial to contrast radiotherapy with radiotherapy and methotrexate given synchronously in head and neck cancer. *Clinical Radiology* 1987; **38**: 575–81.

56 Lo TC, Wiley AL Jnr, Ansfield FJ *et al*. Combined radiation therapy and 5-fluorouracil for advanced squamous cell carcinoma of the oral cavity and oropharynx: a randomised study. *American Journal of Roentgenology* 1976; **126**: 229–35.

57 Shanta V, Krishnamurthi S. Combined bleomycin and radiotherapy in oral cancer. *Clinical Radiology* 1980; **31**: 617–20.

58 Fu KK, Phillips TL, Silverberg IJ *et al*. Combined radiotherapy and chemotherapy with bleomycin and methotrexate for advanced inoperable head and neck cancer: update of a Northern California Oncology Group randomized trial. *Journal of Clinical Oncology* 1987; **5**: 1410–18.

59 Chen RC, Shukovsky LJ. Effects of irradiation on the eye. *Radiology* 1976; **120**: 673–5.

60 Peters LJ, Harrison ML, Dimery IW *et al*. Acute and late toxicity associated with sequential bleomycin-containing regimens and radiation therapy in the treatment of carcinoma of the nasopharynx. *International Journal of Radiation Oncology, Biology, Physics* 1988; **14**: 623–33.

61 Weissberg JB, Son YH, Papac RJ *et al*. Randomised clinical trial of mitomycin C as an adjunct to radiotherapy in head and neck cancer. *International Journal of Radiation Oncology, Biology, Physics* 1989; **17**: 3–9.

62 Vermund H, Kaalhus O, Winther F, Trausjo J, Thorud E, Itarang R. Bleomycin and radiation therapy in squamous cell carcinoma of the upper aerodigestive tract: a phase III clinical trial. *International Journal of Radiation Oncology, Biology, Physics* 1985; **11**: 1877–86.

63 Adelstein DJ, Sharan VM, Earle AS *et al*. Simultaneous radiotherapy and chemotherapy with 5-fluorouracil and cisplatin for locally confined squamous cell head and neck cancer. *Monographs/National Cancer Institute* 1988; **6**: 347–51.

64 Adelstein DJ, Sharan VM, Earle AS *et al*. Simultaneous versus sequential combined technique therapy for squamous cell head and neck cancer. *Cancer* 1990; **65**: 1685–91.

65 Merlano M, Corvo R, Margarino G *et al*. Combined

chemotherapy and radiation therapy in advanced inoperable squamous cell carcinoma of the head and neck: the final report of a randomised trial. *Cancer* 1991; **67**: 915–21.

66 SECOG. An interim report from Secog participants. A randomised trial of combined multi-drug chemotherapy and radiotherapy in advanced squamous cell carcinoma of the head and neck. *European Journal of Surgical Oncology* 1986; **12**: 289–95.

67 Merlano M, Rossok R, Sertoli MR *et al*. Sequential versus alternating chemotherapy and radiotherapy in Stage III–IV squamous cell carcinoma of the head and neck: a phase III study. *Journal of Clinical Oncology* 1988; **6**: 627–32.

68 Merlano M, Vitale V, Rosso R *et al*. Treatment of advanced squamous-cell carcinoma of the head and neck with alternating chemotherapy and radiotherapy. *New England Journal of Medicine* 1992; **327**: 1115–21.

69 Sullivan RD, Miller E, Sykes P. Antimetabolite–metabolite combination in cancer chemotherapy. Effects of intra-arterial methotrexate and intra-muscular citrovorum factor in human cancer. *Cancer* 1959; **12**: 1248–57.

70 Molinari R. Present role of intra-arterial regional chemotherapy in head and neck cancer. *Drugs in Experimental and Clinical Research* 1983; **IX**: 491–504.

71 Baker SR, Wheeler R. Intra-arterial infusion chemotherapy of head and neck cancer. *Cancer Treatment Research* 1984; **22**: 301–45.

72 Mortimer JE, Taylor ME, Schulman S *et al*. Feasibility and efficacy of weekly intra arterial cisplatin in locally advanced (stage III and IV) head and neck cancer. *Journal of Clinical Oncology* 1988; **6**: 969–75.

73 Cheung DK, Regan J, Savin M, Gibberman V, Woessner W. A pilot study of intra-arterial chemotherapy with cisplatin in locally advanced head and neck cancers. *Cancer* 1988; **61**: 903–8.

74 Richard JM, Kramar A, Molinari R *et al*. Randomised EORTC head and neck co-operative group trial of preoperative intra arterial chemotherapy in oral and oropharynx carcinoma. *European Journal of Cancer* 1991; **27**: 821–7.

75 Creagen ET, Woods JE, Rubin J, Schaid PJ. Cisplatin-based chemotherapy for neoplasms arising from salivary glands and contiguous structures of the head and neck. *Cancer* 1988; **62**: 2313–19.

76 Pazdur R, Ajani JA, Patt YZ *et al*. Phase II study of fluorouracil and recombinant interferon alpha-2a in previously untreated colorectal cancer. *Journal of Clinical Oncology* 1990; **50**: 3473–86.

77 Bowman A, Fergusson RJ, Allen SG *et al*. Potenti-

ation of cisplatin by alpha-interferon in advanced non-small cell lung cancer (NSCLC): A Phase II study. *Annals of Oncology* 1990; **1**: 351–3.

78 Rosenberg SA, Lotze MT, Yang JC *et al*. Experience with the use of high-dose interleukin-2 in the treatment of 652 cancer patients. *Annals of Surgery* 1989; **210**: 474–84.

79 Cortesina G, de Stenfani A, Galeaxi E *et al*. Interleukin-2 injected around tumour drainage lymph nodes in head and neck cancer. *Head and Neck* 1991; **13**: 125–31.

80 Gore ME, Riches P, Maclennan K *et al*. Phase I study of intra-arterial interleukin-2 in squamous cell carcinoma of the head and neck. *British Journal of Cancer* 1992; **66**: 405–7.

81 Lotan R, Clifford JL. Nuclear receptors for retinoids: mediators of retinoid effects on normal and malignant cells. *Biomedicine and Pharmacotherapy* 1991; **45**: 145–56.

82 Sacks PG, Oke V, Amos B, Vasey T, Lotan R. Modulation of growth, differentiation and glycoprotein synthesis by β all-trans-retinoic acid in a multicellular tumour spheroid model for squamous carcinoma of the head and neck. *International Journal of Cancer* 1989; **44**: 926–33.

83 Jelten AM, Kim JS, Sacks PG *et al*. Inhibition of growth and squamous-cell differentiation markers in cultured human head and neck squamous carcinoma cells by β-all-trans-retinoic acid. *International Journal of Cancer* 1990; **45**: 195–202.

84 Hong WK, Endicott J, Itri L *et al*. 13-cis-retinoic acid in the treatment of oral leukoplakia. *New England Journal of Medicine* 1986; **315**: 1501–5.

85 Lippman SM, Batsakis JG, Toth BB *et al*. Comparison of low-dose isotretinoin with beta carotene to prevent oral carcinogenesis. *New England Journal of Medicine* 1993; **328**: 15–20.

86 Stich HF, Mathew B, Sankaranarayanam R, Nair MK. Remission of pre-cancerous lesions in the oral cavity of tobacco chewers and maintenance of the protective effect of β-carotene or vitamin A. *American Journal of Clinical Nutrition* 1991; **53**: 2985–3045.

87 Hong WK, Endicott J, Itri LM *et al*. Prevention of second primary tumours with isotretinoin in squamous-cell carcinoma of the head and neck. *New England Journal of Medicine* 1990; **323**: 795–801.

88 de Vries N, van Zandwijk N, Pastorino U. The Euroscan study. *British Journal of Cancer* 1991; **64**: 985–9.

89 de Flora S, Bennicelli C, Zanachi P *et al*. *In vitro* effects of *N*-acetylcysteine on the mutagenicity of direct-acting compounds and procarcinogens. *Carcinogenesis* 1984; **6**: 1735–9.

10 Thermal surgery for oral malignancy

PF Bradley

The underlying concept

The ability of temperature extremes to destroy or alter tissue has been known to man since the earliest times. Subzero temperatures can cause so-called 'frostbite' whilst temperatures above the coagulation point of proteins result in 'burns'. Thermal surgery employs these effects in a carefully controlled manner: the use of temperatures below freezing point constituting cryotherapy while heating effects are obtained by the use of lasers normally functioning in the infrared range of wavelengths. These modalities may be utilised to destroy tissue in the context of premalignant lesions and malignant lesions, and for palliation. They do this by exerting three main effects:

(1) *A cold-induced coagulative necrosis*. This is the end result of cryosurgery. Cryodestruction of normal or benign neoplastic tissue normally requires the attainment of a temperature of at least −15°C (the temperature at which intracellular ice forms[1]) while total ablation of malignant tumour tissue calls for some degree of overkill at a level of −50°C.[2]

(2) *Heat-induced tissue coagulation*. To coagulate tissue proteins requires a temperature of approximately 60°C.[3] Lasers in the near and mid infrared wavelengths are best suited for this in that they show significant tissue penetration.

(3) *Thermal vapourisation or excision of soft tissues*. This effect requires the attainment of the temperature of at least 100°C at which point intracellular water boils disrupting tissue in a plume of steam and carbon particles. It is best shown by the CO_2 laser which functions in the far infrared so that its wavelength is maximally absorbed with minimal penetration. It pro-

duces a minor degree of coagulation at the excision margins which is necessary for haemostasis. Similar effects but with deeper degrees of coagulation may be produced by mid and near infrared lasers.

The use of thermal surgery requires a rather different attitude of mind from conventional surgery when applied to premalignant and malignant disease. Conventional excisional surgery tends to treat the lesion from without inwards in that it aims to remove a margin of normal tissue as well as the tumour itself; this is to ensure that microscopic neoplastic extensions (minimal residual disease: MRD) are excised along with the clinically apparent lesion. Thermal surgery can be employed in this manner as when the CO_2 laser is used to carry out excision – in this instance it acts like a scalpel but in addition has a haemostatic effect on small vessels less than 0.5 mm in diameter and also seals most lymphatics. Commonly however, thermal surgery acts from within outwards when it is asked to carry out cold coagulation, heat coagulation or vapourisation. The surgeon works from the centre of the abnormality outwards rather as the neurosurgeon employs his ultrasound apparatus to destroy central nervous system growths from their centre centrifugally. This has the consequence that there is a greater risk of retaining MRD although there is some evidence that cold coagulation induces local immune effects which can favour the rejection of microscopic deposits[4] – it is possible that heat coagulation may also have this property although much less research has been carried out into this aspect.[5] Therefore in order to produce a cure, thermal surgery is best suited to the treatment of localised exophytic tumours rather than endophytic ones. Ultrasound[6] and nuclear magnetic resonance imaging methods[7] show promise of improved staging of oral malignancy in the future, which would be most helpful in case selection.

Thermal surgery will really come into its own when more certain methods of dealing with MRD are available. Already it can be meaningfully combined with radiotherapy and cytotoxic medication.[8] In the future it may be utilised together with such means as photodynamic therapy,[9] improved interstitial irradiation (e.g. I^{125} seeds[10]) or monoclonally generated antibodies.[11] There is significant benefit in terms of pain and functional deficit. It is possible to save infiltrated bone as by the use of *in situ* liquid nitrogen spray or extracorporeal freezing (nerve and blood vessels may be retained in a similar manner). Tissue regeneration is remarkably enhanced after thermal coagulation. When the body spontaneously separates the coagulated slough there is a powerful stimulus to cellular division, hyperplasia and apparent hypertrophy; this may well be associated with concomitant cytokine release.

It should be pointed out that lasers may also be utilised in the future in relation to malignancy surgery in non-thermal adjunctive roles. These include photo-ablative mechanisms for cold cutting of bone (e.g. Excimer laser[12]), photo-acoustic forces to explode soft or hard tissue (e.g. Q-switched infrared lasers[13]) or photochemical effects as in photodynamic therapy[9] described in Chapter 11.

Individual usage of thermal modalities

The most commonly used thermal modalities will be described and are summarised in Table 10.1. It is only possible in the scope of this chapter to describe basic principles briefly but comprehensive descriptions are available elsewhere.[14,15]

Cryosurgery

For the management of oral premalignant and malignant disease liquid nitrogen apparatus (employing a 'phase change' mechanism) is deemed best in view of its greater potency compared with nitrous oxide machines (employing the 'throttled gas' or Joule Thomson effects). This offers a very simple and effective method of treating T1 and early T2 exophytic squamous cell carcinomas of the oral cavity. (Fig. 10.1) It can often be accomplished under local anaesthesia alone, or combined with intravenous sedation, and indeed the vasocon-

strictor action of the local anaesthetic potentiates ice ball formation. Suitably large tumour probes are normally used and freezing is undertaken until the lesion plus an adequate periphery is subjected to a cell-lethal temperature; freezing should be repeated once after thawing.[1] Gage and Bradley[16] have laid down the principles of this use and suggest the attainment of a temperature of $-50°C$ for oral malignant tumours. Thermocouples can be inserted into the peripheral tissue to ensure that this temperature is reached or alternatively a simple 'two-thirds' rule can be adopted; approximately two-thirds of the inner diameter of the visible ice ball will be at a temperature of $-50°C$ or below. About three-quarters of the diameter will be at $-15°C$, which is the temperature at which most normal tissue and benign neoplastic cells necrose. Gage has pointed out that underlying bone may be treated with good effect; it may persist exposed in the mouth for some months afterwards but gives very little in the way of symptoms. After sloughing of the soft tissue lesion at about 1 week multiple biopsies may be undertaken to ensure that full ablation of the lesion has taken place as advocated by Benson.[17] Gage[18] reported on the 5 year survival following cryosurgery for oral carcinoma in a group of 82 patients. Overall survival at 5 years was 56 per cent (Stage 1, 83 per cent; Stage 2, 50 per cent; Stage 3, 10 per cent), which compares favourably with conventional methods of treatment although the numbers of patients were small. Over half the deaths were due to unrelated disease. A recent Chinese paper describes 50 patients with tongue malignancies for whom there was 95 per cent local cure rate.[19] Careful case selection was undertaken in that patients with tumours infiltrating deeper than an estimated 2 cm or those with lymph node metastases in the neck were excluded.

Cryosurgery may also be used to destroy localised areas of leukoplakia or erythroplakia. However, it is not well suited for the therapy of widespread premalignant lesions. First, it is rather tedious treating large areas in that two freezes should be carried out for each area; second, there is some suggestion from animal studies in the hamster cheek pouch that the irritant effects of cryotherapy could have a promoter action on peripheral unablated leukoplakia,[20] although it is not at all certain as to how fully such results should be extrapolated to the human situation.

Interesting work is being carried out on the extracorporeal freezing of segments of bone infiltrated by tumour which can then be re-implanted at the site of origin.[21] The bony segment is hollowed out prior to treatment to act as a bone tray which can be filled with autogenous cancellous bone chips. Quadruple freezing in baths of liquid nitrogen is necessary in this method under very careful control. The length of contained inferior alveolar nerve should be left in the segment so that it can be anastomosed at the time of re-implantation to allow return of sensation in the soft tissues. This method must still be regarded as experimental but there is now a small group of successful long term cases.[22,23]

CO$_2$ Laser

This laser functions in the far infrared range at 10.6 microns wavelength which is maximally absorbed by water in tissue. It can be used to vapourise superficial lesions such as leukoplakias or erythroplakias.[24] In general, however, modern practice encourages the use of the laser as a form of haemostatic scalpel allowing excision of premalignances (Fig. 10.2) or exophytic T1 and early T2 squamous cell carcinomas (Fig. 10.3).[25] The

Table 10.1 Thermal modalities for oral malignancy/premalignancy

Modality	Specification	Delivery	Oral indications	Problems
Cryosurgery Cold coagulation (−50°C)	Liquid nitrogen apparatus best (phase change)	Probes Spray Extracorporeal	Simple method T1 and early T2 SCC (exophytic) Early bone involvement	Prediction of effect Possible promotor action on premalignant field change if used incompletely
CO$_2$ Laser Vapourisation or cutting (>100°C)	10.6 microns wavelength (μm) (Far infrared)	Mirrors (articulated arm) Wave guides Non-contact	Low morbidity excision premalignancies Excision/biopsy exophytic T1 and early T2 squamous cell carcinoma Hemiglossectomy Adhesive microvascular/ microneural repair potential	Class 4 laser precautions (cornea at risk) Haemostasis may not be fully adequate in very vascular areas e.g. posterior tongue (combination lasers allow blending with Nd-YAG)
Nd-YAG Laser Coagulation (>60°C) ± central vapourisation Cutting with coagulation	1.06 μm (Near infrared)	Fibre contact or non-contact (but can be blended with CO$_2$ via articulated arm (combination laser)	Coagulation of very vascular lesions or near major blood vessels Excision in vascular areas (post-tongue) as contact probe or blended with CO$_2$ (combination laser)	Class 4 precautions (retina at risk) Inadvertent scatter Oedema – more than CO$_2$ and potentially than cyrosurgery
Holmium YAG Laser Cutting with moderate coagulation Removal of bone in small amounts	2.1 μm (Mid infrared)	Fibre usually contact	Excision in vascular areas (post tongue/ tonsillar fossa/nasal cavity) Coagulation small vascular lesions e.g. hereditary haemorrhagic teleangiectasia Excision bone in small amounts (*Note:* Erbium YAG laser at 2.94 μm is more effective with bone)	Class 4 (retina at risk)

laser excision provides good haemostasis in most oral tissues in that it coagulates vessels below 0.5 mm and its use is accompanied by a remarkable lack of after pain, oedema and scarring in the majority of patients. It is the ideal method of excision biopsy of such oral lesions. A handpiece is advocated for most oral uses as it is much easier to manipulate in the mouth than the alternative method of linkage with an operating microscope (although this has a use in lesions of the posterior pharyngeal wall where the longer focal length is helpful). CO_2 laser hemiglossectomy[26] has established itself as the method of choice for this operation in that no suturing is necessary which might enclave tumour remnants; nor is flap replacement indicated which may tether tongue movements.

Recurrence rates after excision of leukoplakia have been reported to be as low as 9 per cent in one series,[27] which is an improvement on a series reported using cryosurgery where a recurrence rate of 18 per cent was noted.[28] This study utilised laser vapourisation but results may be improved still

Table 10.1   *continued*

Modality	Specification	Delivery	Oral indications	Problems
KTP Laser	0.532 μm (visible green)	Fibre usually contact	Similar indications in soft tissue to Holmium YAG. Usually in combination Laser with Nd-YAG	Class 4 (retina at risk)
Adjunctive: Tunable dye Non-thermal, photic in combination with sensitiser (PDT)	0.63 μm (visible red) for HPD	Fibre	Potentially could be used after CO_2 laser excision to deal with minimal residual disease (MRD) by photodynamic therapy	Skin sensitisation Class 4
Low level lasers Non-thermal, bio-stimulative	Helium neon 0.63 μm Gallium Aluminium Arsenide 0.83 μm	Fibre Fibre	Possible aid to healing/ regeneration/pain control	More research necessary to predict effect Class 3B
Excimer Non-thermal Photo-ablative	0.19–0.5 μm (ultraviolet)	Usually fibre	The potential for cold cutting of calcified tissues of bone and tooth	Expensive, bulky apparatus DNA effects possible (0.248 and 0.308 μm) Poor haemostasis Class 4
Erbium YAG Cutting of calcified tissue	2.94 μm (Mid infrared)	Mirrors (articulated arm)	Will cut bone and tooth (some risk of cracking phenomena)	Ablation rates rather slow Needs water coolant
TEA CO_2 Laser Transversely excited atmospheric	10.6 μm (Far infrared)	Mirrors (articulated arm)	Early stage of development Potential for bone and tooth	Still under investigation for optimal pulse characteristics

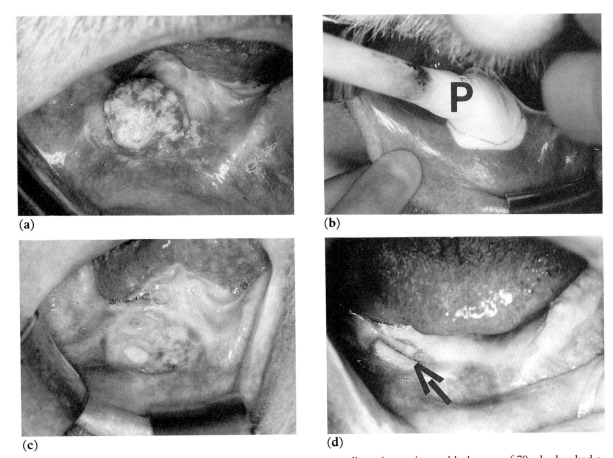

(a)

(b)

(c)

(d)

Fig. 10.1 The use of cryosurgery to treat a recurrent squamous cell carcinoma in an elderly man of 79 who has had a previous resection of lower alveolus and floor of mouth (with skin grafting) several years previously. The patient was infirm and unsuited for further surgery; radiotherapy would have had a poor outlook in a previously operated area with a diminished blood supply such as this. (a) Recurrent squamous cell carcinoma in skin grafted area. (b) Freezing the lesion with a liquid nitrogen probe (P). A double freeze employed using the two-thirds rule. (c) Slough separation at 2 weeks post-treatment. The area may be rebiopsied at this stage (Benson's Histologically Guided Cryosurgery). (d) Healed area at 3 months. An area of non-vital alveolar bone (arrow) is shown exposed to the mouth. This is quite common in such cases and will normally heal spontaneously after some months. No recurrence at 2 years post-operative.

further by the use of excisional techniques. There is as yet no large series of malignant oral tumours so treated, although most authors report favourable impressions. One study of 51 tumours cites a recurrence rate of 20 per cent,[29] while a second report gives the 5 year survival for squamous cell carcinoma of the tongue as 100 per cent for T1N0, 67 per cent for T2N0 and 50 per cent for more advanced tumours.[30]

Nd-YAG Laser

The neodymium yttrium aluminium garnet (Nd-YAG) laser can be used to carry out a thermal coagulation of oral soft tissue tumours using its near infrared wavelength of 1.06 microns which combines maximal tissue penetration with minimal absorption (i.e. the opposite of the CO_2 laser). Tissue coagulation requires temperatures around 60° C; it is possible to observe the coagulative effect quite accurately by naked eye in that the tissue is seen to whiten and shrink. This method has special application to benign vascular tumours such as haemangiomas (Fig. 10.4) and would be particularly suitable for malignancies with a marked vascular element.

The laser can be used in a contact or non-contact

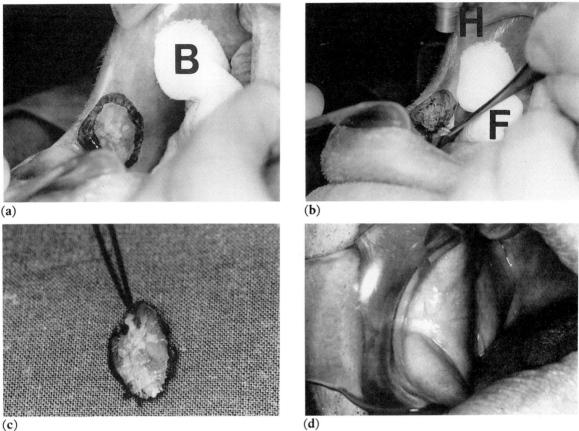

Fig. 10.2 Excision of a premalignant candidal leukoplakia with the CO_2 laser. Such a lesion has an approximate 25 per cent chance of becoming malignant. Preliminary treatment with antifungal agents had been unsuccessful. (a) A peripheral cut around the lesion, which is situated on the inner aspect of the lip, has been made with the laser to establish the correct depth. Note the wet swab acting as a beam stop (B). (b) Excision under way. The laser handpiece (H) is seen held at an angle to the lesion so that the beam can be used like a surgical scalpel. The lesion is being gently retracted by a pair of non-toothed forceps (F). (c) The excised specimen is shown which can be submitted for histology. There is minimal peripheral damage (about 200 microns) which should not hinder microscopic examination in any way. (d) The healed area at 6 weeks. Healing occurs with a normal soft texture mucosa. There is no danger of enclaving any neoplastic cells.

method – in either case it is commonly fibre-delivered. In this it differs from the CO_2 laser for which fibres have not as yet been developed (although flexible wave guides are available). The CO_2 wavelength is delivered by a series of mirrors housed in an articulated arm. A contact Nd-YAG probe can be used for excisional purposes and is useful in very well vascularised areas such as the posterior tongue. This utilises a sapphire end as a 'hot tip' rather than using the radiation itself to cut. There is also the potential to implant fibres into a tumour to carry out 'interstitial hyperthermia'. Alternatively combination lasers are now available where this wavelength may be blended with the

CO_2 wavelength through a handpiece (combination lasers[31]).

Clinical experience and animal experimental work has shown that the Nd-YAG laser produces significantly more oedema than the CO_2 laser and potentially more than with cryosurgery.[32] It should therefore be used with caution in regions such as the posterior tongue where airway problems may become apparent.

The first significant series of malignant tumours of the oral and maxillofacial region treated by Nd-YAG laser has recently been reported from China (30 cases[33]). Of the tumours 26 (87 per cent) disappeared clinically after the coagulative treatment

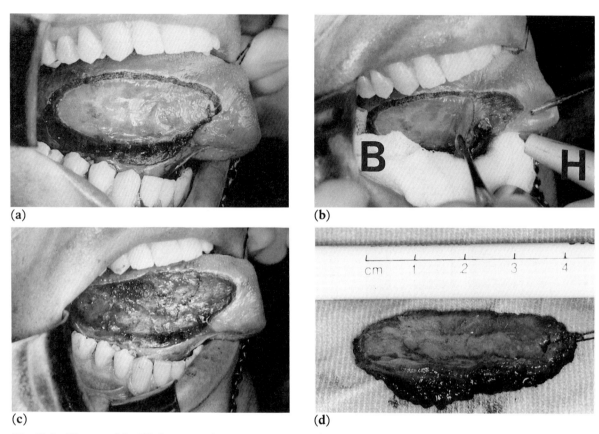

Fig. 10.3 The use of the CO_2 laser to excise an area of early micro-invasive squamous cell carcinoma of the lateral tongue in a young man of 24 years. The laser has an advantage over interstitial radiotherapy in an area of field change. Fifteen watts of power in continuous mode was used (approximately 10 watts continuous wave would be used for superficial cheek and lip lesions whereas 20–30 watts would be used for a hemiglossectomy). (a) Area of excision outlined with a peripheral depth cut. (b) Excision under way. The laser handpiece (H) is seen held at its focused distance. In order to achieve efficient cutting it is important to apply traction to the lesion and this is being carried out with a pair of non-toothed forceps. A wet swab is seen used as a beam stop (B) to protect neighbouring tissues from inadvertent exposure to the beam. (c) The excision bed is seen. The CO_2 laser coagulates vessels of 0.5 mm and below which gives good haemostasis in the anterior and mid-tongue. Larger vessels may however be encountered more posteriorly requiring the use of a defocused beam, diathermy or alternatively blending CO_2 with neodymium-YAG wavelength in a combination laser. (d) The excised specimen is seen which can be submitted for frozen section of its margins if deemed necessary and eventual full histological examination.

and there was no recurrence in the 2–4 year follow up period. Tumours with a diameter of less than 4 cm without deep infiltration and bone involvement were selected for treatment. Also there was one very large lip carcinoma of 7 × 4.5 cm which was successfully managed.

Holmium YAG laser/Ergium YAG/KTP

This laser functions in the mid-infrared range at 2.1 microns. It allows cutting with more moderate coagulation than with Nd-YAG and also the removal of bone in small amounts. It is usually employed as a contact method using fibre delivery. It appears potentially suitable for excisional purposes in vascular areas such as the posterior tongue or tonsillar fossa or nasal cavity: it is being successfully used, for example, for tonsillectomies. It can also be used for coagulation of small vascular lesions such as those in hereditary haemorrhagic telangiectasia. Bone may be excised in small amounts (as in endoscopic laser surgery for example) but this is

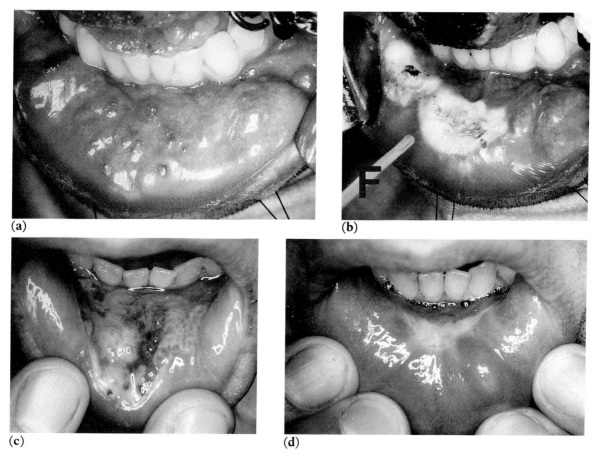

Fig. 10.4 Coagulation of a large angiomatous lesion of the lower lip with the neodymium-YAG laser. (a) Lower lip everted to show the extensive lesion, which shows a positive 'sign of emptying'. (b) Coagulation with the Nd-YAG laser using a fibre (F) in a non-contact method. The area of coagulation shrinks and whitens as can be seen. (c) Situation at 2 weeks when the thermally coagulated slough has separated. Whereas CO_2 laser therapy is associated with remarkably little pain, the patient should be warned after Nd-YAG treatment that there may be some discomfort at about 2–7 days postoperatively, which is adequately managed with non-steroidal anti-inflammatory agents. (d) The eventual healing of the lower lip is seen at 6 weeks. There is more scarring than one would anticipate with the CO_2 laser in view of the deeper degree of coagulation necessary with Nd-YAG in order to combat the highly vascular nature of the lesion. The price is worth paying however in that a successful result has been obtained with such a difficult clinical problem and function is very acceptable.

clinically not very applicable to malignancy surgery. It is of interest here that the Erbium YAG laser at 2.94 microns is a much more effective method of bone cutting although there may be some risk of cracking phenomena.[34,35]

The KTP (Potassium Titanyl Phosphate) is a recently available wavelength at 0.532 microns in the visible green. Like holmium it allows soft tissue cutting with more peripheral coagulation than CO_2 but less than Nd-YAG. It usually comes as a combination laser with Nd-YAG; indeed, the radiation is produced by a frequency doubling crystal of KTP from the basic 1.06 micron wavelength.

Adjunctive lasers

There are a number of laser wavelengths, which do not depend on thermal mechanisms, that may be useful as adjuncts in treatment of oral premalignant and malignant lesions in the future. The *Tunable dye laser* tuned to 0.63 microns is employed in combination with porphyrin sensitising agents (other agents will require their own specific wavelengths) as described in Chapter 11. Its successful use in photodynamic therapy has been described recently in a series of head and neck tumours.[36] This method could potentially be used after for example CO_2 laser excision to deal with MRD.

Low level lasers (LLL) such as the *Helium Neon* at 0.63 microns and the *Gallium Aluminium Arsenide* at 0.83 microns possess, it is claimed, biostimulative effects,[37,38] and as such could possibly aid in regeneration and pain control after excisional surgery. More research is necessary to be able confidently to predict such effects as yet. LLL acupuncture techniques are being developed which again could aid in pain relief.[39] Photo-ablative lasers such as the *Excimer wavelengths*, which function in the 0.19–0.35 microns ultraviolet wavelengths, have the potential of cold cutting calcified tissues such as bone and tooth.[12,40] They could be useful for approach procedures such as mandibulotomy. At the moment the apparatus is very bulky and expensive, while ablation rates are low. The Transversely Excited Atmospheric (TEA) CO_2 laser is currently showing promise for more rapid cutting of calcified tissues.[41]

Palliative uses

All methods of thermal surgery may be used for palliation of recurrent oral malignancies, particularly after the failure of conventional treatment such as excisional surgery or radiotherapy. Cryosurgery tends to produce rather too much oedema to be optimally useful although it may be combined with diathermy or CO_2 laser excision of the main tumour bulk with good effect and even occasional cure.[42] The effect of cryosurgery upon involved nerve branches may help in pain relief.[43] CO_2 lasers allow vapourisation of exophytic masses particularly if utilised with ultrapulsing or super pulsing.[44] The coagulative effects of more deeply penetrating wavelengths such as Nd-YAG may be useful in tumours causing problems by haemorrhage. Nd-YAG in high power can also be used to cause central vapourisation in addition to peripheral coagulation.[45] Patients may gain useful symptomatic relief from debulking of tumours by these techniques. The combination CO_2: Nd-YAG laser is proving valuable in this role.

The future

Thermal surgery already provides a range of useful techniques for the management of oral premalignant and malignant lesions. It allows interesting new regimes of therapy. Thermography is providing a useful laboratory method for understanding the spread of critical isotherms in thermal surgery,[46,47] for example the cell-lethal $-50°C$ in cryosurgery or $60°C$ for full tissue coagulation and $100°C$ for vapourisation effect in laser therapy. Thermal surgery's full potential will be realised in the future when better imaging techniques are established for tumour staging and when perfected means of treating MRD are available. These methods lend themselves well to combination with other modalities. For example, there is evidence that cryosurgery and cytotoxic therapy may act synergistically.[48] Anecdotal cases already show that remarkable results may be achieved occasionally by such combinations.[49] Careful study should allow predictable results to be obtained in the future.

One must not forget potential uses of lasers in repair techniques after malignancy resections; low power CO_2 radiation produces a sticky exudate which can be utilised in vascular and nerve anastomosis[50] particularly if combined with adjunctive adhesives.[51]

There is an intriguing report of low reactive level laser therapy (multi-wavelength diode cluster) being used in a small group of eight malignant ulcers for pain relief and to inhibit growth.[52]

The author advises oncologic surgeons of the head and neck region to 'watch this space carefully'.

References

1 Smith J, Fraser J. An estimation of tissue damage and thermal history in the cryolesion. *Cryobiology* 1974; **11**: 139–43.

2 Gage A. What temperature is lethal for cells? *Journal of Dermatologic Surgery and Oncology* 1979; **5**: 456–60.

3 Steger AC, Lees WR, Walmsley K, Bown SG. Interstitial laser hyperthermia: a new approach to local destruction of tumours. *British Medical Journal* 1989; **299**: 362–5.

4 Ablin RJ, Bradley PF. Immunologic aspects of cryosurgery. In Bradley PF ed. *Cryosurgery of the Maxillofacial Region*, Volume 1. Boca Raton, FL: CRC Press, 1986: 77–99.

5 Helpap B. Morphologic and cell kinetic investigations of the cryolesion (and thermolesion). In: Breitbart

EW, Dachow-Siwiec E eds. *Clinics in Dermatology*, Volume 2. New York: Elsevier, 1990: 5–29.

6 Onik G. Ultrasonic-guided hepatic cryosurgery in the treatment of metastatic colon carcinoma. *Cancer* 1991; **67**: 4. 901–7.

7 Takashima S, Ikezoe J, Harada K *et al*. Tongue cancer: correlation of MR imaging and sonography with pathology. *American Journal of Neuroradiology* 1989; **10**: 4. 419–24.

8 Benson JW. Combined therapy for intraoral cancer and histologically monitored cryosurgery. In: Bradley PF ed. *Cryosurgery of the Maxillofacial Region*, Volume 2. Boca Raton, FL: CRC Press, 1986: 31–54.

9 Carruth JAS. Photodynamic therapy. In: Carruth JAS, Simpson GT eds. *Lasers in Otolaryngology*. Cambridge: Chapman & Hall, 1988: 167–75.

10 Rao G, Kan PT, Howells R. Interstitial volume implants with I-125 seeds. *International Journal of Radiation Oncology, Biology, Physics* 1981; **7**: 431–8.

11 Wawrzynczak EJ, Thorpe PE. Monoclonal antibodies and therapy. In: Franks LM, Teich N eds. *Introduction to the Cellular and Molecular Biology of Cancer*. Oxford: Oxford Science Publications, 1986: 378–405.

12 Frentzen M, Koort HJ. Lasers in dentistry. *International Dental Journal* 1990; **40**: 323–32.

13 Koningsberger R. Endoscopically controlled laser lithotripsy in the treatment of sialolithiasis. *Laryngo-rhino-otologie* 1990; **69**: 322–3 (English abstract).

14 Bradley PF ed. *Cryosurgery of the Maxillofacial Region*, Volumes 1 and 2. Boca Raton, FL: CRC Press, 1986.

15 Bradley PF, Frame JW eds. *Lasers in the Oral Cavity*. In press.

16 Gage A, Bradley PF. Basic technique and monitoring. In: Bradley PF ed. *Cryosurgery of the Maxillofacial Region*, Volume 1. Boca Raton, FL: CRC Press, 1986: 123–52.

17 Benson JW. Combined chemotherapy and cryosurgery for oral cancer. *American Journal of Surgery* 1975; **130**: 596–600.

18 Gage AA. Five year survival after cryosurgery for carcinoma of the mouth. *Surgical and Gynecological Obstetrics* 1977; **145**: 189–92.

19 Li-Zi. Cryosurgery of 50 cases of tongue carcinoma. *Journal of Oral and Maxillofacial Surgery* 1991; **49**: 504–6.

20 Pospisil OA, MacDonald DG. The tumour potentiating effect of cryosurgery on carcinogen treated hamster cheek pouch. *British Journal of Oral Surgery* 1981; **19**: 96–104.

21 Bradley PF. The cryosurgery of bone in the maxillofacial region. In: Bradley PF ed. *Cryosurgery of the Maxillofacial Region*, Volume 2. Boca Raton, FL: CRC Press, 1986: 55–91.

22 Bradley PF. A two-stage procedure for reimplantation of autogenous freeze-treated mandibular bone.

Journal of Oral and Maxillofacial Surgery 1982; **40**: 278–84.

23 Bradley PF. *The cryosurgery of bone in the maxillofacial region*. MD thesis. University of London, 1989.

24 Frame JW. Carbon dioxide laser surgery for benign oral lesions. *British Dental Journal* 1985; **158**: 125–8.

25 Bradley PF. The CO_2 laser in the oral cavity: malignant tumours of the oral cavity. In: Oswal VH, Kashima HK, Flood LM eds. *The CO_2 Laser in Otolaryngology and Head and Neck Surgery*. London: Wright, 1988: 121–40.

26 Carruth JAS. Resection of the tongue with the CO_2 laser: 100 cases. *Journal of Laryngology and Otology* 1985; **99**: 887–9.

27 Roodenburg JLN, Panders AK, Vermey A. Precancerous lesions of the oral mucosa. In: Oswal VH, Kashima HK, Flood LM eds. *The CO_2 Laser in Otolaryngology and Head and Neck Surgery*. London: Wright, 1988: 116–20.

28 Poswillo D. Cryosurgery of benign and oral and orofacial lesions. In: Bradley PF ed. *Cryosurgery of the Maxillofacial Region*, Volume 1. Boca Raton, FL: CRC Press, 1986: 153–75.

29 Rhys Evans PH, Frame JW. CO_2 laser surgery in the oral cavity. In: Carruth JAS, Simpson GT eds. *Lasers in Otolaryngology*. Cambridge: Chapman & Hall, 1988: 101–32.

30 Carruth JAS, Rhys-Williams S. Control of malignant disease of the tongue using the CO_2 laser. *Abstracts of British Medical Laser Association Conference*, January 1986: 50.

31 Colles J. Future developments: multi-function laser. In: Oswal VH, Kashima HK, Flood LM eds. *The CO_2 Laser in Otolaryngology and Head and Neck Surgery*. London: Wright, 1988: 188–91.

32 Bradley PF, Elortegui O, Kisnisci R. Comparison of oedema formation after CO_2 laser, ND YAG laser and cryosurgery. *Lasers in Medical Science* 1992; **7**: 97–102.

33 Zhao FY, Zhang KH, Jiang MJ. The use of ND-YAG laser in the treatment of malignant tumours of the oral and maxillofacial regions. *Lasers in Medical Science* 1991; **6**: 209–12.

34 Small IA, Osbsorn TP, Fullert, Hussain N, Kobernick S. Observations of carbon dioxide laser and bone bur in the osteotomy of the rabbit tibia. *Oral Surgery* 1979; **78**: 159–66.

35 Charlton A, Dickinson MR, King TA, Freemont AJ. Erbium YAG and Holmium YAG laser ablation of bone. *Lasers in Medical Science* 1990; **5**: 365–9.

36 Zhao FY, Zhang KH, Jiang MJ. Photodynamic therapy for treatment of cancers in oral and maxillofacial regions: a long-term follow-up study in 72 complete remission cases. *Lasers in Medical Science* 1991; **6**: 201–4.

37 Pourreau-Schneider N. Helium neon laser treatment transforms fibroblasts into myofibroblasts. *American Journal of Pathology* 1990; **137**: 171–8.

38 Gray RJ, Quayle AA, Hall CA, Schofield MA. Physiotherapy in the treatment of temporomanibular joint disorders: a comparative study of four treatment methods. *British Dental Journal* 1994; **176**: 257–61.

39 Ho V, Bradley PF. Thermographic response to laser acupuncture. In: Lynn Powell G ed. *Proceedings of 3rd International Conference on Lasers in Dentistry*. Salt Lake City, UT: University of Utah Printing Services, 1992.

40 Frentzen M. Laser use on calcified tissues. In: Bradley PF, Frame JW eds. *Lasers in the Oral Cavity*. In press.

41 Melcer T, Fancy JC, Helias G, Badiane M. Ablation of mineralised dental tissues by the long-pulse TEA CO_2 laser. In: Lynn Powell G ed. *Proceedings of the 3rd International Congress on Lasers in Dentistry*. Salt Lake City, UT: University of Utah Printing Services, 1992: 227–8.

42 Gage AA. Cryosurgery of advanced tumours. In: Breitbart EW, Dachow-Siwiec E eds. *Clinics in Dermatology*, Volume 2. New York: Elsevier, 1990: 5–29.

43 Barnard D. Cryosurgery of nerve. In: Bradley PF ed. *Cryosurgery of the Maxillofacial Region*. Boca Raton, FL: CRC Press, 1986: 93–118.

44 Bradley PF. Ultrapulse vs continuous mode CO_2 laser on soft tissue. In: Lynn Powell G ed. *Proceedings of 3rd International Conference on Lasers in Dentistry*. Salt Lake City, UT: University of Utah Printing Services, 1992: 155–6.

45 McDonald GA, Strong S. Endoscopic laser surgery of the tracheo bronchial tree. In: Carruth JAS, Simpson GT eds. *Lasers in Otolaryngology*. London: Chapman & Hall, 1988: 93–9.

46 Bradley PF. Thermography as an aid to cryosurgery. *Acta Thermographica* 1977; **2**: 83–7.

47 Bradley PF, Whitnall M. Comparison of ND YAG laser, CO_2 laser and cryosurgery as a means of treatment of lesions of bone in the maxillofacial region. *Abstracts of 5th Annual Conference of British Medical Laser Association* 1987: 42.

48 Cooper AJ, Powell JR, Perry S, Fraser JD. Cyclophosphamide pretreatment in tumour cryotherapy: a murine model. *Cryobiology* 1981; **18**: 577–9.

49 Gage AA. Treatment of malignant soft tissue lesions of oral cavity, pharynx, face and scalp. In: Bradley PF ed. *Cryosurgery of the Maxillofacial Region*, Volume 2. Boca Raton, FL: CRC Press, 1986: 1–30.

50 Ruiz-Razura A. Laser-assisted microsurgical anastomoses in traumatised blood vessels. *Journal of Reconstructive Microsurgery* 1990; **6**: 55–9.

51 Ashton RC, Mehmet C, Oz MD *et al*. Laser assisted fibrinogen binding of vascular tissue. *Journal of Surgical Research* 1991; **51**: 324–8.

52 Humzah MD, Diamantopoulos C, Dyson M. Multiwavelength low reactive laser therapy (LLLT) as an adjunct in malignant ulcers; Case reports. *Laser Therapy* 1993; **5**: 149–52.

11 Photodynamic therapy in the management of tumours of the mouth, jaw and salivary glands

AF Jefferis

Photodynamic therapy (PDT) depends on the ability of some organic photosensitisers to localise in tumours. This renders them photosensitive, i.e. when tumours containing the compound are exposed to light of a suitable wavelength they undergo necrosis. Various photosensitising compounds have been used, notably the porphyrins. Impetus to investigation of this form of therapy has been given by the development of medical lasers, enabling high intensities of light to be delivered at specific wavelengths.

This form of treatment is different from all others conventionally used in cancer treatment in general and in head and neck malignancy in particular. Despite the impressive improvements in established methods of treatment such as surgery (especially reconstruction), radiotherapy and cytotoxic chemotherapy, about 30 per cent of patients with head and neck cancer will die from uncontrolled local disease. Any method of treatment which might improve this is to be welcomed. PDT is currently being investigated to see whether it might have a place in the treatment of head and neck malignancy.

Photosensitisation of living cells

Thoroughout this century there have been investigations into the photosensitising properties of various organic compounds. The earliest observations were made by illuminating paramecia suspended in solutions of various dyes including acridine. When the suspension was exposed to light there was cell death, whereas in the dark the cells remained alive.[1] In 1903 it was reported that painting human basal cell carcinomas with eosin and exposing them to light resulted in tumour regression in three patients.[2]

The use of porphyrins as possible photosensitisers was first explored using sheep red cells. These were shown to lyse in cell suspension when exposed to light in the presence of chlorophyll or haematoporphyrin.[3] It was found that human tumours had a high endogenous porphyrin content which caused them to fluoresce when exposed to blue light.[4] Later the systematic work of Figge *et al.*[5] showed that mice injected with haematoporphyrins selectively concentrated the haematoporphyrins in tissues of the reticulo-endothelial system, healing wounds and tumours.

The preferential tumour localisation of porphyrins had two features that could be relevant to cancer management; it rendered the cells *fluorescent* and *photosensitive*. The fluorescence caused the porphyrin bearing tumours to emit red light when illuminated with blue light.

The photosensitiser

In an attempt to find a potent and specific sensitiser, it was found that when haematoporphyrin was treated with acid and alkali it had better tumour localising properties than haematoporphyrin alone. This so-called 'haematoporphyrin derivative' or *Hpd* has been the most widely used photosensitiser both experimentally and clinically in studies on PDT.[6]

However, Hpd is a complex mixture of materials

with a variable level of activity. Part of the mixture has been found to be inactive *in vivo*. Much work has been carried out to determine the active component, which would appear to be a dimer, dihaematoporphyrin ether or ester.[7]

A partly purified component of Hpd, enriched in dihaematoporphyrin ether (DHE), has been marketed as 'Photofrin 2'.[8] Much of the recent experimental and clinical work has been with this material, which shares some of the disadvantages of Hpd, in that it has an incompletely defined composition and weak excitation by red light.

In an effort to find a pure compound which could be synthesised, and would not be subject to variation after preparation, Berenbaum and colleagues[9] looked at the photosensitising potential of a range of porphyrin derivatives. They compared the ability of a number of porphyrins, para-, meta- and ortho-isomers of meso-tetra(hydroxyphenyl)-porphyrin (p-THPP, m-THPP, o-THPP), the potassium salt of the para compound (K-p-THPP), DHE and Hpd, to sensitise tumours, normal brain and skin to light. Using inbred BALB/c mice and subcutaneous PC6 plasma cell tumour they found that the tissue selectivity of the potassium salt, the para and meta compounds of THPP were 25- to 30-fold more active than Hpd and DHE on a molar basis.

As well as the porphyrins other compounds are being investigated to see whether they have a potential for tumour photosensitisation. Chloro-aluminium sulphonated phthalocyanine (CASP), a pure compound, has certain properties that make it suitable for PDT. These include an action spectrum which is at 675 nm, a wavelength which allows deeper tissue penetration of light than Hpd (see below) and minimal skin photosensitivity.[10] Other compounds being investigated include chlorins,[11] pheophorbide[12] and rhodamine.[13] These compounds are chemically distinct from the porphyrins and are activated at different wavelengths, despite which the main features of their activity are similar. As there is also less general experience of their use, this chapter will be concerned mainly with the use of porphyrins in PDT.

Selectivity of uptake

Systemically administered porphyrins accumulate differentially in different tissues. This was first shown in mice, where injected haematoporphyrin fluoresced in omentum, placentae, embryos and lymphatics as well as in tumour.[5] Simple fluorescence, by itself, is an inadequate measure of tissue concentration, as tissues vary in their transmitting properties both for their activating and fluorescing wavelengths.

In order to establish the concentrations of Hpd in different tissues ^{3}H and ^{14}C labelled Hpd was injected into mice who had either spontaneous mammary cancer or tumours induced by methylcholanthrene. Seven tissues – tumour, liver, spleen, kidney, lung, skin and muscles – were assayed for radioactivity over a 72 hour period. During this time liver, spleen and kidney always had a higher concentration of label than tumour. During the first 24 hours the same applied for lung, but this then fell to levels below tumour concentrations. Skin and muscle levels were always below that of tumour.[14] Further work indicated that the concentrations were high in the stroma of the tumour rather than the tumour cells themselves. The stroma consists of cells of the reticulo-endothelial system, and this is thought to be the reason for the high concentrations in organs such as liver and spleen.[15]

This ability of normal tissues to absorb photosensitisers means that surrounding normal tissues might be damaged when a tumour is illuminated. The consequence of normal tissue damage will differ depending on which site is being treated. Reactions which are harmless at one site may be potentially lethal at others. The reaction of normal tissues should be examined at each site, to try to identify potential hazards. In the rabbit's oral cavity a series of experiments were undertaken using Hpd as a photosensitiser. It was found that a tumour implanted in the tongue could be damaged by PDT. There was also damage to the surrounding muscle, mucosa and blood vessels.[16]

This damage was found to recover over a period of weeks by a mixture of regeneration and scarring. Similar results were found after treating rat striated muscle using m- and p-THPP. Muscle was damaged, but there was complete recovery.[17]

Mechanism of action

In *in vitro* cell systems the cell membrane appears to be the major site of photodamage.[18] However there are other situations where Hpd penetrates the cell wall and cytoplasm, allowing photodamage to ribosomes, cytoplasmic nucleic acids, lysosomes, mitochondria and cytoplasmic proteins.[19] It is conceivable that Hpd may penetrate the nucleus and damage nucleic acids and chromosomes.[20]

Intracellular damage is thought to be mediated through the production of singlet oxygen, an unstable but highly reactive species. This reacts with various target molecules and is cytotoxic as it oxidises sensitive bonds.[21]

The main action of PDT is probably on the vasculature of the tumour. In a series of experiments, mice and rats with different tumours were first sensitised with DHE. The tumour was then illuminated with light at 630 nm, and slowing of the blood flow through the tumour and surrounding vasculature was seen. This slowing became evident at 10 seconds and reached a maximum at 5 mins after illumination. It appears to be dose-dependent.[22] It has also been claimed that if mice bearing tumours are treated with PDT, and the cells are taken from the treated surface and cultured *in vitro*, there is no loss in viability if this is done immediately after exposure to light. However, if the cells are left *in situ* for 1 to 10 hours before removal they show progressive tumour cell death. The rate at which this tumour cell death occurs is the same as occurs if the mouse is killed. This indicates that tumour cell death is dependent on the blood flow of the tumour.[23] Further evidence of interruption of blood flow as the cause of tumour necrosis in PDT has come from the observation that there is sludging of red blood cells in capillaries 24 hours after treatment followed by intimal damage. At between 48 and 72 hours there is angioneogenesis, and the integrity of the vasculature is eventually re-established.[17,18]

Light sources

Several factors influence the choice of the light source.

(1) *The action spectrum of the photosensitiser.* Photochemical processes depend on the wavelength of the exciting light, the so-called 'action spectrum.' Photoreactive molecules absorb certain wavelengths of light preferentially; their absorption spectrum. In simple systems the action and absorption spectra correspond. Hpd, DHE, m- and p-THPP all have major absorption bands at 500 nm, with weaker ones at 630 nm (Hpd and DHE) and 656 nm (m-THPP and p-THPP).

(2) *Tissue penetration of the wavelength of light chosen.* Preferential tissue penetration occurs at the red end of the spectrum and into the near infrared, i.e. between 600 and 1000 nm. It varies from about 0.5 cm at 600 nm to about 2 cm at 1000 nm. The depth of penetration also depends on the nature of the tissue illuminated, and pigmented tissue quenching the light allowing less effective penetration.

Light sources used in photodynamic therapy produce light at 630 nm for Hpd and DHE, 656 nm for THPP and 675 nm for CASP. These wavelengths give preferential tissue penetration and correspond to an absorption band of the photosensitisers.

(3) *The power of the light required.* The light source should be able to deliver light of the wavelength required. Historically this was done with a Xenon arc lamp producing white light, which was then passed through a series of filters. This removed unwanted wavelengths and heat generated by the light source. This method of producing light for PDT has several disadvantages: it is difficult to produce light of a single specific wavelength; it is difficult to filter out all the heat; and the low intensity of light at the activating wavelength means that light has to be administered for long periods.

The use of the laser has overcome these drawbacks.

Laser light

Laser light has four advantages in overcoming the problems arising from the difficulty in providing the exact power of light required:

(1) It is emitted in parallel beams.
(2) It has a wavelength spread which is many orders of magnitude smaller than a non-laser light source.
(3) It is coherent: that is its wavefronts are consistent and can be predicted
(4) It can be transmitted down optical fibres, with little loss in intensity.

Lasers which have been used in PDT are:

(1) the Argon laser, pumping a Rhodamine B dye laser, capable of being tuned over 20–30 nm around 600 nm without significant loss in power;
(2) the Gold vapour laser which has a pulsed emission at 633 nm;
(3) the Copper vapour laser, pumping a Rhodamine

640 dye laser, with outputs tunable to 625 nm and 656 nm.

The light dosage

The power of the light source is measured in watts. The original arc lamps had outputs of hundreds or thousands of watts, but only small amounts, tens of milliwatts, were available at the right wavelengths, as much of the power was wasted in heat. The lasers in current use in PDT produce usable outputs up to 10 watts at the required wavelengths. It has not been finally resolved as to what powers are needed, but the range of powers used are between 5 mW/cm^2 for thin surface lesions and 500 mW/cm^2 for interstitial lesions. Total doses are measured in joules/cm^2 (1 joule = 1 watt/second). The range in PDT is between 20 and 200 joules/cm^2, apart from one report which uses doses up to 1620 joules/cm^2 (see below). Illumination times at 1 watt/cm^2 are 20 seconds for 20 joules and 200 seconds for 200 joules.

Clinical experience

The first use of Hpd in PDT was by Lipson *et al.*[24] They treated a patient with recurrent carcinoma of the breast using a Xenon arc lamp, the spectrum not being specified, and there was evidence of tumour regression. It was not until the mid 1970s that further clinical experience was obtained. Initially all types of advanced tumour were treated.

One of the problems confronting the initial investigators was how to transmit sufficient activating light to the tumour. This was certainly the problem experienced by Kelly and Snell.[25] In an earlier set of experiments they found that transplants of human bladder cancer were photosensitive but that bladder mucosa was not. Two bladders with active cancer, which were to be removed at cystectomy, were treated with Hpd and light. The light came from a mercury vapour lamp and was transmitted down a quartz rod in a cystoscope. The cystoscope became very hot, and although there were areas of necrosis in the resected specimen, it was not clear whether these were the results of photo- or thermal damage.

Other early investigators treated a disparate group of tumours.[26–29] This was the era before the ready availability of dye lasers and fibre-optic light transport systems, and so the tumours treated were all superficial. Most of the patients treated had recurrent breast cancer on the chest wall. The light source was a 5000 watt Xenon arc lamp, giving as filtered light 25 per cent of its emitted spectrum at between 620 and 640 nm. Patients were given between 2.5 and 5.0 mg Hpd. Recurrences on the chest wall were found to be sensitive to this treatment, there being a 97 per cent response rate (34 of 35), response being defined as a reduction of tumour mass by at least 50 per cent. Despite these good response rates, the treatment of breast cancer highlights the limitations of PDT. Seven patients died, all with metastatic disease. At the time of treatment the breast cancer was already metastatic and no purely local form of treatment could be curative. That is not to say that some measure of local control of disease is not desirable in patients with widespread metastases.

Other tumours treated in this pioneering work included both primary tumours (basal cell carcinomas, recurrent squamous cell carcinoma, mycosis fungoides, Kaposi's sarcoma) and secondary deposits (angiosarcoma, parotid carcinoma, chondrosarcoma, colonic carcinoma, endometrial carcinoma, retinoblastoma, liposarcoma and malignant melanoma). In this varied collection of advanced tumours there was a response, biopsy proven necrosis, or reduction in size of more than 50 per cent in 65 of 70 non-pigmented tumours. There was no response in the six pigmented melanomas treated.

Following these initial investigations with a range of tumours, subsequent work has concentrated on evaluating the potential place for PDT in groups of anatomically similar tumours; the bladder,[30] the bronchus,[31] the oesophagus,[32] the peritoneal cavity[33] and the upper aerodigestive tract.[34–37]

Initial reports in the head and neck were promising; Wile *et al.*[34] treated 114 sites of recurrent cancer in 39 patients and observed complete remissions in 25 per cent and partial remissions in another 40 per cent. Several complete remissions lasted at least 1 year with a considerable improvement in the patients' condition. No histological data was reported and the remissions were assessed by clinical criteria alone at 1 month following treatment. Longer follow up does not give such a favourable picture; Schuller *et al.*[35] followed 19 patients and found only two free of disease at 4 months or more. In 15 patients the disease had progressed within 6 weeks of an initial response. This rather gloomy assessment has been echoed by Gluckman.[36] Reviewing the 41 cases which he had treated with PDT over a 5 year period, he found that in those with advanced disease there was no improvement in their condition. Those with early disease who had refused conventional treatment showed a slightly brighter picture; of the eight patients with disease in the oral cavity there were four who had no evidence of disease, while the other four recurred. Of the eight patients with 'condemned mucosa' six were disease-free, one recurred requiring surgery and another died of an intercurrent disease.

At variance with these disappointing results is the work of Zhao *et al.*[37] They reported 114 cases of head and neck malignancy treated with PDT, using Hpd. There were 72 complete remissions. The tumours treated were the oral mucous membrane (63), the upper lip (3), the lower lip (49), the buccal mucosa (5), tongue (4), palate (1), minor salivary gland (1), salivary gland tumour of the hard palate (10) and facial skin (8). The doses they reported are much higher than those used in the rest of the literature, rising to 1620 joules/cm^2. The results were especially favourable for T1 and T2 tumours, with only 6 of 47 recurrences at 3 years. In T3 tumours 6 of 17 recurred. The tumours with which they found most difficulty were those at the posterior third of the tongue and the posterior part of the oral cavity. Although these results are interesting the experience is not directly transferrable. They reported success in the very tumours which conventional treatment usually cures. However it might give some signals for the future, one being that the use of high doses of light might be safer than has hitherto been thought, and there seems to be no specific biological reason why squamous cell carcinoma in the head and neck will not respond to PDT. The other implication of their work is that the hyperthermic effects of laser light may be tumouricidal. The synergistic effect of hyperthermia has been noted by others.[38]

Side effects and morbidity

The main side effects reported in all series is skin photosensitivity for up to 4 weeks following treatment. In a recent report on 180 patients who had received DHE, one in three had cutaneous photosensitivity, regardless of the dose and any advice which they were given.[39]

The main cause of morbidity is local normal tissue necrosis. This is most worrying when there is damage to the local arterial blood supply.

Damage to local blood vessels causing troublesome, even fatal, haemorrhage has been reported.[28,31] In treating the chest there was occasionally chest wall necrosis. Patients experienced pain when large areas of tumour were treated at one time. When large tumours were destroyed the patient experienced malaise and fever in the following month. There was also some hyperpigmentation in the treated area in some patients.

The future

There are good theoretical grounds for investigating the use of PDT in the oral cavity:

(1) the majority of tumours arise from a mucous membrane and are usually situated within a centimetre of a surface accessible to light;
(2) many tumours remain localised;
(3) in the case of tumours which recur after the failure of primary treatment and those which are advanced when first seen, current treatment fails in the majority of cases.

The majority of clinical work so far reported has been undertaken using Hpd and DHE. With the development of pure compounds that are more selective in their localisation in tumours, this form of treatment still holds much promise. The place for it may be as an adjunct to other forms of treatment, for example treating the resection margins after a surgical excision. It has the advantage that it can be used repeatedly at the same site without apparent deleterious effect.

References

1 Raab O. Ueber die wirkung fluorescinder stoffe auf infusorien. *Zeitschrift fur Biologie* 1900; **39**: 524–46.
2 Tappenier H, Jesionek A. Therapeutische versuche mit fluoreszierenden. *Muenchener Medizinische Wochenschrift* 1903; **1**: 2042–3.
3 Hausmann W. Die sensibilisierende wirkung des haematoporphrins. *Biochemische Zeitschrift* 1911; **30**: 276–316.
4 Policard A. Etudes sur les aspects offerts par des tumour experimentales examinee a la lumiere de Woods. *Comptes Rendus Societe Biologie* 1924; **91**: 1423–4.
5 Figge FHJ, Weilland GS, Manganiello OJ. Cancer detection and therapy. Affinity of neoplastic, embryonic and traumatised regenerating tissues for porphy-

rins and metalloporphyrins. *Proceedings of the Society of Experimental Biology and Medicine* 1948; **68:** 640–1.

6 Lipson RL, Baldes EJ, Olsen AM. The use of a derivative of haematoporphyrin in tumour detection. *Journal of the National Cancer Institute* 1960; **2:** 1–8.

7 Berenbaum MC, Bonnett R, Scourides PA. *In vivo* biological activity of the components of haematoporphyrin derivative. *British Journal of Cancer* 1982; **45:** 571–81.

8 Dougherty TJ, Potter WR, Weishaupt KR. The structure of the active component of haematoporphyrin derivative. In: Andreoni A, Cubeddu R eds. *Porphyrins in Tumour Phototherapy.* New York: Plenum Press, 1983: 22–35.

9 Berenbaum MC, Akande SL, Bonnett R *et al.* meso-Tetra(hydroxyphenyl)porphyrins, a new class of potent tumour photosensitisers with favourable selectivity. *British Journal of Cancer* 1986; **54:** 717–25.

10 Stern SJ, Thomsen S, Small S, Jacques S. Photodynamic therapy with chloraluminium-sulfonated phthalocyanine. *Archives of Otolaryngology – Head and Neck Surgery* 1990; **116:** 1259–66.

11 Kessel D, Dutton CJ. Photodynamic effects; porphyrin vs chlorin. *Photochemistry and Photobiology* 1984; **40:** 403–5.

12 Yano T, Uozumi T, Kawamoto K *et al.* Photodynamic therapy for rat pituitary tumour *in vitro* and *in vivo* using Pheophorbide and a white light. *Lasers in Surgery and Medicine* 1991; **11:** 171–82.

13 Castro DJ, Gaskin A, Saxton RE, Reisler E, Nishimura E, To SY. Photodynamic therapy using rhodamine-123 as a new laser dye; biodistribution, metabolism and histology in New Zealand rabbits. *Laryngoscope* 1991; **101:** 158–64.

14 Gomer CJ, Dougherty TJ. Determination of (^{3}H) and (^{14}C) haematoporphyrin derivative in malignant and normal tissue. *Cancer Research* 1979; **39:** 146–51.

15 Bugelski PJ, Porter CW, Dougherty TJ. Autoradiographic distribution of haematoporphyrin derivative in normal and tumour tissue of the mouse. *Cancer Research* 1981; **41:** 4606–12.

16 Jefferis AF, Chevretton EB, Berenbaum MC. Muscle damage and recovery in the rabbit tongue following photodynamic therapy with haematoporphyrin derivative. *Acta Otolaryngologica* 1991; **111:** 153–60.

17 Chevretton EB. *The effect of photodynamic therapy on normal skeletal muscle and intramuscular tumour in an animal model,* MSc thesis. University of London, 1989.

18 Kessel D. Effects of photoactivated porphyrins at the cell surface of L1210 cells. *Biochemistry* 1977; **16:** 3443–9.

19 Spikes JD. Photobiology of porphyrins (abstract). In: *Proceedings of workshop on porphyrin photosensitisation.* Santa Barbara, California 1983.

20 Christensen T. Multiplication of human NHIK 3025

cells exposed to porphyrins in combination with light. *British Journal of Cancer* 1981; **44:** 433–9.

21 Weishaupf KR, Gomer CJ, Dougherty TJ. Identification of singlet oxygen as the cytotoxic agent in photo-inactivation of a murine tumour. *Cancer Research* 1976; **36:** 2326–9.

22 Wieman TJ, Mong TS, Finger VH. Effect of photodynamic therapy on blood flow in normal and tumour vessels. *Surgery* 1988; **104:** 512–17.

23 Henderson BW, Dougherty TJ. Studies on the mechanism of tumour destruction by photoradiation therapy (PRT). In: *Proceedings of the Clayton Foundation symposium on porphyrin localization and treatment of tumours, Santa Barbara, California* 1983.

24 Lipson RL, Baldes EJ, Gray MJ. Haematoporphyrin derivative for detection and management of cancer. *Cancer* 1967; **20:** 2225–7.

25 Kelly JF, Snell ME. Haematoporphyrin derivative, a possible aid in the diagnosis and therapy of carcinoma of the bladder. *Journal of Urology* 1976; **115:** 150–1.

26 Dougherty TJ, Kaufman JE, Goldfarb A, Weishaupf KR, Boyle D, Mittleman A. Photoradiation therapy for the treatment of malignant tumours. *Cancer Research* 1978; **38:** 2628–35.

27 Trenniert Donker A. In: *Proceedings of the UICC workshop on haematoporphyrin derivative for the detection and treatment of cancer, Roswell Park Memorial Institute, Buffalo, New York* 1979.

28 Kennedy JC. In: *Proceedings of the UICC workshop on haematoporphyrin derivative for the detection and treatment of cancer, Roswell Park Memorial Institute, Buffalo, New York* 1979.

29 Forbes IJ, Cowled PA, Leong AS-Y *et al.* Phototherapy of human tumours using haematoporphyrin derivative. *Medical Journal of Australia* 1980; **2:** 489–93.

30 Benson RC Jr, Kinsey JH, Cortese DA, Farrow GM, Utz DC. Treatment of transitional cell carcinoma of the bladder with haematoporphyrin derivative phototherapy. *Journal of Urology* 1983; **130:** 1090–5.

31 Cortese DA, Kinsey JH. Endoscopic management of lung cancer with haematoporphyrin derivative phototherapy. *Mayo Clinic Proceedings* 1982; **57:** 543–7.

32 McCaughan JS, Hicks W, Laufman L, May E, Roach R. Palliation of oesophageal malignancy with photoradiation therapy. *Cancer* 1984; **54:** 2905–10.

33 Sindelar WF, Delaney TF, Tochner Z *et al.* Technique of photodynamic therapy for disseminated intraperitoneal malignant neoplasms. Phase 1 study. *Archives of Surgery* 1991; **126:** 318–24.

34 Wile AG, Coffey J, Nahebedian MY, Baghdassarian R, Mason GR, Berns MW. Laser photoradiation of cancer. An update of the experience of the University of California, Irvine. *Lasers in Surgery and Medicine* 1984; **4:** 5–12.

35 Schuller DE, McCaughan JE, Rock RP. Photody-

namic therapy in head and neck cancer. *Archives of Otolaryngology – Head and Neck Surgery* 1985; **111:** 351–5.

36 Gluckman JL. Haematoporphyrin photodynamic therapy; is there truly a future in head and neck oncology? Reflections on a 5 year experience. *Laryngoscope* 1991; **101:** 36–42.

37 Zhao FY, Zhang KH, Jiang F, Wu MJ. Photodynamic therapy for treatment of cancers in oral and maxillofacial regions; a long term follow up study in 72 complete remission cases. *Lasers in Medical Science* 1991; **6:** 201–4.

38 Matsumoto N, Salto H, Miyoshi N, Nakanshi K, Fukuda M. Combination effect of hyperthermia and photodynamic therapy on carcinoma. *Archives of Otolaryngology – Head and Neck Surgery* 1990; **116:** 824–9.

39 Dougherty TJ, Cooper MT, Mang TS. Cutaneous phototoxic occurrences in patients receiving photofrin. *Lasers in Surgery and Medicine* 1990; **10:** 485–8.

12 Carcinoma of the oral cavity – management of the primary tumour

JM Henk and JD Langdon

Choice of treatment – surgery or radiotherapy?

The principal treatments available for primary tumours remain surgery and radiotherapy. The basic decision to be made is between radical radiotherapy and elective surgery. If the former is chosen surgery is reserved for 'salvage', i.e. for biopsy proven recurrent or residual disease. If surgery is chosen, radiotherapy may be used in an adjuvant manner, either pre- or postoperatively, but the operation remains the fundamental definitive curative procedure. Preferences for one or other policy vary considerably between treatment centres.

Differences in treatment partly reflect differences in resources and expertise, and in the pattern of disease in various parts of the world. It is unfortunately true also that differences in treatment policy reflect referral patterns and the individual opinions of clinicians to whom the patients are initially referred.

Claims are often made for the superiority of one particular treatment policy over another, either on the basis of outcome or quality of life, which are impossible to substantiate. Satisfactory randomised controlled trials are unlikely ever to be performed because of the heterogeneity of oral cancer, the large number of patients needed to obtain a statistically significant result, and the difficulty in obtaining informed consent.

The major argument in favour of initial radical radiotherapy is that some patients will be cured without surgery and therefore will be spared the possible hazards of deformity and disability which may result from a major operation. A proportion of those in whom radiotherapy fails can be treated successfully surgically, whereas the converse is not true – radiotherapy rarely cures a patient who develops a recurrence after initial surgery. Because of the possibility of surgical salvage, long term survival rates of a policy of radical radiotherapy should be no different from those of a policy of elective surgery. Against this it can be argued that salvage surgery after radiotherapy failure is more difficult, hazardous and less often successful than primary surgery. Salvage surgery necessitates operating on heavily irradiated tissues with consequent fibrosis, poor vasculature and a reduced capacity for healing. Recurrences after radiotherapy tend to be deeply infiltrating and the extent can be difficult to define; indeed it is quite common for the superficial part of the tumour to disappear completely and mucosa heal over it, yet malignant cells survive in the deeper part of the tumour and continue to spread in muscle or bone. Furthermore the routes of tumour spread following radiotherapy are unpredictable and no longer follow the usual patterns. Consequently the failure and complication rates of salvage surgery are greater than those of elective surgery.

Many factors must be considered in deciding the optimum management for each individual patient. These include the site, stage and histology of the tumour and the medical condition and lifestyle of the patient. Ideally every patient should be seen at a joint consultation clinic by a surgeon and radiotherapist who assess objectively and agree the optimum strategy of management for that particular individual. The following factors should influence the decision on treatment policy.

Site of origin

The choice of treatment depends on the part of the mouth in which the tumour arises. The management of primary tumours at the various anatomical sites are discussed later in this chapter. In general, surgery is preferred for those tumours arising on or involving the alveolar processes; for other sites surgery and radiotherapy are alternatives.

Stage of disease

A small lesion which can be excised readily without producing any deformity or disability is in general best managed surgically. Surgery is also usually more appropriate for a very large mass or where there is invasion of bone, provided the tumour is operable, because of the low cure rates by radiotherapy in these circumstances. The management of lesions of intermediate stage, i.e. larger T1, most T2 and early exophytic T3 tumours is more controversial, as policies of elective surgery or radical radiotherapy produce generally similar survival rates; hence discussion centres on the likely functional results and morbidity of either approach.

If the primary tumour is so advanced as to be unresectable it is unlikely that any treatment will be successful. Many such tumours are treated with radiotherapy or chemotherapy with a very occasional spectacular response, but often nothing useful is achieved.

When there is involvement of cervical lymph nodes the primary tumour and nodes are normally both treated surgically. However, there is no clear evidence that a primary tumour is less likely to be cured by radiotherapy in the presence of lymph node metastases than in their absence.[1] An acceptable policy in a patient with an intermediate stage primary and a lymph node metastasis is to give external beam radiotherapy to both primary site and neck to a dose of 40–50 Gy, followed by an iridium wire implant to the primary and a neck dissection.

Previous irradiation

It is not advisable to re-treat a tumour arising in previously irradiated tissue. Such a tumour is likely to be relatively radioresistant because of limited blood supply. Also re-irradiation of normal tissue is very likely to result in necrosis.

Field change

Where multiple primary tumours are present, or if there is extensive premalignant change, surgery is the preferred treatment. Radiotherapy in these circumstances is unsatisfactory; irradiation of the entire oral cavity causes severe morbidity and may not prevent subsequent new primary tumours arising from areas of premalignant change. When a second primary occurs within or immediately adjacent to an irradiated area, a second course of radiotherapy carries a high risk of necrosis, while surgery for the second primary will be subject to a higher complication rate because of the previous radiotherapy.

Histology

The histology report on a biopsy specimen has a relatively small influence on choice of treatment. The less common adenocarcinoma and melanoma are relatively radioresistant and therefore should be treated surgically whenever possible. The grade of malignancy of a squamous carcinoma does not normally influence its management, there being little evidence to suggest that a well differentiated primary should be treated differently from a poorly differentiated one. Poorly differentiated tumours are associated with a higher incidence of lymphatic spread and therefore a worse prognosis, but the local response of the primary to treatment is not related to the histological grade (see Chapter 3). There is the additional problem that a biopsy specimen may not be representative of the entire lesion, and so it is unwise to base a treatment decision on the degree of differentiation seen in the biopsy.

A possible exception is the verrucous carcinoma (Fig. 12.1), which is the subject of much controversy. The observation was made by Perez *et al.*[2] that where large lesions of this histological type were treated by radiotherapy recurrences appeared in some cases which were of a much more anaplastic pattern than the original primary, and it became widely accepted that radiotherapy induces 'anaplastic transformation'. However, other authors have claimed that there is no difference in radiation response between verrucous and other types of squamous carcinoma, and that they should be treated similarly. For example, Vidyasagar *et al.*[3] reported 107 cases of oral verrucous carcinoma treated by radiotherapy with the same results as for squamous cell carcinoma. In an extensive review of the literature McDonald *et al.*[4] refer to several patients who developed anaplastic transformation after local excision or biopsy without radiotherapy. It seems probable that some verrucous carcinomas already contain foci of more malignant cells prior to treatment, and that these cells are the ones most likely to survive after radiotherapy and give rise to recurrence. In practice most verrucous carcinomas present at an early stage as superficial exophytic lesions and are suitable for local excision. When they cannot be excised locally the weight of evidence suggests that they can be dealt with safely in the same way as squamous carcinomas of other types, and either surgery or radiotherapy can be chosen as the primary treatment modality according to the site and stage of the lesion and the condition of the patient.

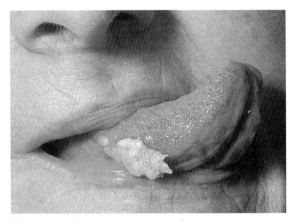

Fig. 12.1   Verrucous carcinoma of tongue.

Age

The patient's age is often quoted as an important factor which must be taken into account when deciding on a course of management. With a young patient there is the fear that if radiotherapy is given it may induce a malignancy in years to come; in fact this risk is very small compared with the mortality of the disease itself. Elderly patients tend to be poor surgical risks, but on the other hand they also tend to do badly with radiotherapy, especially external radiotherapy, and often deteriorate and may die as a result of the debility and poor nutritional status induced by the irradiation. Elderly patients are more likely to be treated by radiotherapy than by surgery, but this is not necessarily always wise. Chronological age *per se* should not necessarily be regarded as a contra-indication to

surgery. Each patient should be assessed according to general medical fitness for a particular treatment. If the patient is elderly, in very poor general condition and with advanced disease, it may be better not to attempt any specific anticancer measures.

Personality

The patient's personality and way of life are important factors which must be considered when deciding on the mode of treatment. An attempt should be made to assess how the patient may react to the differing type of trauma associated with surgery or radiotherapy. Surgery for advanced disease inevitably results in some degree of deformity and difficulty with feeding, however skilled the reconstruction, so an attempt should be made to assess the possibility of rehabilitation and the chance of resuming a normal life. In general men are more likely than women to resume normal activity after a major head and neck operation.

The alcoholic patient who continues smoking has a high risk of postradiation complications, and in some cases it may be preferable to treat by surgery rather than radical radiotherapy. A patient who is thought unlikely to attend regularly for follow up because of personality, alcoholism or other reasons is best treated primarily by surgery, because where radical radiotherapy is employed careful follow up and early institution of salvage surgery in the event of recurrence is essential. Treatment for recurrence after surgery is usually of little or no avail so that failure to attend for follow up is less likely to prejudice survival after surgery than after radiotherapy.

The problem of the excision biopsy

Very small lesions can often be cured by excision biopsy. For example Stell *et al.*[5] described a series of 20 patients so treated, representing 6.4 per cent of a large series of oral carcinoma. In all cases the excision margins were clear histologically and no patients developed local recurrence, although two developed lymph node metastases, which emphasises the importance of careful follow up even for small lesions.

The problem arises when a radiotherapist is presented with a patient for whom the diagnosis of intra-oral carcinoma has been established by excision biopsy and for whom the histology report indicates involved or inadequate excision margins. Radiotherapy has an excellent chance of eliminating the small population of residual cells in such a case.[6]

However, the patient referred after an excisional biopsy can present difficulties to a radiotherapist who did not see the original lesion. Often by the time the patient arrives in the radiotherapist's clinic the mouth appears normal, with not even the scar of excision visible, and there may be no clear record of the exact size and position of the lesion. Very good results can undoubtedly be obtained by excisional biopsy plus radiotherapy, but in order to achieve these it is important that the radiotherapist sees the patient prior to excision, or is presented with an accurate description of the lesion, preferably with the aid of a photograph.

Carcinoma of the lip

Carcinoma of the lip most commonly arises at the vermilion border of the lower lip away from the line of contact with the upper lip. Only 15 per cent arise from the central third and commissure regions, and 5 per cent from the upper lip.

Initially the tumours tend to spread laterally rather than infiltrating deeply; eventually, if uncontrolled, they can spread into the anterior triangle of the neck and invade the mandible. Lymph node metastases occur late.

Both surgery and radiotherapy are frequently employed and are highly effective methods of treatment, each giving cure rates of about 90 per cent.[7]

For these reasons the choice of treatment for an individual patient will often depend on available resources and the personal preferences of the clinicians involved. In the short term the cosmetic appearance is better after radiotherapy than after surgery. However, as years go by surgical scars tend to fade whereas late radiation atrophy becomes more prominent, so in the long term the cosmetic results of good surgery are better than those of radiotherapy. Surgery should definitely be preferred for young patients because of the long term cosmetic result, and also because of the slight risk of radiation-induced tumours. Surgery is also preferable in those patients for whom there is a continued exposure to a risk factor, e.g. farmers and fishermen who are still actively at work. For a small lesion surgery which requires only 1 or 2 nights in hospital is generally considered more convenient than a course of radiotherapy involving a number of outpatient attendances. The patient who dislikes surgery or who is unfit for general anaesthetic can be treated equally effectively with radiotherapy. Radiotherapy should also be considered for larger lesions in older patients, where surgery would involve a more extensive procedure and a longer period of hospitalisation.

Surgery

Up to one-third of the lower lip can be removed with a V or W shaped excision with primary closure. This method is suitable for tumours up to 2 cm in diameter. The residual defect is reconstructed by approximating and suturing the borders in three layers; mucosa, muscle and skin. Particular attention should be paid to the correct alignment of the vermilion junction. This simple procedure can readily be performed under local anaesthetic on an outpatient basis. Initially the lip will appear tight, but this improves after about 3 months.

If more than one-third of the lip is removed, primary closure results in microstomia.[8] Therefore for more extensive lip resections it is necessary to utilise local flaps for reconstruction. For large central defects of the lower lip, particularly in patients who do not have ageing wrinkled faces, the 'step-ladder' approach of Johanson[9] gives excellent cosmesis as the reconstruction advances symmetrical bilateral flaps from the lower third of the face (Fig. 12.2). This results in a 'mini facelift' and the scars are concealed in the labiomental groove around the chin point. For defects more laterally, in the lower lip, the upper lip and particularly involving the commissure, Fries' 'universal procedure' gives excellent functional results with acceptable cosmesis especially in the ageing face.[10] With this technique, lateral facial flaps are developed following full thickness incisions in the cheeks parallel to the branches of the facial nerve. These flaps are then advanced into the lip defect with the sacrifice of Burrows' triangles to prevent piling up of the facial tissues. The majority of lower lip cancers are caused by ultraviolet radiation and often the entire vermilion border will show actinic changes. Whenever these changes are seen a total lip shave should be undertaken in addition to resection of the primary tumour. The resection is reconstructed either by advancing labial or buccal mucosal flaps or, if such tissue is inadequate, by the use of a pedicled anteriorly based tongue flap. After 3 weeks the pedicle is divided and the flap finally set into the lip.

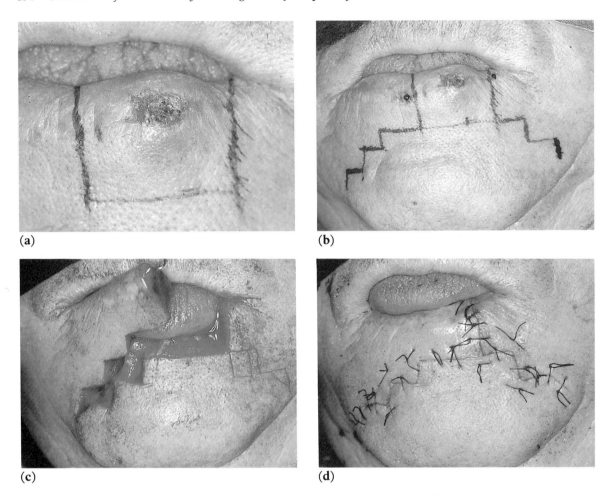

Fig. 12.2 (a) Advanced carcinoma of the lip with excision margins marked. (b) The resulting defect requires local advancement flap for reconstruction. (c) The step-ladder technique described by Johanson *et al.*[9] is being used. (d) Appearance immediately following reconstruction.

Radiotherapy

There are four possible methods of radiotherapy for carcinoma of the lip.

X-ray therapy

This is the simplest and most often used method. The oral cavity is shielded by a piece of lead slipped into the labial sulcus behind the tumour. An external lead cutout is usually used to define the area to be treated, and a single anterior field employed, the energy being chosen according to the thickness of the lesion, usually 100–140 kV. We usually give a dose of 50 Gy in 15 fractions over 3 weeks. Some radiotherapists prefer longer fractionation sched-

ules, claiming better cosmetic results, but there is no clear evidence for this and treatment over 4 weeks or more becomes very taxing on the patient and in terms of convenience and cost compares unfavourably with surgery. Fewer fractions can be used for elderly or infirm patients who have difficulty travelling to hospital. Dick[11] reported a series of 163 patients treated with 140 kV X-rays to a dose of 38.5 Gy in 7 fractions over 8 days. There was local failure in only seven patients. The late cosmetic results were good for 80 per cent of patients.

Electron beam therapy

Carcinoma of the lip can be treated by electron beam in the 8–10 MeV energy range using a similar technique to that described for X-rays. The aperture in a lead cutout should be slightly larger than in the case of X-rays because of fall-off of dosage at the edge of the beam. The same dose and fractionation are employed.

Electron beam therapy requires more elaborate apparatus than does X-ray therapy and has only minimal advantages. Dose distribution through the lip differs slightly, being more uniform in the case of electron therapy with a 10 per cent lower dose on the skin surface (Fig. 12.3). This may give a better cosmetic effect and is more appropriate in the case of a tumour situated on the mucosal surface.

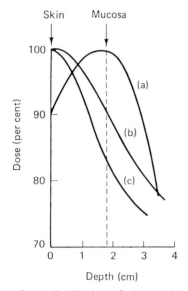

Fig. 12.3 Dose distribution of electron beam and X-irradiation of carcinoma of the lip: (a) 8 MeV electron beam; (b) 250 kV X-rays; (c) 140 kV X-rays.

Surface applicator

The double mould loaded with radium was a popular method of treatment in some radiotherapy centres in the past, and a better cosmetic result was claimed compared with X-ray therapy. It caused appreciable radiation exposure to staff and is now obsolete, having been superseded by electron beam therapy.

Interstitial therapy

An interstitial implant is another very effective way of treating carcinoma of the lip but is complicated and time-consuming. It still has its advocates but

has little or no advantage over electron beam therapy.

Outcome

All methods of radiotherapy give high local control rates at this site. The chance of success with radiation depends on the size of the primary tumour. del Regato and Sala[12] reported radiotherapy failure in none of 96 patients where the primary was under 2 cm in diameter, and in 13 of 142 (9 per cent) where the primary was over 2 cm.

The local recurrence rate after surgery is equally low. For example, MacComb *et al.*[13] reported a 2.5 per cent recurrence rate for carcinoma of the lip up to 2 cm in diameter and a 26 per cent recurrence rate for larger tumours. The incidence of lymph node metastases from carcinoma of the lip overall is about 15 per cent. Distant metastases are exceedingly rare. Failure to control lymph node metastases in the neck accounts for nearly all of the mortality from lip carcinoma. Relative survival rates are, on average, a little in excess of 90 per cent.[13]

Tongue

Surgery

Surgery is the treatment of choice for early lesions suitable for simple intra-oral excision, for tumours on the tip of the tongue, and for advanced disease when surgery should be combined with postoperative radiotherapy (Fig. 12.4). For intermediate

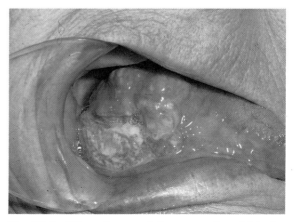

Fig. 12.4 T3 carcinoma of the tongue for which the preferred treatment is surgery and postoperative radiotherapy.

stage disease surgery and radiotherapy have similar outcomes (Fig. 12.5), and the choice between the two depends upon the factors enumerated above, under the heading of 'Choice of treatment'. When performing surgical excision of less than one-third of the tongue, formal reconstruction is not necessary. Indeed the best results are obtained by not attempting to close the defect or to apply a split skin graft. The base of the residual defect should be fulgurated and then allowed to granulate and epithelialise spontaneously. Such treatment is relatively pain-free and results in an undistorted tongue. When available a CO_2 laser may be used for the partial glossectomy. The postoperative course is relatively pain-free, oedema is minimal and healing occurs with minimal scarring.

Any tongue carcinoma exceeding 2 cm in diameter requires at the very least a hemiglossectomy. Many such tumours will infiltrate deeply between the fibres of the hyoglossus muscle. Extensive tongue lesions often involve the floor of the mouth and alveolus. Under any of these circumstances a major resection is indicated. Access is best via a lip split and mandibulotomy. The pull-through procedure is not recommended as it is very difficult to achieve adequate excision in all three dimensions with a limited access. As the resection opens the submandibular space the resection should include a dissection of the neck on the same side as the tumour. The type of neck dissection will depend upon the node status of the patient (see Chapter 13). A rim resection of the mandible is indicated if the tumour reaches the alveolus. Such extensive defects require reconstruction with distant flaps. If the volume of the tongue defect does not exceed two-thirds of the original tongue a radial forearm free flap with microvascular anastomosis gives a reasonable functional result. For very large volume defects, for total glossectomy or for deeply infiltrating tumours when the resection extends to the hyoid bone more bulky flaps are required to fill in the dead space and prevent food pooling. The authors favour a pectoralis major muscle flap without skin as the best method.[14] Whenever it is possible, without compromising the resection, at least one of the hypoglossal nerves should be preserved. If this is done, most patients will eventually relearn to swallow and will establish reasonable speech.

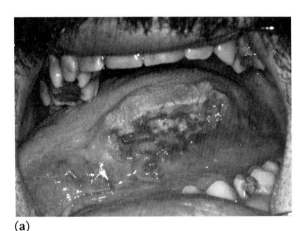

(a)

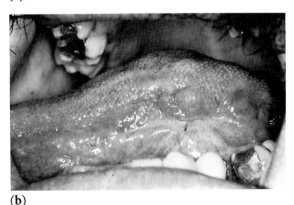

(b)

Fig. 12.5 (a) T2 carcinoma of the lateral border of the tongue. (b) Appearance 2 years after treatment by combined external radiotherapy and iridium-192 implant.

Radiotherapy

Radiotherapy is appropriate for most intermediate stage tumours, i.e. those unsuitable for simple intra-oral excision but with a good prospect of a radiation cure. These include some larger T1 lesions, most T2 and some earlier exophytic T3 tumours. As the results of interstitial irradiation are considerably better than those of external beam irradiation alone (see Chapter 8) only those lesions suitable for all or part of the treatment to be given by an interstitial implant are treated by radiotherapy. If an implant is not feasible because of the position or size of the lesion then surgery and postoperative radiotherapy are preferred. Well differentiated carcinomas not more than 2 cm in diameter can be treated solely by an implant. In all other cases elective irradiation of the regional lymph nodes should be given at the same time. Our experience is that elective nodal irradiation is associated with improved probability of survival.[15] For anteriorly situated lesions the primary can be treated entirely by implant and the lymph nodes irradiated separately. With more posterior lesions there is an inevitable overlap between the radiation fields treating the nodes and the implanted volume, so we combine the two modalities giving 40 Gy over 4 weeks in 20 fractions to both the primary and nodes *en bloc*, adding a further 10 Gy external beam radiation to the nodes, followed by an implant to the primary tumour delivering a further 35 Gy over 3 days. The interval between the external beam radiation and the implant are kept as short as possible so that the total treatment time does not exceed 6 weeks (see Chapter 8).

More advanced disease is normally treated surgically, but in the patient who is unfit for surgery, or refuses operation, radiotherapy is the only curative option. The choice is between external beam radiation alone, in which case a dose of approximately 70 Gy in 35 fractions or equivalent is required, or alternatively if the patient is fit for an implant, 50 Gy can be given by external beam radiotherapy with a boost implant of 25–30 Gy.

Radiotherapy techniques

Most tumours on the lateral border are suitable for a single plane implant. If a double plane implant is thought necessary it indicates an infiltrating tumour which is probably better treated surgically.

An anteriorly placed tumour on the lateral border is best implanted using a hairpin and single pin inserted longitudinally, especially as such tumours tend to involve the under surface of the tongue going towards the base of the frenulum (Fig. 12.6). A tumour further back on the lateral border is implanted using two hairpins in tandem (Fig. 12.7).

Carcinomas on the dorsum of the tongue are rare. If superficial they can be treated by a single plane implant (Fig. 12.8) using iridium hairpins, but there is a risk of underdosage posteriorly so this technique is only suitable for anteriorly placed lesions. A lesion on the dorsum of the tongue close

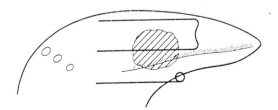

Fig. 12.6 Method of implanting a carcinoma on the junction of anterior middle third of the lateral border of tongue with iridium hairpins.

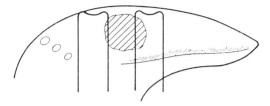

Fig. 12.7 Method of implanting a carcinoma of the middle third of the tongue with iridium-192 hairpins inserted vertically.

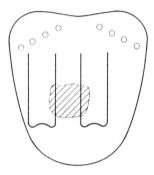

Fig. 12.8 Single plane implant to treat a superficial carcinoma of the dorsum of the tongue.

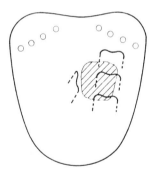

Fig. 12.9 Volume implant for a carcinoma of the dorsum of the tongue.

to the valate papillae, or any lesion with infiltration into the muscle, is better treated by a volume implant using short iridium hairpins positioned vertically (Fig. 12.9).

Radical external beam radiotherapy is rarely indicated as the sole treatment for carcinoma of the tongue. Sometimes it is the only possibility in advanced disease where the patient is unsuitable for major surgery or in earlier disease where the patient is unfit for either surgery or interstitial therapy. In the case of a T1 or T2 tumour confined to the lateral border of the tongue the fields need encompass only the ipsilateral submandibular and upper deep cervical nodes, so anterior and lateral fields with wedge filters can be used (Fig. 12.10). All other cases require lateral parallel opposed fields to the oral cavity and upper neck nodes on both sides and it is advisable to irradiate the lower half of the neck on both sides using an anterior field with mid-line shielding. Similar field arrangements are used for tumours treated by combined external beam and interstitial irradiation as described above (Fig. 12.11).

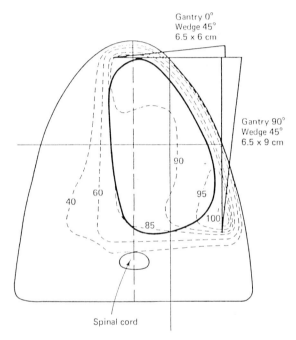

Fig. 12.10   Isodose plan for external radiotherapy of a carcinoma of the lateral border of the tongue.

Outcome

Survival rates for carcinoma of the oral tongue *per se* are difficult to assess because population studies of survival based on ICD (International Classification of Diseases) codes usually include the posterior third of the tongue, which is more accurately included under the heading of oropharyngeal carcinoma and has a worse prognosis than carcinoma of the oral tongue; therefore they tend to underestimate true survival rates. On the other hand many reports of results of treatment include oral tongue with floor of the mouth, at which site carcinoma has a slightly better prognosis.

It is disappointing that despite improved surgical

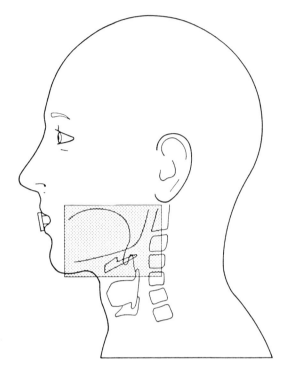

Fig. 12.11   Field arrangement for treatment of an advanced carcinoma of the tongue.

techniques and efforts at earlier diagnosis survival rates in developed countries have scarcely improved at all over the past 40 years. Relative survival rates in the USA stayed virtually constant from 1950 to 1973.[16] Hindle and Nally[17] compared relative survival rates in the UK from 1962 to 1967 with those of 1980 to 1984; there was a reduction in mortality for cancer of the tongue in males from 0.79 to 0.65 but for oral cancer overall the mortality showed an increase. In the USA 5 year relative survival rates were reported to be 36.8 per cent in men and 45 per cent in women from 1974 to 1976. These figures improved for the period 1981 to 1986 to 42.8 per cent and 49.1 per cent respectively.[18]

The most frequent cause of death in carcinoma of the tongue is failure to control lymph node metastases in the neck. The second commonest site of ultimate failure is in the tongue itself. Distant metastases are relatively rare but are being seen more frequently with more radical and improved methods of treatment of the primary tumour and of the lymph nodes.

There are many reports of results of large series treated by radiotherapy.[19–21] In general the local control of the primary tumour is high in T1 and

Table 12.1 Results of treatment of carcinoma of tongue by iridium-192 implantation ± external beam therapy at the Royal Marsden Hospital, 1977–86

Stage	No. treated	5 year crude survival (%)	5 year local control (%)
T1	18	67	89
T2	22	60	78
T3	15	37	20

T2 stages, especially when interstitial irradiation is used, but low in T3 and T4. Results for one centre in the UK are shown in Table 12.1.

Surgical results tend to report tongue and floor of mouth together and it can be difficult to judge results for the individual sites.[22] Typical results for carcinoma of the tongue were reported by Strong in 1979.[23] Of 314 patients reported nearly all were treated by primary surgery. The determinate 5 year survival was reported to be 69 per cent in Stage 1, 53 per cent in Stage 2 and 37 per cent in Stage 3.

Retrospective comparisons between results of primary surgery and primary radiotherapy tend to favour the former,[24,25] but it is difficult to know from such reports how the patients were selected for treatment and whether the surgery and the radiotherapy series were comparable, especially in terms of performance status. Patients in poor medical condition tend to get treated only by external beam radiotherapy and do badly, weighting survival figures in favour of surgery.

Floor of the mouth

Surgery

Floor of mouth cancers spread to involve the under surface of the tongue and the lower alveolus at a relatively early stage. Therefore surgical excision will nearly always include partial glossectomy and marginal resection of the mandible. The resultant defect must always be reconstructed with either a local or a distant flap. It is totally unacceptable to advance the lateral margin of the residual tongue to the buccal mucosa as this causes very severe difficulties with speech and mastication. Small tumours of the floor of the mouth that do not show deep infiltration can be treated by simple excision. It is important that a centimetre margin of normal-appearing mucosa be excised around the tumour.

The resulting defect can either be left to granulate if a CO_2 laser was used for the excision, or fulgurated if diathermy excision was used. Alternatively, if the defect is large it can be repaired using bilateral nasolabial flaps tunnelled into the mouth and interdigitated anteriorly. The submandibular duct should be identified proximally, well clear of the distal margin of the excision and brought out into the floor of mouth or lingual gutter posteriorly.

For larger lesions and those involving the ventral tongue and/or the alveolus, surgical access is gained via a mid-line or lateral (anterior to the mental foramen) mandibulotomy and lip split. As these extensive tumours have a high incidence of nodal involvement the resection is undertaken in continuity with an ipsilateral neck dissection.

Recent work has demonstrated the pattern of bone invasion by carcinoma of the floor of the mouth.[26] Invasion in the edentulous mandible is almost exclusively via deficiencies in the cortical bone of the alveolar crest. In the dentate mandible invasion is usually via the periodontal ligament and is nearly always above the insertion of the mylohyoid muscle. Once tumour has invaded the mandible it soon enters the inferior dental canal and perineural spread occurs anteriorly and posteriorly. Consequently in many cases the continuity of the mandible can safely be maintained provided a marginal resection is carried out which includes the inferior dental canal from the lingula to the mental foramen.

When there is evidence of gross tumour invasion of the bone, resection of the mandible is mandatory. In order to avoid functional and cosmetic deformity, the present authors advocate immediate primary reconstruction. The choice lies between reconstruction with vascularised bone (see Chapter 7), a free corticocancellous graft or an alloplastic system usually supplemented with bone mush.

In the past many attempts have been made to develop alloplastic materials – usually metals or polymers – as systems for mandibular reconstruction. Such systems were thought to be useful in the era when delayed reconstruction of the jaws was advocated. All these systems ultimately failed, with ulceration of the alloplastic implant either through the lining of the oral cavity or through the overlying skin. Occasionally it may be useful to temporarily bridge an incontinuity defect of the mandible with a titanium plate if for some reason immediate bony reconstruction is not possible.

Titanium mesh trays, available commercially in various configurations or custom made, can be used for immediate reconstruction. The tray is trimmed to size and attached to the remaining bone with bicortical screws. The tray is then packed with compressed bone mush usually harvested from the iliac crest. This tissue has great osteogenic potential. The tray and bone mush are then wrapped in a well vascularised muscle flap. Patel and Langdon[27,28] have reported considerable success with this technique, and indeed in younger patients with good jaw function bone has regenerated to reform the resected mandible. The key seems to be that the reconstruction trays are sufficiently rigid to maintain mandibular continuity and yet sufficiently flexible so as not to result in stress shielding in the healing bone.

The resulting soft tissue defect is reconstructed with distant flaps. The choice of flap depends on the volume of the defect. A radial forearm flap is thin and pliable and drapes very nicely into the contours of the tongue, floor of mouth and alveolus. When more bulk is required a pectoralis major muscle flap without skin is brought up through the neck.

Johnson and Langdon,[29] following a prospective study of 11 muscle flaps used for intra-oral reconstruction, have suggested that for oral cavity defects it might be better to leave the raw pectoralis major muscle to undergo spontaneous epithelialisation. The advantages of this are that ultimately the reconstruction is covered by oral mucosa and not skin and that the donor site defect is minimised when a skin paddle is not raised with the muscle flap.

Radiotherapy

Larger T1 and T2 tumours of the floor of the mouth that do not involve the alveolar periosteum or are without deep infiltration into the musculature of the tongue are suitable for treatment by radiotherapy, which will usually give a better functional result than surgery (Fig. 12.12). As in the case of carcinoma of the tongue, a superficial well differentiated T1 tumour can be treated by interstitial therapy alone, but most cases are better treated by combination with external beam radiotherapy. Forty Grey is given to the primary site and 50 Gy to the nodal drainage areas, which should include the entire cervical chain on both sides because there can be direct spread down fast pathways in the anterior neck to lower deep cervical nodes. The field arrangement for radiotherapy combined with implant is shown in Fig. 12.13.

A variety of interstitial techniques are available.

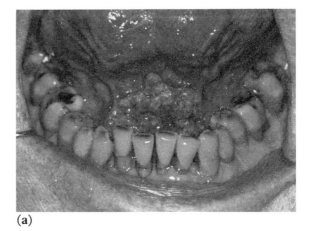

(a)

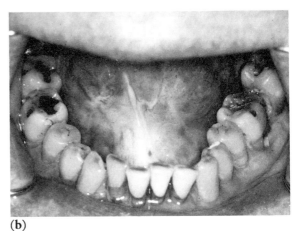

(b)

Fig. 12.12 (a) T2 carcinoma of the floor of the mouth. (b) Appearance 2 years after treatment by combined external beam and interstitial irradiation.

If there is sufficient room radioactive sources are implanted directly into the floor of the mouth, using either short iridium hairpins (Fig. 12.14) or rigid caesium needles held in place by an applicator as described by Marcus *et al.*[30] The former involves less discomfort for the patient but it is more difficult to achieve accurate positioning of the sources. If there is insufficient room in the floor of the mouth, owing to tongue-tie or tethering by the tumour, the sources must be inserted through the substance of the tongue, using either rigid caesium needles or fine iridium wire in loops of plastic tube inserted through the skin in the submental region. Both methods restrict mobility of the tongue while the implant is in position, so feeding via a nasogastric tube may be required.

As an alternative, an intra-oral applicator can be

used to treat an anterior superficial lesion in an edentulous patient. This was a popular technique some years ago, using 140 kV X-rays. Disadvantages are high bone absorption of radiation and difficulty in positioning the applicator accurately. The former can be avoided by the use of an electron beam instead of X-rays, as described by Wexler *et al.*,[31] but even so the technique is rarely used.

Some patients may be unsuitable for either an implant or surgery because of medical contraindications, in which case external radiotherapy must be used alone. A localised volume can be irradiated using oblique fields with wedged filters (Fig 12.15).

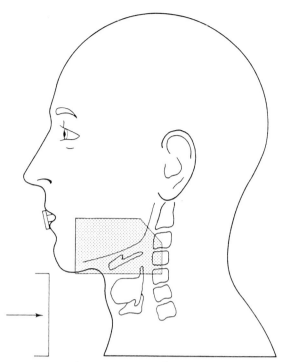

Fig. 12.13 Field arrangement for radiotherapy of a T2 carcinoma of the floor of the mouth.

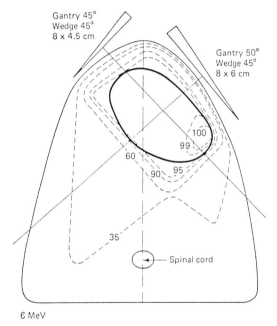

Fig. 12.15 Isodose plan for external radiotherapy of a carcinoma of the floor of the mouth.

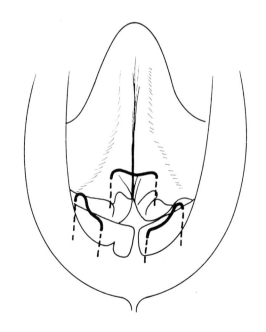

Fig. 12.14 Technique for implantation of a carcinoma of the mid-line floor of mouth using iridium-192 hairpins 2 cm long.

Outcome

In contrast to the possible slight improvement in results of treatment of carcinoma of the tongue in recent years, survival rates from floor of mouth appear to be deteriorating. However, the prognosis remains better than that of carcinoma of the tongue. Five year relative survival rates in the USA declined from 53.3 per cent in males and 63.3 per cent in females in the period 1974 to 1976 to 49.8 per cent in males and 59.2 per cent in females in the period 1981 to 1986.[18] A similar worsening of results has been observed in the UK.[17] It is not clear whether this decrease is real or the result of a trend towards more accurate reporting of the primary site, especially in advanced disease.

The results of external radiotherapy are generally poorer than those of interstitial radiation. For example, Fu *et al.*[32] reported 2 year local control rates of 81 per cent for T1, 65 per cent for T2 and 38 per cent for T3 treated by external beam. By contrast, in a small UK series of T2 tumours treated by combined implant and external beam there were no local failures.[33] Mazeron *et al.*[34] reported a control rate of 93.5 per cent for T1 and 80 per cent for T2 without gingival extension using interstitial therapy as the sole treatment.

Surgical results are similar to those of interstitial radiotherapy for lesions suitable for the latter treatment. In more advanced disease local control is higher with surgery. For example, Million and Cassisi,[35] reported a small series of patients treated by excision including rim resection of the mandible; local control was 81 per cent in T2 and 75 per cent in T3.

Buccal mucosa

Surgery

Lesions strictly confined to the buccal mucosa should be excised widely including the underlying buccinator muscle, followed by a quilted split skin graft. For more extensive lesions with more complicated three-dimensional shapes, i.e. lesions extending posteriorly to the retromolar area, maxillary tuberosity or tonsillar fossa, reconstruction with a free radial forearm flap is advisable; this adapts very well to such shapes and remains soft and mobile postoperatively.

In situations where a free flap is not appropriate alternatives are the buccal fat pad or the forehead flap.

The buccal fat pad has proved to be a useful local flap for the reconstruction of small intra-oral defects up to 3 × 5 cm.[36] This well-vascularised flap can be left raw to epithelialise spontaneously and is used to reconstruct maxillary defects, hard and soft palate defects and cheek and retromolar defects. For large defects at these sites its use can be combined with the temporalis muscle flap.

The use of the forehead flap, an axial flap based on the superficial temporal artery, was first described by McGregor in 1963.[37] It is a very reliable flap able to reach most areas within the mouth in-

cluding the anterior floor of the mouth. However, it is now rarely used because it results in a very obvious cosmetic defect at the donor site; it is a two stage procedure requiring division of the pedicle at 3 weeks; and it requires the creation of a tunnel, either deep or superficial, to the zygomatic arch when the flap is needed in the oral cavity.

Radiotherapy

Radiotherapy is the treatment of choice for T1 and T2 tumours not suitable for simple excision and primary closure (Fig. 12.16).

Irradiation by an interstitial technique gives the best results provided there is at least a clear centimetre of normal mucosa between the margin of the tumour and the alveolobuccal sulci superiorly and

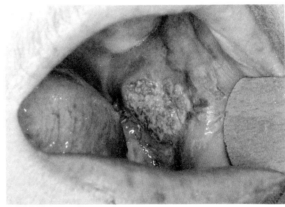

(a)

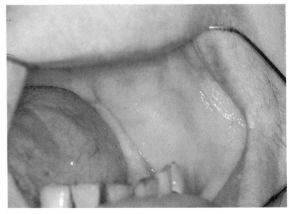

(b)

Fig. 12.16 (a) Carcinoma of the buccal mucosa. (b) Appearance 1 year after treatment by implantation using iridium-192 wire introduced in plastic tubes.

inferiorly, or the retromolar trigone posteriorly. The cheek is suitable only for a single plane implant which should be positioned to lie immediately below the mucosa within the muscle layer. The sources may be inserted either intra-orally through the buccal mucosa or externally through the skin.

The percutaneous method usually permits more accurate and uniform dosage. The sources introduced in this way cause less discomfort than when inserted intra-orally; the only disadvantage is a risk of formation of small scars at the points of entry. Rigid needles containing caesium or radium were formerly used, but have now been largely superseded by fine iridium wire in plastic cannulae which has the advantage of afterloading (Fig. 8.6, p. 111). Iridium hairpins should not be used because the crosspieces or loops will lie against the skin and produce skin necrosis.

The disadvantage of the intra-oral route is that it is of necessity performed with the patient's mouth open so that the tissues of the cheek are stretched. When the mouth is closed the sources will tend to crowd together, especially anteriorly, so it is more difficult to perform an accurate implant to deliver a uniform dosage. If the intra-oral route is favoured either rigid needles or iridium hairpins can be used.

When the tumour is too close to the bone for interstitial therapy the treatment must be by either external beam irradiation or surgery. Where the bone is not involved it is reasonable to treat by external beam radiation in the first instance, reserving surgery for failure. This can be done by a single electron field, or anterior and lateral wedged fields from a supervoltage machine (Fig. 12.17). The latter is preferable if it is desired to treat the ipsilateral neck nodes at the same time.

Outcome

Early tumours of the buccal mucosa generally have a better prognosis than carcinoma of the floor of the mouth or tongue. The incidence of lymph node metastases is lower and local control rates are high. Failure of local control of T1 tumours by either surgery or radiotherapy is rare. The results of radiotherapy for T2 tumours are usually good, but most series contain small numbers. Fletcher[38] reported a 91 per cent local control rate of 3 years in a series of 33 patients. MacComb et al.[13] in a small series quoted survival rates of 64 per cent for T1, 70 per cent for T2, 33 per cent for T3 and 29 per cent for T4 buccal carcinoma treated by surgery alone. Cherian et al.[39] reported an overall 5 year survival rate of 45 per cent from buccal mucosa carcinoma

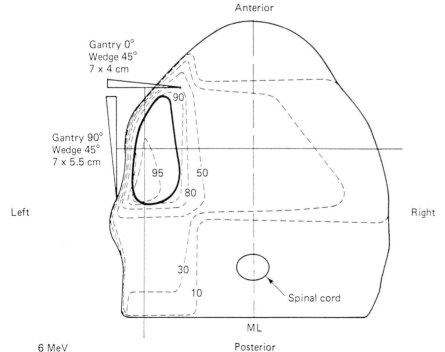

Fig. 12.17 Isodose plan for radiotherapy of a carcinoma of the buccal mucosa. ML, mid-line.

treated in India and claimed that the survival in the same country from a surgical policy was identical.

Carcinoma arising in areas of submucous fibrosis has a much poorer prognosis. It often presents at an advanced stage because of difficulty with mouth opening resulting in delayed diagnosis. Results of radiotherapy are generally less good, possibly because there is a poor blood supply and consequent tumour hypoxia.

Lower alveolus

Surgery

In general, surgery is the treatment modality of choice for all alveolar carcinoma, except for patients unfit for surgery. Access is achieved via a lip split approach. Now that the patterns of bone invasion are better understood the continuity of the mandible can often be preserved by performing a marginal resection. If bone invasion is so extensive that the mandible must be resected in continuity, primary reconstruction should always be undertaken as the results are always better than those of delayed reconstruction.

Several techniques are available for immediate reconstruction of the mandible. Historically, free corticocancellous grafts harvested from the iliac crest or rib grafts have been used. Provided there is a good water-tight cover to the graft, results can be very satisfactory, although it is difficult to reconstruct the chin prominence with this technique. Boyne[40] and Leake[41] have advocated the use of cancellous bone from the ilium packed into mesh trays preformed to match the resected part of the mandible. The early dacron trays did not prove successful, but the titanium trays currently available have given excellent results in the present authors' hands[42] (Fig. 12.18). Of 22 trays inserted only one has been lost due to infection, despite the fact that most patients in the series have received postoperative radiotherapy.

Microvascular tissue transfer is currently in vogue for immediate mandibular reconstruction. The radial forearm flap with a section of the radius, the compound groin flap based on the deep circumflex iliac vessels, and free fibula flaps have all been advocated. A problem with the radial flap is that the harvested bone, although restoring mandibular continuity, is barely adequate for prosthetic reconstruction.

Soft tissue cover for all these reconstruction tech-

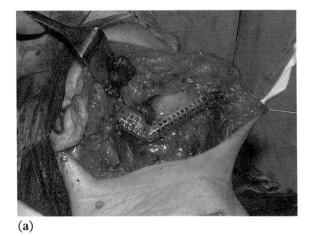

(a)

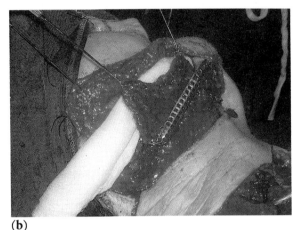

(b)

Fig. 12.18   (a) Mandible reconstructed with a titanium mesh tray. (b) The titanium mesh tray has been packed with bone mush and is being wrapped in a vascularised muscle flap.

niques is critical. With microvascular free flaps the associated skin is used. For cancellous bone mush in titanium trays, and for corticocancellous grafts, the pectoralis major muscle-only flap is most useful.[14,43] The pedicle is brought up through the neck and the flap introduced into the floor of the mouth. The flap is then wrapped around the bone graft and sutured back onto itself on the labial aspect using vicryl™ sutures. Thus the bone graft is totally enveloped in well vascularised soft tissue. The mucosal resection margins are then sutured to the exposed muscle at their appropriate sites and the bare muscle allowed to epithelialise spontaneously. Such flaps withstand immediate postoperative radiotherapy, and the subsequent insertion of osseo-integrated implants has not proved to be a problem.

Radiotherapy

The results of radiotherapy for carcinoma of the alveolus tend to be poorer than those of radiotherapy for carcinomas at other sites in the oral cavity. There are three reasons for this:

(1) Interstitial techniques are not possible, and surface applicators give an inadequate penetration of radiation into the deeper parts of the bone. A very small superficial tumour can be treated by iridium wire in plastic tubes looped over the alveolus as described by Alcock *et al.*[44] Otherwise the only effective method of radiotherapy for most lesions is external beam.
(2) Tumour invading bone tends to have a poor blood supply and so is hypoxic and consequently relatively radioresistant.
(3) When the tumour is invading bone, even if it is successfully eradicated by radiotherapy, subsequent osteoradionecrosis is likely.

In general the only patients who should be treated by radical radiotherapy are those who refuse or are unfit for surgery.

Occasionally a surprisingly good result is obtained even in a patient with extensive bone involvement. A 'wedged pair' technique is used, irradiating a wide margin of bone around the lesion, including the submandibular nodes on the same side (Fig. 12.19).

Outcome

In very selected early disease a local control rate of 81 per cent from radical radiotherapy was reported by Fletcher.[38] More realistic assessment of the outcome of radiotherapy can be gathered from the results from the Christie Hospital, Manchester reported by Porter in 1971.[45] In this series 132 patients were treated; local control rates at 2 years were 32 per cent and 60 per cent for patients with and without evidence of bone involvement respectively; successful salvage surgery was performed in only 12 patients. An important point emerging from the Christie series is that local recurrences were often seen between 2 and 5 years, more so than at other sites in the oral cavity, reflecting the fact that residual tumour cells can grow more slowly in necrotic or poorly vascularised bone and therefore take longer to manifest a frank recurrence.

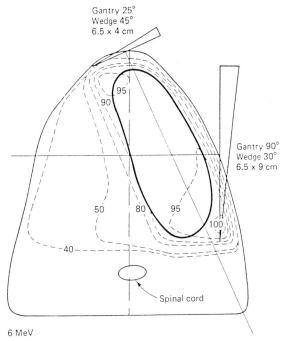

Fig. 12.19 Isodose plan for radiotherapy of a carcinoma of the lower alveolus.

Fayos[46] reported a local recurrence rate of 36 per cent in 55 patients treated. There is nothing to suggest that results of radiotherapy have improved in recent years in tumours at this site. Neutron therapy has been tried and possibly improved local control rates but at the expense of unacceptable morbidity.

The best surgical results reported are those from the MD Anderson Hospital which obtained a 95 per cent local control rate and a 43 per cent 5 year crude survival in a series of 51 patients, 28 of whom were treated by partial thickness resections and 23 by segmental resections.[47]

Retromolar trigone

The retromolar trigone is defined as the anterior surface of the ascending ramus of the mandible. It is roughly triangular in shape with the base being superior behind the third upper molar tooth and the apex inferior behind the third lower molar.[48]

Tumours at this site may invade the ascending ramus of the mandible. They may also spread upwards in soft tissue to involve the pterygomandibular space, which can be difficult to detect clinically or radiologically (Fig. 12.20).

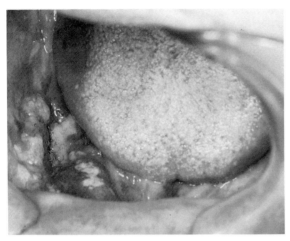

Fig. 12.20 Carcinoma arising on the retromolar trigone.

Surgery

A lip split and mandibulotomy are needed to gain access to the retromolar region. Small defects can often be reconstructed with a masseter or temporalis muscle flap.[49] Larger defects are best reconstructed with a free radial forearm flap which can be made to conform very well to the shape of the defect at this site.

Radiotherapy

For early lesions not invading bone and without node involvement, radiotherapy seems to give high local control rates with a lower morbidity than surgery and therefore is probably the treatment of choice. Contralateral lymph node involvement is rare, so treatment is given by a 'wedged pair' technique (Fig. 12.21) including the ipsilateral upper deep cervical nodes. The volume irradiated should include the potential sites of spread into the pterygomandibular space.

Outcome

Most series report a local control rate of about 85 per cent for T1 tumours and between 60 and 80 per cent for T2. The results for T3 tumours are poor; for example, a figure of 27 per cent local control was reported by Wang.[50] The series reported from the MD Anderson Hospital, consisting of 110 patients treated between 1965 and 1977, suggested that local control and survival rates were similar with surgery and radiotherapy for T1 and T2 tumours, but surgery was preferable for T3 and T4. The overall 5 year survival rate was only 20 per cent because many of the patients were elderly and in poor general health. There was a high mortality from both second primary cancers and intercurrent disease.[51]

Hard palate and upper alveolus

These sites are considered together as they are closely adjacent and both are rare sites of origin of primary squamous carcinoma. A squamous carcinoma presenting at either of these sites is more likely to have arisen in the maxillary antrum than in the oral cavity. An exception is on the Indian subcontinent where carcinoma of the hard palate is seen in association with reverse smoking.[52] Tumours of minor salivary glands are much commoner than squamous carcinomas on the hard palate. The vast majority of squamous carcinomas which present in the upper gum or hard palate arise from the maxillary antrum.

The extent of the disease should always be thoroughly investigated by examination under anaesthetic supplemented by computed tomography (CT) and/or magnetic resonance imaging (MRI).

Most lesions at this site involve bone and require surgical treatment. Radiotherapy alone is suitable only for small early superficial tumours.

Surgery

A tumour confined to the hard palate, upper alveolus and floor of the antrum can be resected by conventional partial maxillectomy. A more extensive tumour confined to the infrastructure of the maxilla requires total maxillectomy.[53] If the preoperative investigations indicate extension of disease into the pterygoid space or infratemporal fossa a more extensive procedure is necessary. The chance of obtaining a cure by surgery alone is small and postoperative radiotherapy is essential. A combined anteroposterior or lateral facial approach is required.[54–56] If the tumour extends superiorly to involve the dura then a combined neurosurgical procedure will be required.[57]

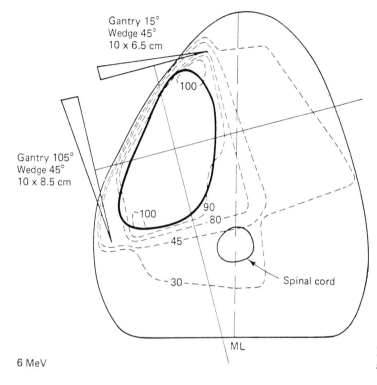

Gantry 15°
Wedge 45°
10 x 6.5 cm

Gantry 105°
Wedge 45°
10 x 8.5 cm

100

100

90

80

45

30

Spinal cord

ML

6 MeV

Fig. 12.21 Isodose plan for radiotherapy of a carcinoma of the retromolar trigone.

Following a maxillary resection the resulting cavity should be grafted to ensure rapid healing and to prevent contracture of the overlying soft tissues.

Recently the use of autogenous keratinocyte grafts has been described.[58,59] With this technique sheets of oral keratinocytes are grown in the laboratory from small oral biopsies harvested 2 to 3 weeks pre-operatively. These sheets are then applied to raw mucosal surfaces at the time of resection and result in accelerated healing and a mucosal lining in the oral cavity. This technique has proved to be particularly useful in grafting maxillectomy cavities where the use of split skin causes particular problems with crusting and cavity hygiene.

The defect created by surgery will require either reconstruction or a prosthesis. Various techniques have been described for reconstruction; Obwegeser[60] described a technique using split ribs. More recently the temporalis muscle flap has been advocated.[61,62] The temporalis muscle flap is a simple technique and has the advantage that it carries with it its own blood supply. It must be remembered that if such a reconstruction is to be undertaken subsequently it is essential that at the time of the original maxillectomy the coronoid process of the mandible is not excised, because if it is resected the blood supply to the mobilised temporalis muscle will have been compromised and the flap will necrose. More recently Tideman[63] has described a modification of this system for reconstruction of the upper jaw.

In general the authors are not in favour of reconstruction following maxillectomy for squamous cell carcinoma. If reconstruction is attempted it becomes much more difficult to inspect the cavity for tumour recurrence and to remove mucus crusts which form. Furthermore it is doubtful if the end result is any better than that of a well constructed hollow box obturator, or an obturator stabilised by osseo-integrated fixtures (see Chapter 19).

The main argument in favour of reconstruction is that some patients have difficulty psychologically in accepting the maxillectomy cavity and for them it may be an advantage to close off the cavity. In this case we would advocate the use of the temporalis muscle flap, but it is essential that if reconstruction is to be undertaken part of the posterior nasal septum should be resected so as to provide an opening through which the maxillectomy cavity can be inspected. For smaller posteriorly sited palatal defects the buccal pad of fat[64] or a masseter muscle flap may be used to close the defect.[49] Composite free transfer grafts from the radius, ilium or fibula have also been used to reconstruct large maxillectomy defects but as yet their long term success has not been proven.

Radiotherapy

Radical radiotherapy is generally suitable for only small superficial lesions. The tumour and the surrounding 1.5 cm margin should be irradiated by external beam using a wedged pair technique. The incidence of lymph node metastases is low so elective nodal irradiation is not indicated. Most commonly the time for radiotherapy is postoperative.

Outcome

There are few series and none large enough to give any meaningful survival figures. The largest series was reported by Evans and Shah.[65] This series contained a total of 62 patients treated between 1960 and 1975, nearly all surgically. Determinate 5 year survival rates were reported varying from 75 per cent in Stage 1 to 8 per cent in Stage 4. Chung et al.[66] reported 32 patients treated by radiotherapy. The patients were fairly evenly distributed between the four T stages; the determinate 5 year survival rate was 59 per cent.

References

1 Mendenhall WM, Parsons JT, Amdur RJ *et al.* Squamous cell carcinoma of the head and neck treated with radiation therapy: the impact of neck stage on local control. *International Journal of Radiation Oncology, Biology, Physics* 1988; **14:** 249–52.

2 Perez, CA, Kraus FT, Evans JC. Anaplastic transformation in verrucous carcinoma of the oral cavity after radiation therapy. *Radiology* 1966; **86:** 108–15.

3 Vidyasagar MS, Fernandes DJ, Kasture DP *et al.* Radiotherapy and verrucous carcinoma of the oral cavity. *Acta Oncologica* 1992; **31:** 43–7.

4 McDonald JS, Crissman JD, Gluckman JL. Verrucous carcinoma of the oral cavity. *Head and Neck Surgery* 1982; **5:** 22–8.

5 Stell PM, Wood GD, Scott MH. Early oral cancer: treatment by biopsy excision. *British Journal of Oral Surgery* 1982; **20:** 234–8.

6 Ange DW, Lindberg RD, Guillamondegui OM. Management of squamous cell carcinoma of the oral tongue and floor of mouth after excisional biopsy. *Radiology* 1975; **116:** 143–6.

7 Bailey BJ. Management of carcinoma of the lip. *Laryngoscope* 1977; **87:** 250–60.

8 Langdon JD, Ord RA. The surgical management of lip cancer. *Journal of Cranio-Maxillo-Facial Surgery* 1987; **15:** 281–7.

9 Johanson B, Aspelund E, Breine U, Holmstrom H. Surgical treatment of non-traumatic lower lip lesions with special reference to the step technique. *Scandinavian Journal of Plastic and Reconstructive Surgery* 1974; **8:** 232–40.

10 Fries R. Advantages of a basic concept in lip reconstruction after tumour resection. *Journal of Maxillofacial Surgery* 1973; **1:** 13–18.

11 Dick DAL. Clinical and cosmetic results in squamous cancer of the lip treated by 140kV radiation therapy. *Clinical Radiology* 1962; **13:** 304–8.

12 del Regato JA, Sala JM. The treatment of carcinomas of the lip. *Radiology* 1959; **73:** 839–47.

13 MacComb WS, Fletcher GH, Healey JG. Carcinoma of the lip. In: MacComb WS, Fletcher GH eds. *Cancer of the Head and Neck*. Baltimore, MD: Wilkins & Wilkins, 1967: 89–151.

14 Johnson MA, Langdon JD. Is skin necessary for intra-oral reconstruction with myo-cutaneous flaps? *British Journal of Oral and Maxillofacial Surgery* 1990; **28:** 299–301.

15 Dearnaley D, Dardoufas C, A'Hern RP, Henk JM. Interstitial irradiation for carcinoma of the tongue and floor of mouth: Royal Marsden Hospital experience 1970–86. *Radiotherapy and Oncology* 1991; **21:** 183–90.

16 American Cancer Society. *1981 Cancer Facts and Figures*. New York: American Cancer Society, 1981.

17 Hindle I, Nally F. Oral cancer: a comparative study between 1962–67 and 1980–84 in England and Wales. *British Dental Journal* 1991; **170:** 15–20.

18 US Department of Health and Human Services Public Health Service. *Cancers of the oral cavity and pharynx: a statistics review monograph 1973–87*. Atlanta, GA, and Bethesda, MD: Centers for Disease Control and National Institutes of Health, 1992.

19 De Croix Y, Ghossein NA. Experience of the Curie Institute in treatment of carcinoma of the mobile tongue. *Cancer* 1981; **47:** 496–502.

20 Mazeron JJ, Crook JM, Marinello G *et al.* Prognostic factors of local outcome for T1, T2 carcinomas of the oral tongue treated by iridium-192 implantation. *International Journal of Radiation Oncology, Biology, Physics* 1990; **19:** 281–5.

21 Lefebvre JL, Coche-Dequeant B, Castelain B *et al.* Interstitial brachytherapy and early tongue squamous cell carcinoma management. *Head and Neck* 1990; **12:** 232–6.

22 Hemprich A, Müller RP. Long-term results in treating squamous cell carcinoma of the lip, oral

cavity and oropharynx. *International Journal of Oral and Maxillofacial Surgery* 1989; **18**: 39–42.

23 Strong EW. Carcinoma of the tongue. *Otolaryngological Clinics of North America* 1979; **12**: 107–14.

24 Robertson AG, McGregor IA, Flatman GE *et al*. The role of radical surgery and post-operative radiotherapy in the management of intra-oral carcinoma. *British Journal of Plastic Surgery* 1985; **38**: 314–20.

25 White D, Byers RM. What is the preferred method of treatment for squamous carcinoma of the tongue? *American Journal of Surgery* 1980; **140**: 553–5.

26 McGregor IA, McGregor FM. In McGregor IA, McGregor FM eds. *Cancer of the Face and Mouth.* Edinburgh: Churchill Livingstone, 1986: 401–5.

27 Patel MF, Langdon JD. Titanium mesh osteosynthesis – a fast and adaptable method of semi-rigid fixation. *British Journal of Oral and Maxillofacial Surgery* 1991; **29**: 316–24.

28 Patel MF, Langdon JD. The use of titanium mesh trays for immediate reconstruction after mandibular resection. *British Journal of Oral and Maxillofacial Surgery* 1991; **29**: 412.

29 Johnson MA, Langdon JD. Is skin necessary for intra oral reconstruction with myocutaneous flaps? *British Journal of Oral and Maxillofacial Surgery* 1990; **28**: 299–301.

30 Marcus RB, Million RR, Mitchell TP. A pre-loaded custom-designed implantation device for stage T1–2 carcinoma of the floor of the mouth. *International Journal of Radiation Oncology, Biology, Physics* 1980; **6**: 111–13.

31 Wexler MC, Tobochnik N, Spiegler P, Herman MW. Characteristics of an intra-oral cone for electron beam therapy with an 18 MeV linear accelerator. *International Journal of Radiation Oncology, Biology, Physics* 1982; **8**: 2001–4.

32 Fu KK, Lichter A, Galante M. Carcinoma of the floor of the mouth: an analysis of treatment results and the sites and causes of failure. *International Journal of Radiation Oncology, Biology, Physics* 1976; **1**: 829–37.

33 Henk JM. Treatment of oral cancer by interstitial irradiation using iridium-192. *British Journal of Oral and Maxillofacial Surgery* 1992; **30**: 355–9.

34 Mazeron JJ, Grimard L, Raynal M *et al*. Iridium-192 curietherapy for T1 and T2 epidermoid carcinomas of the floor of the mouth. *International Journal of Radiation Oncology, Biology, Physics* 1990; **18**: 1299–306.

35 Million RR, Cassisi NJ. *Management of Head and Neck Cancer: A Multidisciplinary Approach.* Philadelphia, PA: JB Lippincott, 1984: 264.

36 Samman N, Cheung LK, Tideman H. The buccal fat pad in oral reconstruction. *International Journal of Oral and Maxillofacial Surgery* 1993; **22**: 2–6.

37 McGregor IA. The temporal flap in intra-oral cancer. *British Journal of Plastic Surgery* 1963; **16**: 318–35.

38 Fletcher GH. *Textbook of Radiotherapy*, 3rd edn.

Philadelphia, PA: Lea and Febiger, 1980.

39 Cherian T, Sebastian P, Iqbal Ahmed M *et al*. Evaluation of salvage surgery in heavily-irradiated cancer of the buccal mucosa. *Cancer* 1990; **68**: 295–9.

40 Boyne PJ. Autogenous cancellous bone and marrow transplants. *Clinical Orthopaedics* 1970; **73**: 199–209.

41 Leake DL. Mandibular reconstruction with a new type of alloplastic tray. *Journal of Oral Surgery* 1974; **32**: 23–6.

42 Patel MF, Langdon JD. The use of titanium mesh trays for immediate reconstruction after mandibular resection. *British Journal of Oral and Maxillofacial Surgery* 1991; **29**: 316–24.

43 Phillips JG, Falconer DT, Postlethwaite K, Peckitt N. Pectoralis muscle flap with bone graft in intra-oral reconstruction. *British Journal of Oral and Maxillofacial Surgery* 1990; **28**: 160–3.

44 Alcock CJ, Paine CH, Weatherburn H. Interstitial radiotherapy in treatment of superficial tumours of the lower alveolar ridge. *Clinical Radiology* 1984; **35**: 363–6.

45 Porter EH. The local prognosis after radical radiotherapy for squamous carcinoma of the alveolus and of the floor of the mouth. *Clinical Radiology* 1971; **22**: 139–43.

46 Fayos JV. Carcinoma of the mandible; results of radiation therapy. *Acta Radiologica* 1973; **12**: 378–86.

47 Byers RM, Newman R, Russell N, Yue A. Results of treatment for squamous carcinoma of the lower gum. *Cancer* 1981; **47**: 2236–8.

48 Lederman M. Cancer of the oral cavity: observations on classification and natural history. *International Journal of Radiation Oncology, Biology, Physics* 1980; **6**: 1559–65.

49 Langdon JD. The masseter muscle cross-over flap: a versatile flap for reconstruction in the oral cavity. *British Journal of Oral and Maxillofacial Surgery* 1989; **27**: 394–9.

50 Wang CC. *Radiation Therapy for Head and Neck Neoplasms: Indications Techniques and Results.* Chicago, IL: Yearbook Medical Pubishers, 1990: 151.

51 Byers RM, Fields RS, Anderson B *et al*. Treatment of squamous carcinoma of the retro-molar trigone. *American Journal of Clinical Oncology* 1984; **7**: 647–52.

52 Ramula C, Raju MVS, Venkataratham G. Nicotine stomatitis and its relation to carcinoma of the hard palate in reverse smoking of chuttas. *Journal of Dental Research* 1973; **52**: 711–12.

53 Crockett DJ. Surgical approach to the back of the maxilla. *British Journal of Surgery* 1963; **50**: 819–21.

54 Wilson JSP, Shaw H, Cleatus S. Surgical approaches to the temporal and pterygoid regions. *Journal of the Royal Society of Medicine* 1980; **73**: 744–5.

55 Brusati R, Raffaini M, Bozzetti A. Jaeger's juga extended incision to approach the pterygomaxillary region. *International Journal of Oral and Maxillofacial Surgery* 1989; **18**: 298–301.

56 Brown AMS, Lavery KM, Millar BG. The transfacial approach to the postnasal space and retromaxillary structures. *British Journal of Oral and Maxillofacial Surgery* 1991; **29**: 230–6.

57 Grime PD, Haskell R, Robertson I, Gullan R. Transfacial access for neurosurgical procedures: an extended role for the maxillofacial surgeon. II Middle cranial fossa, infratemporal fossa and pterygoid space. *International Journal of Maxillofacial Surgery* 1991; **20**: 291–5.

58 Langdon JD, Leigh IM, Navsaria HA, Williams DM. Autologous oral keratinocyte grafts in the mouth. *Lancet* 1990; **335**: 1472–3.

59 Langdon JD, Williams DM, Navsaria HA, Leigh IM. Autologous keratinocyte grafting for intra-oral reconstruction. *British Dental Journal* 1991; **171**: 87–90.

60 Obwegeser HL. Late reconstruction of large maxillary defects after tumour resection. *Journal of Maxillofacial Surgery* 1973; **1**: 19–29.

61 Bradley P, Brockbank J. The temporalis muscle flap in oral reconstruction. *Journal of Maxillofacial Surgery* 1981; **9**: 139–45.

62 Phillips JG, Peckitt WS. Reconstruction of the palate using bilateral temporalis muscle flaps. *British Journal of Surgery* 1988; **26**: 322–5.

63 Tideman H, Samman N, Cheung LK. Immediate reconstruction of maxillectomy: a new method. *International Journal of Oral and Maxillofacial Surgery* 1993; **22**: 221–225.

64 Fujimura N, Nagura H, Enomoto S. Grafting of the buccal fat pad into palatal defects. *Journal of Cranio-Maxillo-Facial Surgery* 1990; **18**: 219–22.

65 Evans JF, Shah JP. Epidermoid carcinoma of the palate. *American Journal of Surgery* 1981; **142**: 451–5.

66 Chung CK, Johns ME, Cantrell RW, Constable WC. Radiotherapy in the management of primary malignancies of the hard palate. *Laryngoscope* 1980; **90**: 576–84.

13   Management of the regional lymph nodes

JM Henk and JD Langdon

The oral cavity and salivary glands have a rich lymphatic drainage; approximately one-third of all the lymph nodes in the body are found in the neck. Most types of malignant oral and salivary gland tumours frequently spread to the lymph nodes of the neck. Uncontrolled nodal metastases are the commonest cause of treatment failure in oral cavity carcinoma. The management of the neck remains controversial, especially in those patients with no palpable lymph node metastases at presentation.

Mechanism of lymphatic metastases

Anatomical and pathological studies suggest that lymph node metastases occur as a result of emboli of tumour cells passing along lymph vessels and lodging in the regional nodes, where they subsequently grow.[1] Lymphatic permeation, or 'in transit' metastases of tumour cells growing in lymph vessels in an intermediate position between the primary and the first drainage lymph nodes have not been found in untreated patients, with the possible exception of adenoid cystic carcinoma.

McKelvie[2] examined block dissection specimens histologically to study the pattern of spread of squamous carcinoma in the lymphatic system of the neck. His findings suggest that, initially, tumour emboli appear either in one node, or in one or two adjacent nodes, in the first group draining the primary site. Tumour grows in the first node until it is completely replaced by tumour, at which stage the metastasis is usually palpable on clinical examination. Tumour cells may then be passed to the next group of nodes lower in the neck, where the same process occurs. It is unusual to find only microscopic foci of tumour in both the first and subsequent lymph node stations. This stepwise spread is important in planning the treatment of lymph node metastases; if a patient has palpable lymph node metastases in the upper part of the neck, microscopic nodal involvement lower in the neck is likely; on the other hand, if there are no lymph node metastases palpable microscopic nodal involvement, if present, is likely to be limited to the first group of nodes draining the primary site. However, it must be remembered that there are exceptions to this rule in the case of those parts of the mouth that may drain by so-called 'fast pathways', i.e. lymph vessels that pass directly to nodes low in the neck. This is seen, for example, from the tip of the tongue with direct spread to the jugulo-omohyoid nodes, and where there is involvement of the oropharynx with a possibility of direct spread to the deep mid-cervical nodes or to nodes in the posterior triangle.

Distribution of lymph node metastases

The distribution of lymph node metastases from oral cancer has been extensively documented. The clinical findings in 787 patients were described by Lindberg,[3] and the histological findings in 516 radical neck dissection specimens by Shah *et al.*[4] Clinical and histological findings are generally in agreement.[5]

Metastases occur most commonly in the upper deep cervical and submandibular nodes on the same side as the primary tumour. The more anterior the primary, the more likely is involvement of submandibular nodes.[4] Mid-deep cervical nodes are not infrequently affected. However, involvement of the lower deep cervical nodes is rare; Shah *et al.*[4] found six instances in 192 elective neck dissection specimens. Nodes at higher levels were also involved in three of these cases. Involvement of posterior triangle or submental nodes is exceedingly rare, and invariably associated with involvement of other nodal areas.

Contralateral node metastases are rare at presentation. They occurred in only 6 per cent of Lindberg's series. They are almost invariably associated with ipsilateral involvement. They may appear subsequent to treatment of ipsilateral nodes, especially where the primary was near the mid-line.[4]

The distribution of lymph node metastases from salivary gland tumours has not been so extensively documented. Parotid tumours spread initially to pre-auricular or upper deep cervical nodes. Submandibular gland tumours spread to submandibular, upper deep cervical and mid-deep cervical nodes.

Incidence of lymph node metastases

The likelihood of lymph node metastases depends on the size, site and histological type of the primary tumour.

Size

The larger the primary tumour, the more likely are lymph node metastases. Lindberg[3] reported that, at presentation, 12 per cent of patients with tumour of 2 cm diameter or less (T1) were found to have lymph node metastases. The incidence rose to 30 per cent for T2, i.e. primary 2–4 cm diameter, and to 50 per cent for T3, i.e. tumours more than 4 cm. In the case of the massive T4 tumours, the incidence of nodal metastases was even higher.

Site

As a general principle, the more posterior the lesion in the mouth, the more likely are lymph node metastases. For instance, Lindberg[3] found a 45 per cent incidence from primary tumours of the retromolar trigone and anterior faucial pillar, compared with 35 per cent from the tongue and 30 per cent from the floor of the mouth. The incidence from lower alveolus tumours is similar to that for the floor of the mouth, while it is a little lower in the case of buccal mucosa and hard palate primaries. The lowest incidence is from carcinoma of the lip where it is between 10 and 15 per cent.

Histology

In the case of squamous carcinoma of the oral cavity, the instance of lymph node metastases is related to the degree of differentiation. Langdon et al.[6] found that the better differentiated the primary, the less likely were lymph node metastases; in their series, the incidence was 17 per cent in verrucous carcinoma, 26 per cent in well differentiated squamous cell carcinoma, 33 per cent in moderately differentiated squamous cell carcinoma, and 50 per cent in poorly differentiated squamous cell carcinoma. In most other reported series the incidence of nodal metastases in verrucous carcinomas is considerably lower.

In major and minor salivary gland tumours, histology is the most significant factor determining the likelihood of lymphatic spread. Low grade tumours have a low incidence of nodal involvement. In high grade tumours, there is a high incidence, especially in undifferentiated carcinoma, adenocarcinoma and squamous cell carcinoma. In muco-epidermoid tumours the risk of lymph node involvement depends on histological grade; the incidence is low in grades 1 and 2 and higher in grade 3.[7]

Adenoid cystic carcinoma is generally believed to spread to lymph nodes rather rarely. It has been suggested that node involvement occurs only by direct lymphatic permeation, and that tumour emboli to the nodes do not occur,[8] but others have described unequivocal lymph node metastases low in the neck with no evidence of intervening lymphatic permeation.[9] An overall incidence of node involvement of 15 per cent has been described in several large series.[10,11] Stell et al.[9] found that the risk of node involvement was significantly higher in males and from poorly differentiated tumours.

Diagnosis of lymph node metastases

Clinical examination

Clinical examination remains the most important method of detecting lymph node metastases in the neck.

The neck must be examined at presentation and at least once a month during the first year after treatment. If the intervals are longer than 1 month, there is a risk of a previously undetected metastasis becoming large or extending outside the capsule of the node, or of other nodes becoming involved; all of which are associated with a worsening prognosis. An involved node may even become fixed and inoperable. When a year or so has elapsed after the initial treatment, the follow up intervals can be extended gradually, because most lymph node metastases occur in the first year, and any becoming manifest after the first year are likely to be slow growing, so that there is a diminishing risk of failure to detect the neck disease at a curable stage. Examination of the neck is best carried out with the patient seated. Initially, the neck should be inspected from both the front and the back for asymmetry and any visible swelling. Palpation is best carried out initially from behind, feeling both sides simultaneously, and from above downwards, beginning by running the fingers along the mental and submandibular regions, palpating behind the angle of the jaw and then both anterior and posterior triangles down to the clavicle. The submandibular spaces should be palpated bimanually with one finger in the floor of the mouth. Examination of the deep cervical lymphatic chain is facilitated by using two hands, the fingers of one gently retracting the sternomastoid muscle backwards while the fingertips of the other hand hooked around the front of the neck can palpate the region of the carotid sheath. In this way a node nestling behind the carotid sheath may be rolled forwards and become palpable, although it was not felt during the initial simultaneous palpation of both sides of the neck.

An attempt should be made to distinguish involved from uninvolved nodes. At the earliest stage a lymph node metastasis is small, firm and usually almond-shaped and non-tender. As it grows it becomes larger and rounder but remains mobile for a variable period, depending on its growth rate. Eventually it becomes fixed to the adjacent structures such as the carotid sheath or muscle. With continued growth it becomes fixed and painful, and eventually involves the skin, finally fungating.

Uninvolved nodes may be palpable for a variety of reasons, and are often difficult to distinguish clinically from metastases. Reactive hyperplasia frequently occurs in the nodes draining a tumour-bearing site, perhaps as a direct response to the tumour itself, but more likely in most cases as a result of secondary infection of the lesion. Reactive nodes are typically soft and mobile, often tender, and subside with treatment of the primary. Nodes palpable because of old infection, for example, tuberculosis, are very hard, discrete and mobile; calcification may be demonstrated on X-ray.

Some non-lymphoid structures in the neck may be mistaken for secondary lymph nodes. The carotid bulb is often palpable as an apparently discrete rounded structure, and in the elderly a tortuous carotid artery has a knobbly feel. These structures can be distinguished by their pulsation; but it is very important for the examiner consciously to feel for pulsation, otherwise this sign may not be elicited. The transverse process of the atlas vertebra is palpable just behind the angle of the jaw, especially in a patient with a thin neck, and should not be confused with an upper deep cervical lymph node. The submandibular salivary gland is often enlarged, especially after radiotherapy or if a tumour involves the submandibular duct. If the patient is aware of a submandibular swelling, he will be able to tell the clinician if there is any fluctuation in size, especially in relation to eating. If there is no such history, it is important to attempt to distinguish an enlarged submandibular salivary gland from a submandibular lymph node. The salivary gland is situated just above and in front of the cornu of the hyoid bone and is usually lower and more posterior in position than a submandibular lymph node. It is usually smooth and rounded on bimanual examination and can be balloted, but when chronically inflamed it may be less clearly demarcated and mistaken for a partly fixed lymph node metastasis.

Imaging

Clinical examination remains the most important method of detecting lymph node metastases in the neck. Studies correlating clinical findings with subsequent histological examination of lymph nodes removed at dissection reveal that the sensitivity of clinical examination is usually between 60 per cent and 70 per cent.[12,13]

Computerised tomography (CT) is the most widely used imaging technique for investigation of the neck in patients with oral and salivary gland tumours. The sensitivity of CT scanning alone is very similar to that of clinical examination.[12,13] However, it can often detect nodes which have not proved to be palpable (Fig. 13.1), especially posterior to the internal jugular vein and in the parapharyngeal space. Hence the sensitivity of the two investigations combined is higher than either alone, and can be over 90 per cent. Nodes above 1 cm in diameter are usually regarded as suspicious of malignancy in head and neck cancer patients; however, reactive nodes can be up to 2 cm in diameter,

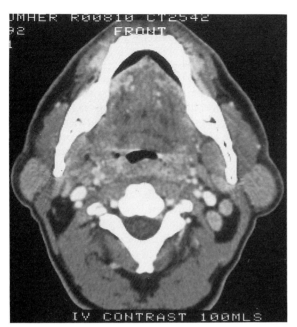

Fig. 13.1 Computed tomography scan showing a nodal metastasis which was not found upon clinical examination.

especially in the jugulodigastric region.[14] There is therefore a significant false-positive rate, so that the specificity of CT is around 75 per cent. A greater value of CT is in the assessment of the extent and position of gross nodal disease, especially deep to the carotid artery, and hence in assessing operability.

Ultrasound scanning has been shown to increase the rate of detection of nodal metastases compared with clinical examination alone.[15] This technique is simple and relatively cheap, and can be used to guide fine-needle aspiration biopsy of impalpable nodes.

Magnetic resonance imaging (MRI) with gadolinium enhancement also improves the detection rate of nodal metastases,[16] but it is not yet clear whether it is superior to CT in this respect. Other methods of detection of occult nodal metastases which have been tried include lymphography, thermography and isotope scanning, but none has proved reliable.

Cytology

Aspiration cytology is a useful confirmatory test to increase the accuracy of diagnosis of nodal metastases. In experienced hands, the accuracy of cytology is high and there is no evidence that inserting a fine needle into the lymph nodes spreads the disease or worsens the prognosis. False-positive results are virtually never obtained; inevitably, there is a proportion of false-negative results even in the best hands, as the needle tip may fail to locate the actual tumour cells within a node. Accordingly, a positive result can be taken as definite evidence of nodal involvement and treatment proceeded with on this basis. In the event of a negative result, the absence of nodal metastases cannot be assumed.

Histology

Some reports have shown that a previous open biopsy of a neck node increases the risk of both local recurrence and metastases after neck dissection.[17] However, more recent reports have failed to show any deleterious effect of open biopsy provided radiotherapy is part of the treatment.[18,19]

It is probably wise to avoid open biopsy if possible. When an involved lymph node is suspected but aspiration cytology is negative, the best policy is to prepare the patient for neck dissection and begin by removing the involved node for frozen section. It is unusual for cytology to be negative in a patient with an inoperable neck mass, but in such a case, there is no evidence that biopsy prior to radiotherapy adversely affects the prognosis.

Surgical treatment

Crile[20] first described the classical block dissection of the neck in 1906. This operation removes the lymph nodes from one side of the neck: in the process the sternocleidomastoid muscle, the internal jugular vein, the spinal accessory nerve, the submandibular salivary gland, the lower pole of the parotid and the lobe of the thyroid on the same side are also removed in one block of tissue. Because of the considerable morbidity associated with the procedure several modifications have been described and their terminology has been confusing. The classification described by Suen and Goepfert[21] will be used here.

(1) Standard Radical Neck Dissection (as described by Crile[20]) in which all node levels are dissected and none of the above structures are preserved.
(2) Modified Radical Neck Dissection which is identical to the above except that the spinal accessory nerve is preserved.

(3) Functional Neck Dissection in which all node levels may be dissected, but the sternocleidomastoid muscle, internal jugular vein and spinal accessory nerve are preserved.
(4) Selective Neck Dissection in which only selective nodes are dissected such as in the submandibular triangle dissection, supra-omohyoid dissection, anterior neck dissection and posterior neck dissection.

Standard radical neck dissection

Whenever clinically palpable neck disease is present it is likely that further extension of disease has already taken place although as yet it is not palpable. In such circumstances anything less than a radical neck dissection risks leaving disease in the neck. Other indications for radical neck dissection are nodal involvement of other than first echelon nodes, neck disease arising after successful management of the primary, the development of clinically positive nodes after previous neck irradiation and when a fixed node in the neck becomes mobile following radiotherapy.

The radical neck dissection has many important advantages – it is a straightforward procedure, there is a low risk of leaving disease in the neck and it is a relatively rapid operation – but it also has important disadvantages. All patients will have some degree of trapezius muscle dysfunction with shoulder droop and pain and limitation of movement. There will be some cosmetic deformity of the neck following loss of the sternocleidomastoid muscle although this is partially alleviated when the pedicle of a pectoralis major or latissimus dorsi flap is brought through the neck. Bilateral simultaneous radical neck dissection cannot safely be undertaken as it results in gross venous congestion of the brain and face.

Modified radical neck dissection

This procedure is identical to the standard radical neck dissection except that the spinal accessory nerve is preserved. This means that the posterior triangle cannot be thoroughly cleared but for oral cavity carcinomas the incidence of nodal disease in the posterior triangle is very low.

Functional neck dissection

The morbidity of this procedure is considerably lower than for radical neck dissection. However,

the procedure is technically more difficult, the operation takes longer and almost always the yield of nodes in the specimen is less than for radical neck dissection.[22] Whenever clinically palpable nodes are present and therefore there is a risk of extracapsular spread of disease the procedure is unsafe as there is inevitably a higher risk of leaving disease behind in the neck. Indications for functional neck dissection are therefore for elective neck dissection when indicated (see below) and for the less involved side when simultaneous bilateral neck dissection is indicated. Although there have been many descriptions of functional neck dissection, there are basically two techniques. These are the anteroposterior approach advocated by Bocca and Pignataro and the anterior approach developed by Ballantyne.[23] The present authors find the latter approach the most straightforward although radical clearance of the posterior triangle is difficult.

Selective neck dissection

Supra-omohyoid neck dissection removes nodes in the submandibular, submental, upper deep cervical and mid-deep cervical regions, together with the submandibular salivary gland and some adjacent soft tissue. This operation should not be used for the treatment of involved lymph nodes. As stated above, involvement of nodes in the upper part of the neck is often associated with microscopic deposits in lower neck nodes. The operation is often employed for elective neck dissection in a patient with a primary in the anterior part of the oral cavity and a clinically negative neck. It may also have a place in the management of bilateral nodes but is otherwise not recommended.

Suprahyoid dissection removes nodes only in the submental and submandibular regions. It is inadequate as a cancer operation and is not recommended.

Neck incisions

Crile used a long vertical incision, but many surgeons now prefer modified incisions which cross the carotid artery at right angles, thereby reducing the risk of carotid artery exposure and rupture postoperatively.[24]

Many incisions have been described, each surgeon arguing the advantages of his own preference. The choice of flaps is governed by three factors:

(1) Whatever flap design is favoured it must give

adequate exposure to enable a thorough neck dissection to be completed.

(2) The flaps should be of such a design that they will remain well vascularised and heal satisfactorily. This is particularly important in previously irradiated necks.

(3) Whenever possible flaps should be designed so that at the completion of surgery the carotid artery and its bifurcation are adequately covered.

In the irradiated patient a double horizontal incision as described by McFee is safest (Fig. 13.2). The first incision begins over the mastoid process, coming down to the horn of the hyoid bone and then passing upwards to the point of the chin. The second incision is 2 cm above the clavicle starting laterally at the anterior border of the trapezius and ending medially at the mid-line (Fig. 13.3).

In the non-irradiated patient a Y-type incision such as that of Morestin may give better access for the inexperienced surgeon (Fig. 13.4). The upper part of the incision is like that of the McFee incision. A vertical limb then starts from the midpoint of this incision and runs downwards in a Z-shaped course to the mid-clavicular point. With subsequent scar contraction the Z contracts to a straight line, thus avoiding webbing in the neck. In practice access with the McFee incision is very good and we advocate its use in all situations except when bilateral neck dissection is to be undertaken. In this situation a utility flap on each side joining at the mid-line is safest and gives adequate access (Fig. 13.5).

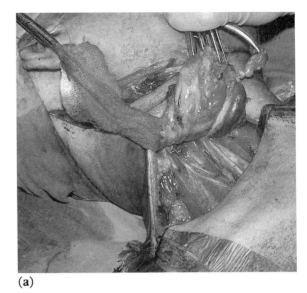

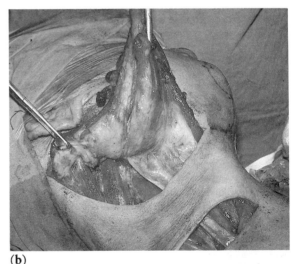

(a)

(b)

Fig. 13.3 (a) and (b) Radical neck dissection in progress showing the excellent access gained through the McFee incision.

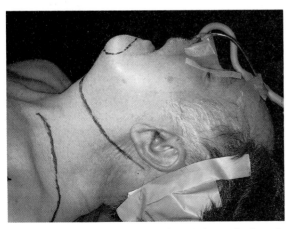

Fig. 13.2 McFee incision preferred for radical neck dissection.

Outcome

Results of neck dissection vary considerably between different reported series. Local recurrence rates as low as 15 per cent and as high as 55 per cent have been reported. The chance of success depends on three factors: the size of the nodal metastases;[25] the number of nodes involved by tumour, more than three nodes involved indicating a poor prognosis;[26] and the presence or absence of spread

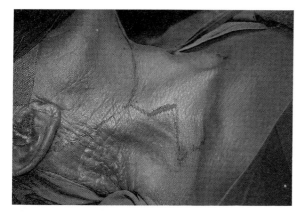

Fig. 13.4 Conventional Morestin-type incision.

of malignancy beyond the capsule of the nodes.[27] Most recurrences occur within 6 months of operation: recurrence after 12 months is rare.[6,28]

Recurrence rate in the neck is related to control of the primary tumour, as it is possible for a recurrent primary to infiltrate once again into the side of the neck which has been completely cleared of all malignancy at the initial treatment. It is important to take the primary control into account when assessing the results of a method of treatment of lymph node metastases, whether it be by surgery alone, radiotherapy or some combination of treatment modalities. The results of treatment of the neck can only be assessed accurately in those patients in whom the primary disease is controlled.

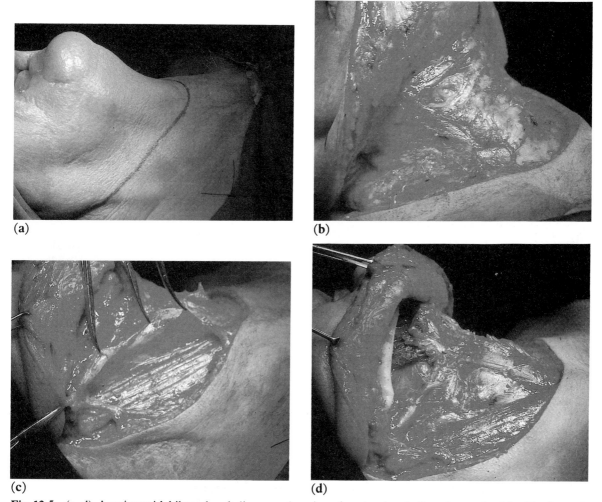

(a)

(b)

(c)

(d)

Fig. 13.5 (a–d) A patient with bilateral neck disease undergoing a functional neck dissection on the right side. Access is via a 'utility' flap, using the anterior approach according to Ballantyne.[23]

Many reported series fail to take primary control into account, which makes assessment of the results difficult or impossible.

Although many authors[22,29,30] now advocate functional and selective neck dissections even for N1 disease, relying on postoperative radiotherapy to effect a cure, the present authors do not accept this approach. On general principles it is wrong to compromise a curative operation: more evidence based on prospective trials is needed before functional neck dissection can be accepted to give results as good as those of the classical operation, so the authors' policy remains to perform a radical neck dissection whenever palpable disease is present in the neck.

Radiotherapy

Radiosensitivity of nodal metastases

For many years there was a widely held belief that metastases in lymph nodes were inherently more radioresistant than the primary tumours from which they were derived, and thus that neck nodes were not amenable to radiotherapy and should always be treated surgically. This concept was derived from experience of the management of oral cancer in the 1930s and 1940s when it was a more common disease. During this period, it was standard practice to treat many of the primary lesions, especially in the tongue, by radium needle implants, with good results. However, it is not possible to treat lymph node metastases in the neck solely by radium needles, and the only external radiotherapy available at that time was orthovoltage X-rays with which it was difficult to administer adequate dosage to the neck. Consequently, results of irradiation of neck metastases were poor, and so they came to be regarded as unsuitable for radiotherapy because of 'radioresistance'. Nevertheless, Martin[31] was able to report a series of 146 patients with oral cancer having nodal metastases where the nodes were treated by a combination of radium needle implant and orthovoltage X-rays; a 5 year survival of 27 per cent was obtained in the series of 146 patients, compared with a 25 per cent 5 year survival in a historical group of similar cases, where the nodes were treated by block dissection.

The advent of supervoltage radiotherapy in the 1950s made it possible to deliver a homogenous dose of radiation to both primary and lymph nodes *en bloc*. There are several reported series, summarised by Henk,[32] of patients treated by radical supervoltage external radiation in this way. The results demonstrate that a lymph node metastasis is not necessarily more radioresistant than its primary. The likelihood of control by radiotherapy is related to the size of the lesion, whether it be a primary or a metastasis. It is most usual either to control both the primary and the nodes, or to fail with both. Node failure with primary control is no commoner than the converse; it occurs usually in a patient with a small primary and a large node. The use of supervoltage radiation to the primary does, however, tend to give lower primary control rates compared with interstitial therapy (see Chapter 8), so that in practice node failure is still more common than primary failure in patients treated solely by radiotherapy. The reason why surgery is nearly always the preferred treatment for nodal metastases, but not necessarily for the primary, is that the success rate of surgical salvage for postradiotherapy recurrence is high in the case of the primary tumour but low in the case of nodes.

Technique

The technique of irradiating lymph nodes simultaneously with the primary tumour is described in the previous chapter. If treatment is to nodal areas alone, the entire lymphatic drainage of the oral cavity can be covered by a single anterior field from a linear accelerator, as the lymph node involvement is mostly in the anterior half of the neck. It is rarely necessary to add an opposing posterior field except in a patient with an unusually broad neck or where there is involvement of the posterior triangle. The chin should be well extended so that the submandibular and upper deep cervical nodes can be included in the field without the beam passing through the mouth (Fig. 13.6). A central lead strip shields the mid-line structures.

For elective nodal irradiation for subclinical disease, a dose of 50 Gy over 5 weeks is adequate.[33] A similar technique is used for postoperative radiotherapy after neck dissection, in which case 60 Gy is advisable. For control of clinically involved nodes treated solely by radiotherapy, the ultimate dose is 65–70 Gy; a similar technique is used to deliver to 50 Gy followed by a boost to the involved nodes, ideally using a lateral electron field of appropriate energy.

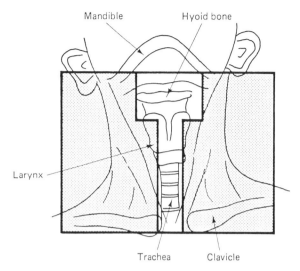

Mandible   Hyoid bone

Larynx

Trachea   Clavicle

Fig. 13.6 Anterior field for irradiating lymph nodes of the neck.

Management of the clinically negative neck – stage N0

There is no doubt that in a proportion of patients with oral cancer the regional lymph nodes contain occult foci of cancer cells at the time of presentation, although no lymph nodes may be palpable. This can be inferred from the experience that many patients develop lymph node metastases at an interval after successful treatment of the primary, and in the absence of any recurrence at the primary site. Confirmation of the existence of occult metastases has been established by histological examination of block dissection specimens where microscopic foci of cancer cells have frequently been found. It therefore seems logical that removal or treatment of the regional lymph nodes may be expected to improve cure rates. On the other hand, it may be argued that treatment of the nodes in all patients is unnecessary, and may in fact be harmful because the nodes are a barrier to the spread of the disease, and may be producing specific immune defences against the tumour.

There is a continuing debate about whether or not elective treatment should be given to the clinically negative neck in oral cancer. The arguments in favour of treatment are as follows:

(1) There is a high incidence of histologically involved nodes in N0-stage patients undergoing elective neck dissection. Sako et al.[34] reported

a 28 per cent incidence of histologically positive nodes in 123 patients with squamous cell carcinoma at various head and neck sites who underwent elective neck dissection without palpable lymph nodes. The incidence from primaries in the oral cavity may be even higher. Southwick[35] summarised several reports with an incidence up to 60 per cent.

(2) The survival rate is significantly lower in patients who develop nodal metastases.

(3) The recurrence rate after neck dissection is higher in those cases with more advanced disease where there is extracapsular extension of tumour or multiple nodes involved.

(4) By waiting until microscopic foci develop into palpable masses, some patients will be given the opportunity to reach the bad prognostic stage above.

(5) Some patients may fail to attend regularly for follow up, increasing the likelihood of the disease reaching a bad prognostic stage or even becoming inoperable.

(6) Neck dissection or neck irradiation carry a low morbidity.

(7) Nodal failure is the most frequent cause of death in many reported series. For example, Pierquin et al.[36] reported that in 61 patients with carcinoma of the tongue and floor of the mouth in whom the primary was treated by interstitial irradiation, there was a 5 year survival rate of only 51 per cent, despite a 95 per cent local control rate of the primary tumour.

(8) Some retrospective reviews have reported a higher survival rate in patients managed by elective nodal treatment, compared with a watch policy. Roux-Berger et al.[37] reviewing cases of carcinoma of the tongue, reported a 5 year survival of 22 per cent in patients undergoing elective neck dissection and 11 per cent in patients undergoing therapeutic dissection. Piedbois et al.[38] compared 110 patients undergoing elective neck dissection with 120 managed by a watch policy and therapeutic neck dissection reserved for nodal relapse; although there was no overall difference in survival, a multivariate analysis revealed that elective neck dissection was a significantly favourable prognostic factor. Similarly, Dearnaley et al.[39] found elective neck irradiation to be a significantly favourable factor.

The arguments against elective neck treatment may be summarised as follows:

(1) The overall incidence of histologically positive nodes in elective neck dissection specimens seems to exceed the incidence of subsequent lymph node metastases in patients in whom the neck is dissected. Accordingly, it is possible that some microscopic foci of tumour are destroyed by the body's own defences and never develop into overt metastases.

(2) Removal of regional lymph nodes removes a barrier to the spread of the disease and destroys nodes which may be producing an immunological response against the primary tumour. Removal of these nodes is therefore likely to increase the risk of primary recurrence and distant metastases. This is almost certainly a spurious argument as animal experiments, e.g. those of Pilch *et al.*,[40] show that in those instances where the animal mounts an immunological response to its tumour, the clones of specifically sensitised lymphoid cells are distributed systemically by the time a tumour is clinically evident.

(3) The primary tumour may recur or a second primary develop and metastasise to the dissected neck.

(4) Elective treatment is no guarantee against neck recurrence. In the series of elective neck dissections reported by Piedbois *et al.*[38] 13 per cent of the patients developed neck recurrence, despite having no recurrence at the primary site. In a series of 244 elective neck dissections reported by de Croix and Ghossein,[41] the recurrence rate was 8 per cent without primary recurrence; this figure included 7 out of 160 patients for whom no histological evidence of nodal metastases had been found in the neck dissection specimens!

(5) The adverse effects of elective nodal treatment are far from negligible. Piedbois *et al.*[38] reported a 2 per cent mortality from neck dissection. Minor morbidity is frequent, including deformity, stiffness and problems with shoulder function. Elective nodal irradiation can lead to some degree of permanent xerostomia.

(6) No prospective controlled clinical trial has shown any advantage from elective neck treatment. Vandenbrouck *et al.*[42] reported a controlled trial conducted at the Institute Gustav Roussy from 1966 to 1973; it involved patients with carcinomas of the tongue and floor of the mouth where the primary was treated by interstitial irradiation. Eighty patients were randomly allocated to elective neck dissection, or to a watch and wait policy. In the former group, 49 per cent had positive nodes, 13 per cent with extracapsular extension. In the latter group, 47 per cent subsequently developed lymph node metastases, all but one within 15 months of the primary treatment; surgery was performed on 41 per cent. There was no difference in survival or recurrence patterns between the two treatment groups, but with such small numbers confidence intervals are wide. Pointon and Gleave[43] reported a controlled trial of elective neck irradiation in 204 patients with oral cavity carcinoma. The patients were randomly allocated to receive either no neck treatment or nodal irradiation to a dose of 40 Gy in 16 fractions over 3 weeks. Of the control group 25 per cent required subsequent block dissection, compared with 14 per cent of the treated group; this difference was just short of the conventional 5 per cent significance level. There was no difference in survival.

Elective neck dissection

Surgery is the method most often employed for the treatment of the clinically negative neck. The choice of operation is between a functional neck dissection and a supra-omohyoid neck dissection. For aggressive primary disease or tumours in the posterior part of the oral cavity, a functional neck dissection is recommended. For less aggressive disease in the anterior part of the oral cavity a supra-omohyoid dissection may be undertaken.

The effectiveness of elective neck dissection can be judged only from recurrence rates in the neck in patients who do not develop recurrence at the primary site. The failure rate appears to be around 5 per cent. Khafif *et al.*[25] reported two recurrences in 42 patients who underwent elective neck dissection. de Croix and Ghossein[41] reported rather higher figures. Their series contained 160 patients for whom the neck dissection proved histologically negative but, nevertheless, there were still four recurrences (2.5 per cent). Of the 51 patients with three or less nodes histologically involved there were five recurrences (10 per cent), and of the 33 patients with either more than three nodes involved or the presence of extracapsular spread of tumour there were seven recurrences (21 per cent).

Elective neck irradiation

Micrometastases in the neck contain small numbers of cells which may be presumed to be mostly well oxygenated. According to radiobiological theory, such metastases should be controllable by a dose of radiation appreciably lower than that necessary to control a palpable tumour. Unfortunately, quite large deposits may be impalpable; extracapsular extension is a not infrequent histological finding in elective neck dissection specimens. Accordingly, doses only 10–15 per cent lower than maximum tissue tolerance are normally employed. The earliest data on dosage for elective nodal irradiation came from Fletcher[44] and Bagshaw and Thompson.[45] Fletcher reported on patients with unilateral involved nodes who were treated by block dissection; he found that irradiation of the opposite side of the neck reduced the incidence of contralateral neck metastases from approximately 30 per cent to less than 5 per cent; where metastases did appear, the dose given was less than 50 Gy over 5 weeks for elective nodal irradiation of patients staged N0; of 91 patients with carcinomas of the oral cavity, only five developed nodal metastases, all of whom also had recurrence at the primary site.

More recent reviews support the earlier claims of the effectiveness of 50 Gy over 5 weeks in eliminating subclinical neck disease. Mendenhall et al.[46] reported on the incidence of nodal metastases and ultimate neck failure in patients with a controlled primary; of 15 patients without elective neck irradiation, four developed nodes, of whom only one was salvaged surgically; of 25 patients receiving elective nodal irradiation, only one developed nodal metastases and was successfully salvaged by surgery. Rabuzzi et al.[47] irradiated the neck of 33 N0-stage patients: four developed nodal metastases, of whom three also had primary recurrence. These results led Jesse and Fletcher[48] to claim unequivocally that 50 Gy over 5 weeks would prevent metastases occurring in the N0-stage neck. It is possible that the dose used in the trial by Pointon and Gleave[43] was biologically less effective than 50 Gy over 5 weeks. Meoz et al.[33] reported that 20 Gy in five treatments was ineffective.

Meoz et al.[33] also demonstrated the importance of adequate coverage of all the nodal areas at risk; most of their neck failures could be explained by inadequate radiation fields failing to cover adequately all the nodes at risk.

Many of the series reported from the USA show an impressive effect of elective nodal irradiation. However, there is a possible fallacy associated with the question of recurrence of the primary. Those who claim that elective nodal radiation is virtually 100 per cent successful assume that, where there is a recurrence of the primary and nodal metastases appear, the latter are the result of remetastasis to the neck from the recurrent primary. It is, however, possible that recurrence of the primary indicates aggressive or radioresistant disease, where subclinical nodal metastases may survive the radiation; hence the failure rate of elective nodal irradiation may be somewhat higher than many of its advocates claim.

The authors' policy

There is no clear evidence of an overall advantage from elective nodal treatment, or that surgical treatment is superior to radiotherapy or vice versa. Nevertheless, nodal failure remains a significant problem.

We advocate treating each patient individually and choosing whether or not to give nodal treatment according to the likelihood of there being occult nodal disease present, and to the prospects of conducting a watch policy successfully. An optimum watch policy requires follow up examination monthly for the first year after treatment and bi-monthly up to 2 years. With a patient for whom subsequent follow up may be difficult because of unreliability or residence overseas so that regular monthly examination is not feasible, elective neck treatment should be undertaken.

In a patient who is suitable for a watch policy, the choice will depend on the probability of the presence of micrometastases, which depends on the size, site and histology of the primary tumour. A watch policy can be adopted where the risk is relatively low, for example, in carcinoma of the lip, or at other sites where the primary is no more than 2 cm in diameter, or is confined to the mucosa or verrucous in type. Patients with larger primary tumours in the mouth or where the histology is poorly differentiated in type should normally have elective neck treatment.

The choice between neck dissection or irradiation depends on the method of treatment of the primary. In general the morbidity of radiotherapy is lower than that of surgery. However, in many surgical procedures it is necessary to enter the neck for purpose of access. In this situation the normal lymphatic channels will be distorted, making the prediction of lymphatic pathways more difficult, and subsequent scarring in the neck will make palpation difficult and reduce the chances of early diagnosis of lymphatic metastases. For a patient with advanced or aggressive primary disease it is often advisable to perform an elective neck dissection as a staging procedure to decide whether or not the neck should be included in the postoperative radiotherapy field. Where the primary is treated by radiotherapy, we advocate neck irradiation.

Management of the clinically positive neck – stages N1, N2a, N2b, N3

Surgery

Surgery is the preferred treatment for nodal metastases, and in general we favour the operation of radical neck dissection (see above). This method of treatment has the highest rate of success but, nevertheless, there is still an appreciable recurrence rate from surgery alone as described above. The risk of recurrence is greater in patients with larger nodes[25] and where histological findings show multiple node involvement or transcapsular spread.[26,49]

Radiotherapy

As previously stated, lymph node metastases are not necessarily more radioresistant than primary tumours, but they cannot be satisfactorily treated by interstitial irradiation, so control rates tend to be lower. Schneider et al.[50] reported a 2 year local control rate of 81 per cent from radiotherapy of single nodes not exceeding 3 cm in diameter; for single nodes greater than 3 cm, the control rate was 64 per cent. They did, however, exclude from their analysis all patients with recurrence at the primary site, so the true control rate is almost certainly lower than the figures quoted.

Henk[32] reported a 64 per cent 3 year control rate of all unilateral mobile lymph node metastases whether or not the primary was controlled: it is possible that in one or two of these patients a recurrent primary remetastasised to a previously sterilised neck, but this seems rather unlikely.

The above series referred to lymph node metastases from a variety of primary sites. Bartelink et al.[51] found that metastases from oral cavity squamous cell carcinoma responded less well to radiotherapy than metastases from pharyngeal carcinoma. A possible criticism of all the results quoted for control of nodal metastases by radiotherapy is that cytological or histological confirmation of malignancy was not obtained from all patients, so it is probable that in some patients the palpable lymph nodes did not contain tumour. It is a not infrequent experience that such nodes when removed for biopsy or by block dissection prove to be histologically negative; for instance, Sako et al.[34] found that 28 per cent of block dissection specimens from patients with palpable nodes contained no tumour.

There seems little doubt that the results of radiotherapy alone are somewhat inferior to those of surgery alone. Radical radiotherapy with salvage surgery is not advisable as a treatment policy for lymph node metastases, in contrast to the management of oral primary tumours. The major reason is that recurrence in the neck after radiotherapy is not as readily diagnosable as recurrence at the primary site. Recurrence after irradiation may not appear as a discrete lymph node mass, but as diffuse infiltration of the soft tissues, so salvage surgery is less likely to be effective.

Combined treatment

The question then arises, can a combination of surgery and radiotherapy give better results than either modality alone? Pre-operative radiotherapy has been discussed elsewhere in this book. Results of controlled trials leave little doubt that it reduces the local recurrence rate after neck dissection with little or no increase in morbidity,[52] but it can be inconvenient and is not popular. It may have a place in the case of borderline operability, or when the primary is being treated by radical radiotherapy. It is also being advised where there has been a previous biopsy.[19]

Postoperative radiotherapy is much more widely practised than pre-operative radiotherapy, but has not been tested in a controlled trial. Retrospective series certainly strongly suggest that it considerably reduced the risk of local recurrence, especially where there are multiple nodes involved or there is extracapsular extension. For example, in the series reported by de Croix and Ghossein[26] postoperative radiotherapy was given to those patients for whom histological examination of the block dissection specimen revealed involvement of three or more nodes, or extracapsular extension; there were 27 in all. Local recurrence in the neck occurred in only four patients, a lower incidence than would be expected without radiotherapy. A number of other large retrospective series have shown a reduced incidence of local recurrence when postoperative radiotherapy was given.[53,54] Postoperative radiotherapy should always be considered in those patients with histological features associated with a high risk of recurrence, i.e. multiple nodal involvement and extracapsular spread of tumour.

The choice of treatment for the N1 neck depends to some extent on how the primary is treated. The authors adopt the following policy. Where there is advanced inoperable primary disease, the involved node is included in the treatment volume and given a radical dose, because if the primary is controlled by the irradiation, it is likely that the node will be controlled also, and there is no need to perform surgery for the node alone. If the treatment for the primary is external irradiation followed by an implant, the nodes are included in the externally irradiated volume and given a pre-operative dose of 45–50 Gy over 4.5–5 weeks, or the equivalent. A neck dissection is done as soon as possible after removal of the implant. When the primary is treated solely by surgery or interstitial irradiation, the neck nodes are treated by surgery, and subsequent postoperative radiotherapy is given if there is multiple nodal involvement or extracapsular extension. There are rare occasions when the patient proves fit for interstitial irradiation but unfit for major surgery; in these cases, the neck is treated by external beam irradiation.

Influence of positive neck on primary treatment

It has been suggested that the risk of failure of radiotherapy to the primary tumour is greater when lymph node metastases are present. There is very little data on this for oral cancer. Data on supraglottic and oropharyngeal cancer are conflicting, with the weight of evidence in favour of there being no relation between the presence of nodal metastases and primary control.[55]

The presence of nodal metastases need not necessarily influence the choice of treatment for the primary. Usually, if there are nodal metastases, they are treated surgically and it may be more convenient to treat the primary surgically at the same time. However, if it is felt that radiation may give a better functional result than surgery, radio-

therapy to the primary can be combined with a neck dissection.

Inoperable nodal metastases

The operability of lymph nodes may be difficult to assess. Fixity is a difficult physical sign to interpret, and most nodal metastases of 3 cm or less in diameter are removable and should be managed in a similar manner whether or not they appear fixed. Attachment to the carotid sheath certainly need not be a contra-indication to surgery. It may be possible to peel the tumour off the carotid sheath, and, if necessary, the external carotid artery can be removed. Stell and Green[56] reported a median survival of 24 months in a small series of patients in whom nodes were considered fixed but were treated by neck dissection.

CT scanning is a useful adjunct in assessing operability.

The treatment most commonly given to patients with inoperable nodes is external radiotherapy, but results are usually poor with control rates less than 50 per cent and very few 5 year survivors. The addition of chemotherapy (see Chapter 9) or hyperthermia[57] may possibly improve local control but not survival.

In some cases, it may be worth trying to render a fixed mass operable by prior radiotherapy. Jesse and Fletcher[48] advocate pre-operative radiotherapy to a dose of 50 Gy over 5 weeks. If, at the end of the 5 week course of treatment the node becomes mobile, neck dissection is attempted; if not, a further 20 Gy are given by a smaller field to the residual mass. Chemotherapy may also be used for the same purpose, but the response is less predictable than to radiotherapy.

Bilateral metastases

It is rather uncommon for a patient with oral cancer to present with bilateral metastases. Bilateral metastases are usually found where the primary is close to the mid-line, e.g. in the lip or floor of the mouth, and indicate a poor prognosis. It is unwise to perform simultaneous radical neck dissection on both sides of the neck because of the high morbidity and mortality associated with removal of both internal jugular veins. Where surgery is attempted in such a patient, a modified block dissection is done on the side of the neck with the less extensive disease, although some surgeons attempt a jugular vein graft. The value of bilateral dissection has been questioned by Stell and Green,[56] who found that the median survival of all patients with head and neck cancer who had bilateral neck dissection was 6 months, compared with 2 months for untreated patients.

The patient with bilateral nodal metastases often has a large inoperable primary that is best treated by external irradiation, in which case it is logical to treat the nodes also by radiotherapy. There is an exception in the case of carcinoma of the lip, where the primary can be treated separately by surgery or interstitial irradiation; in these cases it is worth considering surgery for the lymph nodes, combined with pre- or postoperative radiotherapy as discussed above.

Nodal metastases subsequent to primary treatment

Provided the patient is followed up at regular intervals after treatment to the primary, it should be possible to detect a lymph node metastasis while it is still relatively small and operable. Aspiration cytology is useful to confirm the presence of carcinoma in a lymph node. If cytology is negative and there is real doubt about the nature of a lump in the neck, an open biopsy is necessary as described above.

The management of a lymph node metastasis depends on several factors, i.e. whether or not the primary tumour is controlled, any previous treatment given to the neck, and the side of the neck involved, as follows.

Untreated neck with primary controlled
Neck dissection should be performed and postoperative radiotherapy given if there is involvement of multiple nodes or extracapsular extension.

Untreated neck with primary recurrent
In these cases, it is necessary to perform a surgical salvage procedure, if possible, to remove the recurrent primary. A neck dissection should be performed in continuity and postoperative radiotherapy given as indicated. If the primary is considered unsuitable for any attempt at radical treatment, there is no point in operating on the neck or giving radical radiotherapy, and only palliative treatment is indicated.

Ipsilateral metastases in the electively treated neck
Metastases in the treated neck are most commonly associated with primary recurrence, and again the primary and nodes should be removed in continuity if at all possible; otherwise, only palliative treatment is indicated. Occasionally, a lymph node metastasis appears without recurrence of the primary in a neck where elective treatment has been given previously. If the treatment was radiotherapy, surgery can be performed with some measure of success, although it is not possible to follow this up by postoperative radiotherapy. If an elective neck dissection has been performed and a node appears in the operated side, the prognosis is very poor; it is most unlikely that further surgery can be done, so the only treatment is radical radiotherapy, but the success rate is low.

Contralateral node metastases
These are metastases which appear on the side of the neck opposite to the primary or to the initial lymph node metastases. They are most often seen after an ipsilateral neck dissection. They sometimes can be treated successfully by a block dissection. Pointon and Jelly[28] reported of 26 patients from the Manchester region who underwent a second block dissection between 1950 and 1969; 14 of the patients survived for 5 years after the second operation. It is advisable to preserve the internal jugular vein and to give postoperative radiotherapy.

Management of neck recurrence

Recurrence of tumour in the treated side of the neck carries a very poor prognosis. However, in some cases, it may be worth trying to obtain local control of the neck disease in order to relieve or prevent the distressing symptoms which such recurrence causes, e.g. pain, bleeding, offensive fungation or contraction.

One possible approach is to remove as much as possible of the recurrent tumour surgically and add radiotherapy. Often, radiotherapy has already been given, so further external beam therapy is not possible. In selective cases, an alternative is interstitial irradiation. At the time of surgery, plastic tubes are inserted into the area of recurrent tumour and subsequently loaded with iridium-192 wires (Fig. 13.7). It has been found that neck skin does not tolerate re-irradiation, so there is a high risk of skin

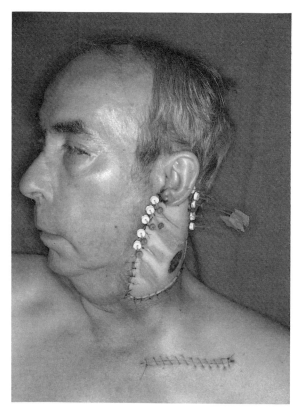

Fig. 13.7 Iridium-192 wire implant for recurrent neck disease.

necrosis. However, the necrosis can be prevented by replacing the neck skin with a pedicled flap[58] (Fig. 13.7).

References

1 Willis RA. *The Spread of Tumours in the Human Body*. London: Butterworths, 1952.

2 McKelvie P. Penetration of the cervical lymph node system by cancer. *Proceedings of the Royal Society of Medicine* 1976; **69**: 409–11.

3 Lindberg R. Distribution of cervical lymph node metastases from squamous cell carcinoma of the upper respiratory and digestive tracts. *Cancer* 1972; **29**: 1446–9.

4 Shah JP, Candela FC, Poddar AK. The patterns of cervical node metastases from squamous carcinoma of the oral cavity. *Cancer* 1990; **66**: 109–13.

5 Sharpe DT. The pattern of lymph node metastases in intraoral squamous cell carcinoma. *British Journal of Plastic Surgery* 1981; **34**: 97–101.

6 Langdon JD, Harvey PW, Rapidis AD, Patel MF, Johnson NW, Hopps R. Oral cancer: the behaviour and response to treatment of 194 cases. *Journal of Maxillofacial Surgery* 1977; **5**: 221–37.

7 Healey WV, Perzin KH, Smith L. Mucoepidermoid carcinoma of salivary gland origin. *Cancer* 1970; **26**: 368–88.

8 Allan MS, Marsh WL. Lymph node involvement by direct extension. *Cancer* 1976; **38**: 2017–21.

9 Stell PM, Cruickshank AH, Stoney PJ, McCormick MS. Lymph node metastases in adenoid cystic carcinoma. *American Journal of Otolaryngology* 1985; **6**: 433–5.

10 Spiro RH, Huvos AG, Strong EW. Adenoid cystic carcinoma of salivary origin. *American Journal of Surgery* 1974; **128**: 512–20.

11 Conley J, Dingman DL. Adenoid cystic carcinoma in the head and neck. *Archives of Otolaryngology* 1974; **100**: 81–90.

12 Feinmesser R, Freeman JL, Noyek AM *et al*. MRI and neck metastases: A clinical, radiological, pathological, correlative study. *Journal of Otolaryngology* 1990; **19**: 136–40.

13 Watkinson JC, Todd CEC, Paskin L *et al*. Metastatic carcinoma in the neck: A clinical, radiological, scintigraphic and pathological study. *Clinical Otolaryngology* 1991; **16**: 187–92.

14 Mancuso AA. Cervical lymph node metastases: Oncological imaging and diagnosis. *International Journal of Radiation Oncology, Biology, Physics* 1984; **10**: 411–23.

15 Baatenburg de Jong, RJ, Rongen RJ, de Jong PC *et al*. Screening from lymph nodes in the neck with ultrasound. *Clinical Otolaryngology* 1988; **13**: 5–9.

16 van der Brekel, MW, Castelijris JA, Croll GA *et al*. Magnetic resonance imaging vs palpation of cervical lymph node metastasis. *Archives of Otolaryngology – Head and Neck Surgery* 1991; **117**: 663–73.

17 McGuirt WF, McCabe BF. Significance of node biopsy before definitive treatment of cervical metastatic carcinomas. *Laryngoscope* 1978; **88**: 594–7.

18 Robbins KT, Cale R, Marvel J *et al*. The violated neck: cervical node biopsy prior to definitive treatment. *Otolaryngology – Head and Neck Surgery* 1986; **94**: 605–10.

19 Parsons JT, Million RR, Cassisi NJ. The influence of excisional or incisional biopsy of metastatic neck nodes on the management of head and neck cancer. *International Journal of Radiation Oncology, Biology, Physics* 1985; **11**: 1447–54.

20 Crile G. Excision of cancer of the head and neck with special reference to the plan of dissection based on 132 operations. *Journal of the American Medical Association* 1906; **47**: 1780–9.

21 Suen JY, Goepfert H. Standardisation of neck dissection nomenclature. *Head and Neck Surgery* 1987; **10**: 75–7 (editorial).

22 Byers RM. Modified neck dissection. A study of 967 cases from 1970 to 1980. *American Journal of Surgery* 1985; **150**: 414–21.

23 Suen JY. Functional neck dissection. In: Ballantyne JC, Harrison DEF eds. *Rob & Smith's Operative Surgery*. London: Butterworths, 1986: 382–7.

24 McKelvie P. Block dissection of the neck. *British Journal of Hospital Medicine* 1976; **16**: 534–6.

25 Khafif RA, Rafla S, Tepper P *et al*. Effectiveness of radiotherapy with radical neck dissection in cancers of the head and neck. *Archives of Otolaryngology – Head and Neck Surgery* 1991; **117**: 196–9.

26 de Croix Y, Ghossein NA. Experience of the Curie Institute in treatment of cancer of the mobile tongue. 1. Treatment policies and result. *Cancer* 1981; **47**: 496–502.

27 Johnson JT, Barnes EL, Myers EN, Schramm VL, Borochovitz D, Sigler BA. The extra capsular spread of tumours in cervical mode metastases. *Archives of Otolaryngology* 1981; **107**: 725–9.

28 Pointon RC, Jelly GO. Block dissection of the neck for squamous cell carcinoma of the mouth and lips. *Proceedings of the Royal Society of Medicine* 1976; **69**: 414–16.

29 Bocca E, Pignataro O, Oldini C, Cappa C. Functional neck dissection: an evaluation and review of 843 cases. *Laryngoscope* 1984; **94**: 942–5.

30 Byers RM, Wolf PF, Ballantyne AJ. Rationale for elective modified neck dissection. *Head and Neck Surgery* 1988; **10**: 160–7.

31 Martin CL. Treatment of cervical lymph metastases with irradiation alone. *Radiology* 1950; **55**: 62–7.

32 Henk JM. Radiosensitivity of lymph node metastases. *Proceedings of the Royal Society of Medicine* 1975; **68**: 85–6.

33 Meoz RT, Fletcher GH, Lindberg RD. Anatomical coverage in elective irradiation of the neck for squamous carcinoma of the oral tongue. *International Journal of Radiation Oncology, Biology, Physics* 1982; **8**: 1881–5.

34 Sako K, Padier RN, Marchetta FC, Pickner JW. Fallibility of palpation in the diagnosis of metastases in cervical nodes. *Surgery, Gynaecology and Obstetrics* 1964; **118**: 989–90.

35 Southwick HW. Elective neck dissection for intraoral cancer. *Journal of the American Medical Association* 1971; **217**: 454–5.

36 Pierquin B, Chassagne D, Baillet F *et al*. The place of implantation in tongue and floor of mouth cancer. *Journal of the American Medical Association* 1971; **215**: 961–3.

37 Roux-Berger JL, Baud M, Courtial J. Cancer de la partie mobile de la langue. Le curage ganglionaire prophylactique est-il justifie? Statistique de la Foundation Curie. *Memoir de L'academic de Chirurgie* 1949; **75**: 120–6.

38 Piedbois P, Mazeron JJ, Haddad E *et al*. Stage I–II squamous carcinoma of the oral cavity treated by iridium-192: is elective neck dissection indicated? *Radiotherapy and Oncology* 1991; **21**: 100–6.

39 Dearnaley DP, Dardoufas C, A'Hern RP, Henk JM.

Interstitial irradiation for carcinoma of the tongue and floor of mouth: Royal Marsden experience 1970–86. *Radiotherapy and Oncology* 1991; **21**: 183–92.

40 Pilch YH, Bard DS, Ramming KP. The role of the regional lymph nodes in the development of host immunological response to tumours. *American Journal of Roentgenology* 1971; **111**: 48–55.

41 de Croix Y, Ghossein NA. Experience of the Curie Institute in treatment of cancer of the mobile tongue. 1. Treatment policies and result. *Cancer* 1981; **47**: 496–502.

42 Vandenbrouck C, Sancho-Garnier H, Chassagne D, Saravane D, Cachin Y, Micheau C. Elective versus therapeutic radial neck dissection in epidermoid carcinoma of the oral cavity: results of a randomised clinical trial. *Cancer* 1980; **46**: 386–90.

43 Pointon RC, Gleave EN. Lymphatic spread. In: Sikora K, Halnan KE eds. *Treatment of Cancer*. London: Chapman and Hall, 1990: 323–7.

44 Fletcher GH. Elective irradiation of sub-clinical disease in cancers of the head and neck. *Cancer* 1972; **29**: 1450–4.

45 Bagshaw MA, Thompson RW. Elective irradition of the neck in patients with primary carcinoma of the head and neck. *Journal of the American Medical Association* 1971; **217**: 456–8.

46 Mendenhall WM, Million RR, Cassisi NJ. Elective neck irradiation in squamous cell carcinoma of the head and neck. *Head and Neck Surgery* 1980; **3**: 15–20.

47 Rabuzzi DD, Chung CT, Sagerman RH. Prophylactic neck irradiation. *Archives of Otolaryngology* 1980; **106**: 454–5.

48 Jesse RH, Fletcher GH. Treatment of the neck in patients with squamous cell carcinoma of the head and neck. *Cancer* 1977; **39**: 868–72.

49 Carter RL, Bliss JM, Soo KC, O'Brien C. Radical neck dissections for squamous carcinomas: pathological findings and their clinical implications with particular reference to transcapsular spread. *International Journal of Radiation Oncology, Biology, Physics* 1987; **13**: 825–32.

50 Schneider JJ, Fletcher GH, Barkley HT. Control by irradiation alone of non-fixed clinically positive lymph nodes from squamous cell carcinoma of the oral cavity, oropharynx, supraglottic, larynx and hypopharynx. *American Journal of Roentgenology* 1975; **123**: 42–8.

51 Bartelink H, Breur K, Hart G. Radiotherapy of lymph node metastases in patients with squamous cell carcinoma of the head and neck region. *International Journal of Radiation Oncology, Biology, Physics* 1982; **8**: 983–9.

52 Strong EW. Pre-operative radiation and radical neck dissection. *Surgery Clinics of North America* 1969; **49**: 271–6.

53 Bartelink H, Breur K, Hart G *et al*. The value of post-operative radiotherapy as an adjuvant to radical neck dissection. *Cancer* 1983; **52**: 1008–13.

54 Vikram B, Strong EW, Shah JP, Spiro R. Failure in the neck following multimodality treatment for advanced head and neck cancer. *Head and Neck Surgery* 1984; **6**: 720–3.

55 Mendenhall WM, Parsons JT, Amdur RJ *et al.* Squamous cell carcinoma of the head and neck treated with radiation therapy: the impact of neck stage on local control. *International Journal of Radiation Oncology, Biology, Physics* 1988; **14**: 249–52.

56 Stell PM, Green JR. Management of metastases to the lymph glands of the neck. *Proceedings of the Royal Society of Medicine* 1976; **69**: 411–13.

57 Areangeli G, Barni E, Civadalli, A *et al.* Effectiveness of microwave hyperthermia combined with ionizing radiation: clinical results on neck node metastases. *International Journal of Radiation Oncology, Biology, Physics* 1980; **6**: 143–8.

58 Stafford N, Dearnaley DP. Treatment of 'inoperable' neck nodes using surgical clearance and post-operative interstitial irradiation. *British Journal of Surgery* 1988; **75**: 62–4.

14 Pathology of salivary gland tumours

JW Eveson

Introduction

Salivary gland tumours are relatively uncommon; according to data from the cancer registries of England and Wales they form 0.3 per cent of all malignant tumours, which is an incidence of 1.4 per 100 000 population. The large majority of salivary gland tumours are primary epithelial neoplasms (94 per cent) and only these tumours will be discussed here.[1] There are striking variations in the frequency of tumours in different salivary glands and the distribution of individual tumour types (Table 14.1). Thus, nearly 75 per cent of tumours arise in the parotid gland but only 15 per cent of these tumours are malignant. On the other hand, tumours of the sublingual gland are a rarity but most are malignant. It is worthwhile noting that nearly half of tumours of minor (oropharyngeal) salivary glands, are likely to be malignant.

Table 14.1 Percentage frequency of primary epithelial tumours of salivary glands modified from Eveson and Cawson[1]

Site	Frequency (%)	Malignant (%)
Parotid	75	15
Submandibular	11	37
Sublingual	0.3	86
Minor	14	46

Adenomas

Pleomorphic adenoma

Pleomorphic adenoma is the most common tumour of both major and minor salivary glands.[1,2] While they can present at any age, the peak incidence is in the fourth and fifth decades and there is a slight female preponderance. They are most common in the parotid gland, particularly the tail, and the palate. The tumour usually forms a painless, slow growing mass which may show episodic bursts of active growth. Occasionally they can become infected or infarcted and then show sudden changes in size and become painful. Significant facial nerve weakness strongly suggests malignant progression.

Microscopically, the tumour is characterised by having variable encapsulation and architectural rather than cellular pleomorphism. The epithelial and modified myoepithelial cells show a variety of configurations and intermingle with a stroma which can be mucoid, myxoid, fibrous or chondroid. The epithelial and myoepithelial components may be arranged in ducts, strands or sheets of cells. The modified myoepithelial cells are usually polygonal with small, dark nuclei and the cytoplasm may be eosinophilic or clear. They may form an outer layer around the duct-like structures or more solid sheets. Two common variants are where the myoepithelial cells are spindle shaped and may resemble a connective tissue neoplasm or the cytoplasm becomes hyalinised and the nucleus is eccentric forming so-called hyaline or plasmacytoid cells. Squamous metaplasia is common and may be extensive, particularly in minor glands, and may simulate a well differentiated squamous carcinoma. Areas of oncocytic metaplasia are common and occasionally the whole tumour may undergo oncocytic change and can then be misdiagnosed as an oncocytoma.[3]

Although the ratio of epithelium to stroma is extremely variable, in the major glands stroma usually forms the bulk of the tumour. Pleomorphic adenoma in minor glands, on the other hand, tends to be more cellular. The most characteristic appearance of the stroma is the formation of mucoid or myxochondroid areas containing scattered epithelial cells which may be stellate and appear to melt into the background.[4] There may be formation of true cartilage and much less commonly osseous metaplasia. Some areas of stroma may show collagenisation and deposition of elastic tissue and this tends to increase as the tumour ages so that extensive areas of hyaline scarring can form. From a microscopical point of view it is very important to examine such scarred areas carefully because these can be the site of maligant progression and foci can be easily missed by casual perusal.

The principal clinical problems associated with pleomorphic adenoma are the tendency of tumours to recur and malignant progression. Recurrence rates in the literature are extremely variable. In the parotids they are approximately 3.4 per cent in 5 years and 6.8 per cent in 10 years with a range of 1–50 per cent, reflecting cases reported before parotidectomy became the treatment of choice.[5] Recurrences in minor glands are now uncommon.

Attempts have been made to subclassify pleomorphic adenomas on the basis of the type differentiation of the epithelial cells and the proportion and differentiation of the stroma.[6] It has been suggested that cell-rich variants have a higher risk of malignant transformation and that cell-poor variants have a greater propensity to recurrence. One of the major problems when subclassifying these tumours, however, is the extremely variable histological appearances within a single tumour mass which would give a high possibility of sampling errors. It is most likely that the signficiant risk of recurrence in parotid pleomorphic adenomas is due to anatomical features which dictate clinical management. The tumours, although usually discrete, show variable or absent capsulation.[7,8] The tumours tend to grow into the capsule (intracapsular invasion) or bulge through it to impinge on adjacent salivary tissue and produce the characteristic macroscopically bosselated appearance (Fig. 14.1). There is often a natural plane of cleavage between the tumour and the capsule which leaves tumour cells embedded in any capsule which is not excised (Fig. 14.2). In addition, some tumours are mucoid and floppy so that they are easily ruptured during removal. It is also likely that many of the cells, embedded as they are in a myxochondroid matrix, do not have stringent nutritional requirements and survive if seeded into the wound during surgery. For the preceding reasons, it becomes obvious that 'enucleation' or localised exicision of parotid pleomorphic adenoma is likely to be fol-

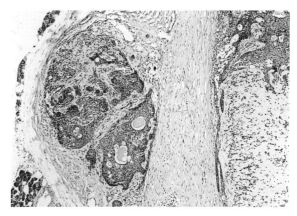

Fig. 14.1 Pleomorphic adenoma showing a nodule of tumour within the capsule. Such apparently separate foci are almost invariably shown to be attached to the main tumour upon serial sectioning. H&E × 60.

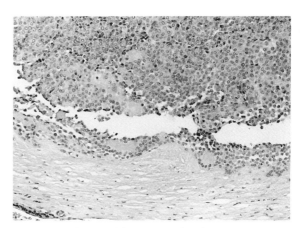

Fig. 14.2 Pleomorphic adenoma showing a natural plane of cleavage just below the capsule producing an artifactual split. H&E × 150.

lowed by recurrence, although the long latent period between surgery and recurrence (often more than 20 years) may lull surgeons into a false sense of security.[9] When tumours recur there are multiple nodules often scattered over a wide area so that surgical eradication can be difficult, mutilating or impossible.[10]

Myoepithelioma

Rarely, tumours consist of myoepithelial cells which may be spindle shaped, plasmacytoid, clear cell or a combination of these.[11-13] The myoepithelial nature of these cells is confirmed by immunocytochemical staining for S-100 antigen, actin, myosin or high molecular weight keratins. The cells usually form solid sheets, or less commonly anastomosing cords, and ductal differentiation is not a feature. The cells are sharply demarcated from the stroma which helps to differentiate them from pleomorphic adenoma which can show areas with similar cellular appearances. Myoepithelioma, however, appears to have more aggressive behaviour than pleomorphic adenoma and there are rare malignant myoepitheliomas.

Warthin's tumour (adenolymphoma; papillary cystadenoma lymphomatosum)

This is the second most common salivary neoplasm. It forms almost exclusively in the parotid gland and accounts for 10–15 per cent of primary epithelial tumours.[14]

The majority of patients are elderly and in the past there was a reported striking male predominance of between 7 and 10 to 1.[15,16] This has fallen steadily[17] and most recent reports show either a slight male preponderance or an equal gender incidence.[18] The reasons for this change are unknown.

Most tumours arise in the lower pole of the parotid where they form painless, discrete soft swellings which may be fluctuant. They rarely exceed 6 cm in diameter. Occasionally tumours become infected or infarcted when pain, increased swelling or facial nerve weakness may be a feature. Bilateral tumours are not rare (5–10 per cent of cases) and sometimes they are multifocal and can arise in association with other salivary gland neoplasms.

There is a thin capsule and the cut surface of the tumours shows cystic spaces lined by papillary ingrowths and containing viscid, brownish fluid.

Microscopy shows cysts lined by a double layer of columnar oncocytic epithelial cells which are palisaded on the luminal aspect and less regular in the basal layer (Fig. 14.3). Mucous metaplasia is common and sometimes florid but ciliated epithelium is focal and rare. The cysts contain amorphous material which may become inspissated and contains cholesterol clefts.

The stroma consists of lymphoid tissue often with germinal centres. There may be a capsule and subcapsular sinus similar to the normal lymph node but sometimes the lymphoid tissue merges with the surrounding salivary gland. The amount of stroma is extremely variable and in some cases the tumour may be virtually free of lymphocytes. Occasionally tumours undergo necrosis and show extensive

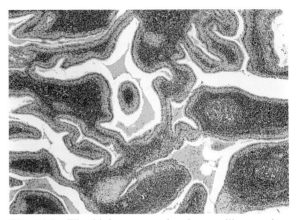

Fig. 14.3   Warthin's tumour showing papillary projections lined by columnar oncocytic epithelium and a densely cellular stroma of small lymphocytes. H&E × 60.

fibrosis and epithelioid granuloma formation so that the appearances can resemble a tuberculous lymph node. In these infected or infarcted Warthin's tumours there can also be extensive squamous metaplasia.[19,20]

Warthin's tumour is benign and complete excision is curative. Recurrences are normally due to multifocal tumours.

Oncocytoma

Oncocytoma is a rare tumour usually seen in the seventh or eighth decade, most commonly in the parotid.[21,22] It consists of a well demarcated mass of polyhedral cells with eosinophilic cytoplasm with vesicular nuclei. The cells form columns or tubules which are separated by fine fibrous septa. Often cells with intensely eosinophilic cytoplasm and hyperchromatic condensed nuclei (so-called dark cells) are scattered amongst the more numerous 'light cells'. Oncocytic metaplasia is seen in a variety of other benign and malignant salivary gland tumours including pleomorphic adenoma, basal cell adenoma and mucoepidermoid carcinoma, and such metaplasia appears to be more common than oncocytoma itself.[3] Rare, clear cell variants of oncocytoma have also been described.[23]

Multifocal nodular oncocytic hyperplasia

This is a rare condition in which multiple non-encapsulated nodules of oncocytic or clear cells form in the parotid gland.[3,24,25] The nodules usually have a lobular distribution but satellite foci may give an erroneous impression of invasion. Multifocal nodular oncocytic hyperplasia can be seen in association with a typical oncocytoma and it is possible that such tumours arise by fusion of hyperplastic nodules.

Canalicular adenoma

Canalicular adenoma consists of columnar cells arranged in anastomosing, bilayered strands.[26,27] The stroma is loose and degenerating and cyst formation is common so that frequently the tumour consists of no more than a mural nodule. Ninety per cent of cases arise in the upper lip and the large majority of the remainder in the buccal mucosa or other minor glands. It is interesting to note that salivary tumours are nearly ten times more common in the upper lip than the lower lip whereas virtually the reverse applies to mucoceles. Therefore, clinicians should have a high index of suspicion that they are dealing with a salivary neoplasm when a patient presents with a cystic swelling in the upper lip.

Sebaceous adenoma

Although sebaceous gland differentiation is common in the parotid and to a lesser extent the submandibular glands, sebaceous tumours are rare.[28] Sebaceous adenomas are cystic or solid circumscribed tumours consisting of nests of sebaceous cells without cellular atypia or invasion. They arise predominantly in the parotid and submandibular glands in elderly patients.

Sebaceous lymphadenoma is a rare variant of sebaceous adenoma which consists of well differentiated sebaceous cells usually arranged in glands with duct formation, lying in a stroma of lymphocytes which may show follicle formation. It is thought that like Warthin's tumour these neoplasms arise in salivary duct inclusions in intra- or paraparotid lymph nodes. Occasionally, they may be associated with miscroscopic foci of Warthin's tumour. Sebaceous adenomas are benign and do not recur after conservative excision.

Basal cell adenoma

Basal cell adenomas form 1–2 per cent of salivary gland tumours, the majority arising in the parotid glands (70 per cent) and the upper lip (20 per cent). The peak age of incidence is in the seventh decade.

Microscopically, the tumours consist of circumscribed or encapsulated masses of isomorphic basaloid cells with distinct basement membrane-like structures. There is no mucoid stromal component which distinguishes these tumours from pleomorphic adenomas. There are four cellular patterns: trabecular, tubular, solid and membranous.

The trabecular and tubular variants are frequently combined and consist of anastomosing cords of uniform dark cells with formation of duct-like structures (Fig. 14.4). The stroma is typically scanty and fibrous but may be cellular and a variant where the stroma is rich in myoepithelial cells has been described.[29] Some, however, believe this variant to be merely part of the spectrum of pleomorphic adenoma.[30] Tubulo-trabecular basal cell adenoma can undergo oncocytic metaplasia and thus resemble an oncocytoma.[3]

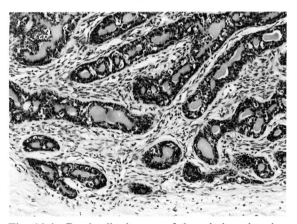

Fig. 14.4 Basal cell adenoma of the tubulo-trabecular type. H&E × 150.

The solid variant consists of compact masses of dark-staining epithelial cells which may have a peripheral row of more palisaded cells and basisquamous whorling of the globular ends of the epithelial islands. The epithelial islands are sharply demarcated from the stroma by a prominant periodic acid-Schiff (PAS) positive basement membrane.

The membranous (dermal analogue) type is a rare but distinctive variant. There is a thick, hyaline basement membrane layer and intercellular hyaline droplets. This tumour may be multifocal and multicentric and in about 10 per cent of cases there is an association with dermal cylindromas (turban tumours) which the tumour microscopically resembles.[31] Malignant transformation of basal cell adenomas to basal cell adenocarcinomas has been reported.[32]

Duct papillomas

These form a rare but distinctive group of tumours. They include:

(1) *Inverted duct papilloma*

These rare tumours resemble the inverted papilloma of the nose and are thought to arise from the excretory ducts of minor glands.[33] They are lined by squamous epithelial cells which proliferate and extend into the surrounding connective tissue. Mucous metaplasia and microcysts lined by squamous or columnar epithelium may be present. Conservative excision appears to be curative.

(2) *Intraductal papilloma*

This very rare tumour arises from the excretory ducts of minor glands where it forms a solitary frond-like mass of fibrovascular connective tissue lined by columnar or squamous epithelium.[34]

(3) *Sialadenoma papilliferum*

This tumour, which resembles syringocystadenoma papilliferum of skin, is most common in the palate.[35,36] It forms an exophytic, painless mass of papillary fronds on the surface but more deeply there are characteristic double-layered, duct-like structures with papillary projections. Local excision is usually curative.[37]

Cystadenomas

Papillary cystadenomas which closely resemble Warthin's tumour but with lack of a lymphocytic stroma are rare and usually form in the parotid.[38] It is probable that a significant number of so-called oncocytic papillary cystadenomas in the larynx are merely oncocytic metaplasia and duct dilatation rather than true tumours.[39] Similar oncocytic metaplasia and duct dilatation can be seen in stomatitis ('cheilitis') glandularis which is a condition of uncertain aetiology that predominantly affects the lips.[40,41]

Mucinous cystadenoma is a rare tumour consisting of a circumscribed mass with cystic spaces lined by mucus-producing cells. There should be no cellular atypia or evidence of invasion and this diagnosis must be made with caution as the malignant counterpart is much more common.

Carcinomas

Acinic cell carcinoma

Acinic cell carcinoma is uncommon and accounts for about 2 per cent of all salivary gland tumours.[1,42] The majority (80 per cent) present in the parotid gland and about 15 per cent arise in the minor glands. They are twice as common in men than women and most are found in the elderly.[43] They are usually well circumscribed macroscopically but gross examination of resection specimens may show multinodularity. Pain and facial nerve involvement are uncommon. They are rarely bilateral.[44]

Acinic cell carcinomas have a wide variety of appearances. They may be circumscribed but this is typically incomplete. The tumours may be solid, or cystic to varying degress. The typical tumour cells closely resemble the serous acinar cells of normal salivary gland. They are large, round or polygonal, and have granular, basophilic and PAS positive cytoplasm although cells showing the latter can be patchily distributed. Cells resembling intercalated ducts can also be present and occasional tumours show clear or vacuolated cells. Cellular atypia and mitoses are uncommon.

These tumours have a wide variety of morphological growth patterns including solid, microcystic, papillary, cystic and follicular. The most typical pattern is the solid and this closely resembles the normal serous cells of the parotid arranged in sheets or ill defined theques. In the microcystic variety there are many clear round spaces between tumour cells. The follicular pattern, which is rare, is seen when the microcystic spaces coalesce and frequently contain eosinophilic, proteinaceous fluid giving the tumour a distinct resemblance to thyroid gland. A papillary cystic pattern is another uncommon variant and, as in other acinic cell carcinomas, there may be concentrically laminated calcifications (psammoma bodies) (Fig. 14.5).

The stroma may be sparse but some tumours show a striking lymphocytic infiltrate which can initially give the impression that the tumour is a secondary in a lymph node.

Acinic cell carcinomas are low grade malignancies but there is a wide range in the reported frequency of local recurrence or metastasis.[45] The morphological form or the predominant cell type do not correlate well with prognosis but, as in other salivary gland malignancies, pain and fixation,

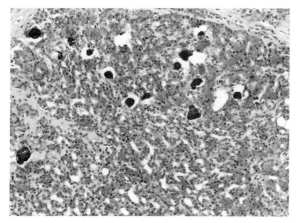

Fig. 14.5 Acinic cell carcinoma showing microcalcifications. H&E × 150.

gross invasion and facial nerve involvement indicate of poor prognosis.[43]

Well differentiated tumours should be treated by total conservative parotidectomy but if the facial nerve is involved it may need to be sacrificed. Poorly differentiated tumours or those showing obvious clinical signs of malignancy will require radical parotidectomy and adjuvant radiotherapy.

Mucoepidermoid carcinoma

Mucoepidermoid carcinomas are characterised by the presence of squamous cells, mucus-producing cells and cells of an intermediate type.

There is a wide variation in the relative frequency of mucoepidermoid carcinoma of the parotid ranging from 1.5 per cent in a large UK survey[1] to 12.3 per cent in an American study.[16] In the minor glands, however, they form about 9 per cent of all tumours.[2]

Clinically, mucoepidermoid carcinomas are typically circumscribed swellings and rarely cause pain or facial weakness. In both major and minor glands there may be a significant cystic component which can confuse the clinical picture.

Macroscopically most tumours, although clinically circumscribed, show invasion and cyst formation and there may be haemorrhage into the cysts.

The proportion of the various cell types and their morphological configuration vary between tumours and often within the same tumour mass. In the cystic tumours, mucous cells predominate but in solid tumours epidermoid and intermediate cells are more common.

Mucous cells are cuboidal, columnar or goblet-like and they can line cysts or form solid masses. When mucous cells are sparse they can be more easily visualised using appropriate stains such as mucicarmine or PAS. The cysts, particularly in minor glands, have a tendency to distend and rupture into the surrounding tissue. This evokes a florid inflammatory response, sometimes with cholesterol clefts and a granulomatous reaction and fibrosis. It is probable that this process results in spread of malignant cells into the surrounding tissue.[46]

The squamous (epidermoid) cells have obvious intercellular bridges but keratinisation, particularly in the form of keratin pearls, is sufficiently uncommon that its presence should make the diagnosis questionable.[47] These may also form solid sheets or line cysts usually together with mucous cells.

Intermediate cells have scanty, faintly eosinophilic cytoplasm and small, dark-staining nuclei.

Hydropic degeneration producing clear cells is not uncommon and occasionally clear cells form the bulk of the tumour so that careful examination may be needed to find evidence of epidermoid differentiation. The clear cells may contain glycogen, typically in the form of droplets rather than granules.

The behaviour of mucoepidermoid carcinomas is unpredictable but even the most histologically benign tumours have the capacity to metastasise. Many attempts have been made to grade these tumours into high and low grades in order to correlate the morphology with behaviour.

High grade tumours correlate with behaviour more reliably than low grade tumours. They are usually large (>4 cm), infiltrative and tend to be solid rather than cystic.[48,49] Haemorrhage, and particularly necrosis, are associated with aggressive behaviour. The tumour shows cytological features of malignancy and usually consists of undifferentiated intermediate cells, or poorly differentiated squamous cells often in an inflamed fibroblastic stroma.[50] Such tumours have a poor prognosis and require radical treatment.

Well differentiated or low grade tumours are usually small (<4 cm) and predominantly cystic. They typically consist of epidermoid and mucous cells and do not show cytological features of malignancy. As mentioned previously, although they are clinically circumscribed, they almost invariably show microscopical evidence of invasion.

The overall survival rate using meta-analysis is about 70 per cent after 5 years and 50 per cent at

10 years.[5] However, for high grade tumours the prognosis is much worse than these figures would suggest.[51]

Total conservative parotidectomy is usually sufficient for low grade tumours. With high grade tumours prognosis is so poor that it is debatable whether radical surgery is appropriate and probably has no advantage over radiotherapy which is obviously less mutilating.

Adenoid cystic carcinoma

Adenoid cystic carcinomas are slow growing but relentlessly progressive tumours. They form about 2 per cent of parotid tumours but are relatively more frequent in the submandibular gland (17 per cent) and the minor glands (13 per cent).

The peak age incidence is in the sixth decade and tumours usually form a slowly enlarging mass. Occasionally growth is more rapid in a pre-existing mass. Pain and tenderness and facial palsy are common manifestations. Ulceration is uncommon but is sometimes seen in intra-oral tumours which are subjected to trauma.[52]

Adenoid cystic carcinomas have a variety of histological features with three predominant growth patterns: cribriform (cylindromatous), tubular and solid.[53-56] Some tumours show combinations of all three growth patterns. The cells are of two types in varying proportions: duct lining cells which are uniform, small and dark-staining, and myoepithelial cells which typically have clear cytoplasm. Mitoses are usually infrequent.

The cribriform variant is the most typical and consists of islands of epithelial cells containing numerous spherical spaces giving a 'Swiss cheese' pattern. These spaces are pseudocysts and consist of proteoglycans and reduplicated basement membrane material. Small, duct-like structures may be present in the more solid areas.

The tubular variant consists of double-layered, duct-like structures with an inner, dark-staining lining cell and an outer, typically clear, myoepithelial cell layer. Similar areas can, however, be seen in pleomorphic adenomas and epithelial–myoepithelial carcinomas which can make diagnosis difficult in limited biopsy material or fine needle aspiration specimens.

The solid variant consists of sheets or islands of dark-staining cells which may show mitoses. There is often central necrosis and artifactual splitting of the tumour islands from the surrounding stroma.

All types of adenoid cystic carcinoma are malig-

nant and can metastasise, often after many years and typically to the lung. The main problem with the tumour is local spread. There is a particular propensity for the tumour to show perineural invasion and spread along nerves, often for considerable distances from the clinically detectable main tumour mass. The tumour can extend widely through bone and again there may be little clinical evidence of the extent of the spread, particularly in the maxilla. In many instances lymph node involvement is through contiguous spread rather than permeation or embolisation.

The overall long term prognosis is poor with many patients dying 15 or 20 years after diagnosis.

The tubular variety has the best prognosis and the solid type has the worst.[57] Site is important, tumours in the submandibular gland and maxilla having a particularly poor prognosis. Tumours with atypical histograms on cytophotometry also have a poor prognosis.[58]

In many, if not the majority of cases, it is probably not possible to eradicate the tumour completely by surgery. Therefore, supraradical and mutilating surgery is not justified. Many treat the tumour by radical resection and postoperative radiotherapy and some tumours appear to respond satisfactorily to radiotherapy alone. Long term survival with pulmonary metastasis is also possible so the presence of lung secondaries does not necessarily preclude vigorous treatment of the primary tumour.

Polymorphous low grade adenocarcinoma

This is a distinctive clinicopathological entity which has only been recognised relatively recently.[59,60] As it was described independently by several workers it has also been termed a lobular carcinoma,[61] terminal duct carcinoma[62] and polymorphous low grade adenocarcinoma of minor glands.[63] It is seen almost exclusively in minor glands but there have been isolated reports of the tumour in major glands, usually supervening on a pleomorphic adenoma.[64] The importance of polymorphous low grade adenocarcinoma is that it has a relatively good prognosis and that it can be readily confused with several other salivary gland carcinomas including adenoid cystic carcinoma and carcinoma arising in pleomorphic adenoma and possibly resulting in inappropriate treatment.

The characteristic histological feature of this

tumour is cytological uniformity and morphological diversity.

Macroscopically the tumour may appear to be circumscribed but there is microscopical evidence of invasion and no defined capsule.

The cells are small to medium in size and have pale, vesicular nuclei with few mitoses. The tumour can show a striking variety of morphological patterns in a single case and these include: lobular (sometimes with a peripheral palisade), papillary, cribriform (sometimes resembling adenoid cystic carcinoma) and trabecular with small duct-like structures. The cells may show concentric targetting or whorling around nerves and sometimes ducts or blood vessels (Fig. 14.6). The stroma is also variable and may show collagenisation, elastosis or mucinosis. Foci of interstitial or stromal haemorrhage are common.

Although there is microscopical evidence of invasion and neurotropism, the polymorphous low grade adenocarcinoma does not show the relentless spread associated with adenoid cystic carcinoma. There is local recurrence in about 20 per cent of cases but regional and distant metastasis is uncommon.

It is unclear whether so-called papillary low grade adenocarcinomas, which also predominantly involve minor glands, are a distinct entity or particularly papillary variants of polymorphous low grade adenocarcinoma.[65,66] However, there is evidence that the former tumours have a worse prognosis with a greater risk of local recurrence and lymph node metastasis.

Epithelial–myoepithelial carcinoma

This tumour has been described under a variety of names and was previously thought to be benign.[67] In the first World Health Organization (WHO) classification,[68] the Armed Forces Institute of Pathology fascicle on salivary gland tumours[46] and many standard pathology texts it is called a clear cell adenoma or a glycogen rich adenoma. It is also termed an intercalated duct carcinoma.

The large majority of tumours are seen in the major glands, particularly the parotid and the peak age of incidence is in the seventh and eighth decades. They usually produce a painless swelling but pain and facial nerve involvement have been reported.

The tumour is composed of two cell types which may be present in highly variable porportions. There are inner, dark-staining, duct-lining cells and outer clear cells (Fig. 14.7). The outer cells stain strongly for glycogen and are positive for S-100 protein, actin and myosin.[69] A myoepithelial origin for these cells is supported by the electron microscopical features.

Sometimes the duct-like structures are widely dispersed in an abundant fibrous stroma or they may be packed together to form sheets. In some tumours clear cells predominate and duct-lining cells may be very infrequent. It is probable that many so-called clear cell carcinomas are epithelial–myoepithelial carcinomas of this type.

The cells are cytologically bland and mitoses are infrequent giving the tumour an histologically innocent appearance. However, the tumour shows local spread and can also show perineural and vascular

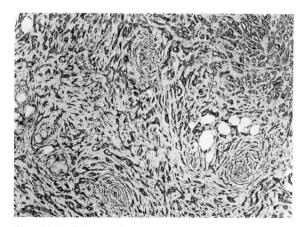

Fig. 14.6 Polymorphous low grade adenocarcinoma showing striking perineural whorling and surviving elements of minor salivary gland within the tumour. H&E × 60.

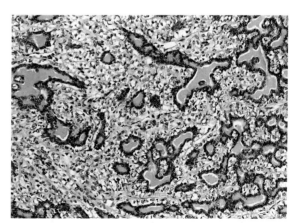

Fig. 14.7 Epithelial–myoepithelial carcinoma consisting of dark-staining inner cuboidal cells and outer clear cells which in areas form solid sheets. H&E × 150.

invasion. Recurrence and metastasis has been reported in about one-third of cases.

Basal cell adenocarcinoma

This is an epithelial neoplasm that has the cytological characteristics of a basal cell adenoma but a morphological growth pattern indicative of malignancy.[70]

There have been few reported cases thus far as it is a relatively recently characterised tumour. It appears to be most common in the parotid and submandibular glands and is extremely rare in the minor glands. There is no gender predilection and most patients are over 50 years of age.

The tumour consists of uniform dark-staining cells which typically form multiple solid islands resembling cutaneous basal cell carcinomas or eccrine cylindromas (Fig. 14.8). The islands often have a distinct, hyalinised basal membrane zone and there may be hyaline material between the cells in the form of droplets. Peripheral palisading of nuclei at the tumour/stroma interface is a variable feature. Occasionally the tumour is trabecular or tubular in type rather than membranous. Cytological features of malignancy can be minimal and occasionally there is squamous differentiation or the formation of small lumina within the tumour islands. The stroma is typically fibroblastic.

The main distinction from benign basal cell adenomas is evidence of invasion which can be into the surrounding gland and commonly involves nerves and vessels.

Basal cell adenocarcinomas are low grade malignancies with a local recurrence rate of about 25 per cent and metastasis in less than 10 per cent of cases.

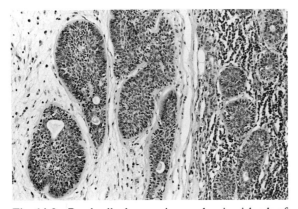

Fig. 14.8 Basal cell adenocarcinoma showing islands of tumour which resemble solid basal cell adenoma but with invasion of adjacent lymphoid tissue. H&E × 150.

Sebaceous carcinoma

This is a very rare tumour composed of sebaceous cells of varying degrees of maturity which arise almost exclusively in the parotid gland.[28,71] They usually form discrete swellings with local invasion or less commonly perineural invasion or metastasis to regional lymph nodes.

The tumour consists of sheets or theques of cells with variable atypia, pleomorphism and mitotic activity. The cytoplasm is usually foamy but there may be foci where it is clear so that the tumour falls into the differential diagnostic spectrum of clear cell salivary neoplasms.

Sebaceous lymphadenocarcinoma is a very rare but distinctive variant where sebaceous carcinoma appears to arise in a sebaceous lymphadenoma.

Sebaceous carcinoma is slow growing and is generally considered to be low grade but in one series a third of the patients died from the disease.[72]

Papillary cystadenocarcinoma

This is a malignant tumour which is characterised by the formation of cysts with papillary endocystic projections. The palate is the most common site.[73] The tumour is composed of single or multiple cystic spaces with papillary projections consisting of narrow fibrous tissue cores covered by cuboidal or low columnar epithelial cells and sometimes goblet-shaped mucous cells.

Some tumours show nuclear pleomorphism and mitoses or obvious invasive growth. However, some are deceptively innocent cytologically and some authorities are reluctant to accept the existence of benign papillary cystic neoplasms of the salivary gland apart from Warthin's tumour or the papillary cystadenoma which resembles Warthin's tumour without lymphoid stroma.

The main differential diagnosis is from polymorphous low grade adenocarcinoma, papillary variants of acinic cell carcinoma and metastases, particularly from the thyroid gland.

Most papillary adenocarcinomas are low grade but very late metastasis has been reported so protracted follow up is essential.

Mucinous adenocarcinoma

This is a rare carcinoma which is characterised by abundant mucus production. Typically there are multiple, mucus-filled cysts lined by cuboidal or columnar mucous cells. Epidermoid and intermediate cells are absent. Too few cases have been reported to make any definitive statement about prognosis.

Oncocytic carcinoma

This is an extremely rare tumour composed of malignant oncocytic cells but it is important to distinguish the tumour from oncocytic metaplasia in other neoplasms such as pleomorphic adenoma and mucoepidermoid carcinoma in particular.

The histological features considered to be important in establishing this diagnosis are controversial. Goode and Corio[74] considered the following to be the main characteristics:

(1) oncocytic features together with dysplasia and features such as mitoses and nuclear pleomorphism;
(2) perineural or vascular invasion;
(3) infiltration of the surrounding tissues or paraparotid lymph nodes.

It would appear from Goode and Corio's review that oncocytic carcinoma is a particularly aggressive form of salivary neoplasm as over half their cases either died from the disease or were alive with residual tumours. However, in a recent review of a large series of oncocytic tumours, apparently aggressive histological features such as perineural or capsular invasion were not always associated with a poor prognosis.[22] Size appears to be an important factor and until further series are reported each tumour should be treated on the basis of the clinicopathological findings.

Salivary duct carcinoma

This is a high grade carcinoma characterised by the formation of relatively large cell aggregates resembling salivary ducts and is similar to the duct carcinoma of the breast.[75–77] The epithelium shows a variety of configurations with cribriform, looping or solid growth patterns, sometimes with central comedo necrosis (Fig. 14.9).

Duct carcinomas are twice as common in men and are seen mainly in the elderly. They are most common in the parotid where they typically form a rapidly growing mass with pain and facial nerve palsy.

Microscopically, the cells are large and eosinophilic and there is usually gross nuclear pelomorphism and frequent mitoses. The stroma is

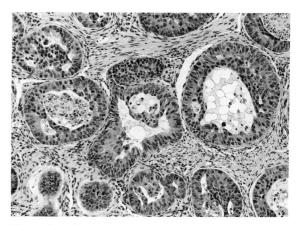

Fig. 14.9 Salivary duct carcinoma showing gross pleomorphism and areas of central necrosis. H&E × 150.

often abundant and is typically fibrous and desmoplastic and sometimes heavily inflamed.

The prognosis is poor as there is usually extensive spread and involvement of the regional lymph nodes at presentation. Most patients do not survive for more than 3 years so the value of mutilating surgery is questionable.

Adenocarcinoma

This designation of adenocarcinoma (not otherwise specified; NOS) is given to carcinomas with glandular, ductal or secretory differentiation which do not fit into the other designated categories of carcinoma. It is likely that as tumours in this group become more accurately defined this category will disappear.[78]

Malignant myoepithelioma (myoepithelial carcinoma)

This rare malignant tumour is composed of atypical myoepithelial cells with increased mitotic activity and aggressive growth.[79,80] As the majority of the reported cases appear to be associated with a preexisting pleomorphic adenoma some regard these tumours as a variant of carcinoma in pleomorphic adenoma. Most tumours have arisen in the parotid gland in patients over 50 years of age.

Like benign myoepithelioma, malignant myoepithelioma can be composed of spindle-shaped cells or rounded cells with eosinophilic cytoplasm of the so-called hyaline or plasmacytoid type. Although there may be mixtures of both cell types, one tends to predominate. They are distinguished from the benign counterpart by evidence of invasive growth, mitotic activity and cellular pleomorphism. In the spindle-cell variety confusion with a soft tissue tumour such as a fibrosarcoma or a fibrohistiocytic neoplasm is possible. Immunocytochemistry may be useful and most malignant myoepitheliomas are positive for keratins, S-100, smooth muscle actin or myosin, and glial fibrillary acidic protein (GFAP).

The tumour appears to be locally destructive but rarely metastasises so that local exicision may be curative.

Carcinoma in pleomorphic adenoma

These tumours show evidence of malignancy, such as a progressive course and infiltrative growth, together with cytological features of malignancy and are in association with a pre-existing pleomophic adenoma.

Carcinoma in pleomorphic adenoma develops in about 5 per cent of pleomorphic adenomas but the incidence of malignancy increases progressively with time so that the risk is about 1.5 per cent after 5 years but increases to nearly 10 per cent after 15 years. The typical history is that of a sudden increase in size, and pain or nerve involvement in a long standing lump or in a multifocal recurrence after unsuccessful surgery. It must be appreciated, however, that even benign pleomorphic adenomas may show episodic burst of growth. The average age at presentation is about 65 years, which is some 20 years after the average age of presentation of benign pleomorphic adenoma.

There are four main subtypes of carcinoma in pleomorphic adenoma:

(1) Non-invasive (dysplastic) carcinoma
(2) Invasive carcinoma
(3) Carcinosarcoma
(4) Metastasising (benign) pleomorphic adenoma

Non-invasive carcinoma

This refers to areas of dysplasia in a pleomorphic adenoma which are 'intracapsular'. Little has been documented about this type of tumour[81] but presumably it represents a precursor phase to frankly invasive tumours and complete excision should be curative. However, this assumption needs to be verified by appropriate clinicopathological studies.

Invasive carcinoma

In this variant there is evidence of both a pre-existing pleomorphic adenoma and frankly invasive carcinoma. Both elements can be extremely variable. The carcinoma can be undifferentiated, poorly differentiated adenocarcinoma, squamous, mucoepidermoid or even adenoid cystic carcinoma. A typical feature is finding several carcinoma types intermingled[46] and this is useful in making the diagnosis, particularly when much, or even all, of the pre-existing pleomorphic adenoma has been obliterated by the malignant component. Sometimes the original pleomorphic adenoma has been virtually replaced by fibrous hyaline scar often with elastosis, and it is essential that such tumours are examined critically as foci of carcinoma can readily be overlooked.

These tumours have a relatively poor prognosis and tend to metastasise to regional lymph nodes in 60 per cent of cases[42]. The 5 year survival rate is about 55 per cent and 10 years is 30 per cent.[5] Those tumours with high grade malignant component, especially when the invasion is beyond 8 mm, have a worse prognosis.

Carcinosarcoma

This is a rare biphasic tumour composed of both carcinoma and sarcoma. The sarcomatous element is usually chondrosarcoma or osteosarcoma.[82,83] The prognosis in the few reported cases of this tumour has been extremely poor.

Metastasising pleomorphic adenoma

This is a cytologically benign, pleomorphic adenoma which shows obvious local invasion and distant metastasis, with both the primary and secondary tumours showing similar 'benign' appearances.[84] These tumours appear to behave as carcinomas despite their bland histology but too few cases have been reported to make a sensible statement about prognosis.

Squamous cell carcinoma

Squamous cell carcinomas of the salivary glands are uncommon and form between 1 and 2 per cent of all salivary gland tumours.[1,41,85] They are seen mainly in the elderly and there is a 2 to 1 male predominance. The majority arise in the parotid gland. Clinically they present as rapidly growing swellings with other features of malignancy such as pain, haemorrhage, necrosis, ulceration and nerve involvement.

Microscopically they are typical squamous cell carcinomas which can range from well to poorly differentiated. However, it is important to distinguish between primary squamous cell carcinoma of the salivary gland and carcinomas of the overlying skin or mucosa or the possibility of a metastasis, particularly from the nasopharynx or lung.

The 5 year survival rate is about 40 per cent and treatment is by radical excision and radiotherapy.

Small cell carcinoma

This is a rare malignant tumour which has similar histology and histochemistry to small cell carcinoma of the lung.

Microscopy reveals small, dark-staining cells which may show smear artifact and extensive necrosis. Two types of small cell carcinoma can be distinguished by electron microscopy and immunocytochemistry. In the neuro-endocrine type there are small, dense-core, endocrine granules and positive staining for neurone-specific enolase and chromogranin. A ductal variety without evidence of neuro-endocrine differentiation has also been described.[86] It is essential in small cell carcinomas of the salivary gland to exclude the possibility of a lung metastasis.

Although these tumours are infiltrative and can metastasise, their prognosis from early reports appeared to be considerably better than that of small cell carcinoma of the lung, with a 46 per cent 5 year survival rate.[86] However, later follow up studies of these patients[87] showed a much poorer long term prognosis.

Undifferentiated carcinoma

This is a malignant epithelial tumour which is too poorly differentiated to be placed in any of the other groups of carcinoma. They constitute about 5 per cent of salivary neoplasms.

A variety of cell types can be seen but spheroidal, large cells or more spindle-shaped cells tend to be predominant.[88] There is no evidence of lobule formation and it may be difficult to distinguish these tumours from lymphomas except by immunocytochemistry. Necrosis may be a feature and usually there are frequent mitoses. A basaloid variant has recently been described.[89]

The prognosis tends to be poor and apart from the microscopy, the size of the primary tumour seems to have a significant impact on prognosis with those tumours over 4 cm in diameter having the worst outlook. The overall 5 year survival rate is about 30 per cent.

A characteristic subtype has been called undiffer-

entiated carcinoma with lymphoid stroma (previously designated as malignant lymphoepithelial lesion of the salivary gland or lymphoepithelial carcinoma). This tumour is seen most commonly in Arctic Eskimos and in Southern China and an association with Epstein–Barr virus has been postulated.[90,91] Microscopically the tumour is characterised by ill defined islands of pale-staining, pleomorphic carcinoma cells which often appear syncytial. There is a benign, lymphoplasmacytic stroma. These tumours are identical to nasopharyngeal carcinoma and it is essential that a metastasis from the nasopharynx is excluded before establishing this diagnosis.

The tumour is aggressive and tends to metastasise to regional lymph nodes or distant organs in up to 80 per cent of patients and over a third of patients die from the disease.

References

1 Eveson JW, Cawson RA. Salivary gland tumours. A review of 2410 cases with particular reference to histological types, site, age and sex distribution. *Journal of Pathology* 1985; **146:** 51–8.
2 Eveson JW, Cawson RA. Tumours of the minor (oropharyngeal) salivary glands: a demographic study of 336 cases. *Journal of Oral Pathology* 1985; **14:** 500–9.
3 Palmer TJ, Gleeson MJ, Eveson JW, Cawson RA. Oncocytic adenomas and oncocytic hyperplasia of salivary glands: a clinicopathological study of 26 cases. *Histopathology* 1990; **16:** 487–93.
4 Lucas RB. *Pathology of Tumours of the Oral Tissues.* Edinburgh: Churchill Livingstone, 1984.
5 Hickman RE, Cawson RA, Duffy SW. The prognosis of specific types of salivary gland tumors. *Cancer* 1984; **54:** 1620–4.
6 Seifert G, Donath K. Classification of the pathohistology of diseases of the salivary glands – review of 2,600 cases in the Salivary Gland Register. *Beitrage zur Pathologie* 1976; **159:** 1–32.
7 Patey DH, Thackray AC. The treatment of parotid tumours in the light of a pathological study of parotidectomy material. *British Journal of Surgery* 1958; **45:** 477–87.
8 Batsakis JG. Recurrent mixed tumor. *Annals of Otology, Rhinology and Laryngology* 1986; **95:** 543–4.
9 Stevens KL, Hobsley M. The treatment of pleomorphic adenomas by formal parotidectomy. *British Journal of Surgery* 1982; **69:** 1–3.
10 Clairmont AA, Richardson GS, Hanna DC. The pseudocapsule of pleomorphic adenomas (benign mixed tumors): the argument against enucleation. *American Journal of Surgery* 1977; **134:** 242–3.
11 bin Yaacob H. Some important aspects of the palatal

pleomorphic adenoma. *Singapore Medical Journal* 1981; **22**: 358–60.

12 Dardick I, Cavell S, Boivin M *et al.* Salivary gland myoepithelioma variants. Histological, ultrastructural, and immunocytological features. *Virchows Archives A, Pathological Anatomy and Histopathology* 1989; **416**: 25–42.

13 Mori M, Ninomiya T, Okada Y, Tsukitani K. Myoepitheliomas and myoepithelial adenomas of salivary gland origin. Immunohistochemical evaluation of filament proteins, S-100 alpha and beta, glial fibrillary acidic proteins, neuron-specific enolase, and lactoferrin. *Pathology Research and Practice* 1989; **184**: 168–78.

14 Eveson JW, Cawson RA. Warthin's tumor (cystadenolymphoma) of salivary glands. A clinicopathologic investigation of 278 cases. *Oral Surgery, Oral Medicine, Oral Pathology* 1986; **61**: 256–62.

15 Chaudhry AP, Gorlin RJ. Papillary cystadenoma lymphomatosum (adenolymphoma). *American Journal of Surgery* 1958; **95**: 923–31.

16 Foote FW, Frazell EL. Tumors of the major salivary glands. *Cancer* 1953; **6**: 1065–133.

17 Dietert SE. Papillary cystadenoma lymphomatosum (Warthin's tumor) in patients in a general hospital over a 24-year period. *American Journal of Clinical Pathology* 1975; **63**: 866–75.

18 Lamelas J, Terry JH Jr, Alfonso AE. Warthin's tumor: multicentricity and increasing incidence in women. *American Journal of Surgery* 1987; **154**: 347–51.

19 Seifert G, Bull HG, Donath K. Histologic subclassification of the cystadenolymphoma of the parotid gland. Analysis of 275 cases. *Virchows Archives A, Pathological Anatomy and Histopathology* 1980; **388**: 13–38.

20 Eveson JW, Cawson RA. Infarcted ('infected') adenolymphomas. A clinicopathological study of 20 cases. *Clinical Otolaryngology* 1989; **14**: 205–10.

21 Hartwick RW, Batsakis JG. Non-Warthin's tumor oncocytic lesions. *Annals of Otology, Rhinology and Laryngology* 1990; **99**: 674–7.

22 Brandwein MS, Huvos AG. Oncocytic tumors of major salivary glands. A study of 68 cases with follow-up of 44 patients. *American Journal of Surgical Pathology* 1991; **15**: 514–28.

23 Ellis GL. 'Clear cell' oncocytoma of salivary gland. *Human Pathology* 1988; **19**: 862–7.

24 Sorensen M, Baunsgaard P, Frederiksen P, Haahr PA. Multifocal adenomatous oncocytic hyperplasia of the parotid gland (unusual clear cell variant in two female siblings). *Pathology Research and Practice* 1986; **181**: 254–9.

25 Ghandur Mnaymneh L. Multinodular oncocytoma of the parotid gland: a benign lesion simulating malignancy. *Human Pathology* 1984; **15**: 485–6.

26 Seifert G, Brocheriou C, Cardesa A, Eveson JW. WHO international histological classification of tumours: tentative histological classification of salivary gland tumours. *Pathology Research and Practice* 1990; **186**: 555–81.

27 Daley TD, Gardner DG, Smout MS. Canalicular adenoma: not a basal cell adenoma. *Oral Surgery, Oral Medicine, Oral Pathology* 1984; **57**: 181–8.

28 Gnepp DR, Brannon R. Sebaceous neoplasms of salivary gland origin. Report of 21 cases. *Cancer* 1984; **53**: 2155–70.

29 Dardick I, Daley TD, van Nostrand AW. Basal cell adenoma with myoepithelial cell-derived 'stroma': a new major salivary gland tumor entity. *Head and Neck Surgery* 1986; **8**: 257–67.

30 Batsakis JG, Luna MA, el Naggar AK. Basaloid monomorphic adenomas. *Annals of Otology, Rhinology and Laryngology* 1991; **100**: 687–90.

31 Herbst EW, Utz W. Multifocal dermal-type basal cell adenomas of parotid glands with coexisting dermal cylindromas. *Virchows Archives A, Pathological Anatomy and Histopathology* 1984; **403**: 95–102.

32 Hyma BA, Scheithauer BW, Weiland LH, Irons GB. Membranous basal cell adenoma of the parotid gland. Malignant transformation in a patient with multiple dermal cylindromas. *Archives of Pathology and Laboratory Medicine* 1988; **112**: 209–11.

33 Clark DB, Priddy RW, Swanson AE. Oral inverted ductal papilloma. *Oral Surgery, Oral Medicine, Oral Pathology* 1990; **69**: 487–90.

34 Abbey LM. Solitary intraductal papilloma of the minor salivary glands. *Oral Surgery, Oral Medicine, Oral Pathology* 1975; **40**: 135–40.

35 Abrams AM, Finck FM. Sialadenoma papilliferum. A previously unreported salivary gland tumor. *Cancer* 1969; **24**: 1057–63.

36 Mitre BK. Sialadenoma papilliferum: report of case and review of literature. *Journal of Oral and Maxillofacial Surgery* 1986; **44**: 469–74.

37 Rennie JS, MacDonald DG, Critchlow HA. Sialadenoma papilliferum. A case report and review of the literature. *International Journal of Oral Surgery* 1984; **13**: 452–4.

38 Tabor EK, Curtin HD. MR of the salivary glands. *Radiology Clinics of North America* 1989; **27**: 379–92.

39 Ferlito A, Recher G. Oncocytic lesions of the larynx. *Archives of Oto-Rhino-Laryngology* 1981; **232**: 107–15.

40 Winchester L, Scully C, Prime SS, Eveson JW. Cheilitis glandularis: a case affecting the upper lip. *Oral Surgery, Oral Medicine, Oral Pathology* 1986; **62**: 654–6.

41 Williams HK, Williams DM. Persistent sialadenitis of the minor glands – stomatitis glandularis. *British Journal of Oral and Maxillofacial Surgery* 1989; **27**: 212–16.

42 Seifert G, Miehlke A, Haubrich J, Chilla R. *Diseases of the Salivary Glands.* Stuttgart: Georg Thième Verlag, 1986.

43 Lewis JE, Olsen KD, Weiland LH. Acinic cell carci-

noma. Clinicopathologic review. *Cancer* 1991; **67:** 172–9.

44 Gnepp DR, Schroeder W, Heffner D. Synchronous tumors arising in a single major salivary gland. *Cancer* 1989; **63:** 1219–24.

45 Ellis GL, Corio RL. Acinic cell adenocarcinoma. A clinicopathologic analysis of 294 cases. *Cancer* 1983; **52:** 542–9.

46 Thackray AC, Lucas RB. *Tumors of the Major Salivary Glands, Atlas of Tumor Pathology.* Washington, DC: Armed Forces Institute of Pathology, 1974.

47 Batsakis JG, Luna MA. Histopathologic grading of salivary gland neoplasms: I Mucoepidermoid carcinomas. *Annals of Otology, Rhinology and Laryngology* 1990; **99:** 835–8.

48 Evans HL. Mucoepidermoid carcinoma of salivary glands: a study of 69 cases with special attention to histologic grading. *American Journal of Clinical Pathology* 1984; **81:** 696–701.

49 Seifert G. *WHO International Histological Classification of Tumours. Histological Typing of Salivary Gland Tumours.* Berlin: Springer-Verlag, 1991.

50 Hamper K, Schimmelpenning H, Caselitz J *et al.* Mucoepidermoid tumors of the salivary glands. Correlation of cytophotometrical data and prognosis. *Cancer* 1989; **63:** 708–17.

51 Jensen OJ, Poulsen T, Schiodt T. Mucoepidermoid tumors of salivary glands. A long term follow-up study. *APMIS* 1988; **96:** 421–7.

52 Spiro RH, Huvos AG, Strong EW. Adenoid cystic carcinoma of salivary origin. A clinicopathologic study of 242 cases. *American Journal of Surgery* 1974; **128:** 512–20.

53 Perzin KH, Gullane P, Clairmont AC. Adenoid cystic carcinomas arising in salivary glands: a correlation of histologic features and clinical course. *Cancer* 1978; **42:** 265–82.

54 Chomette G, Auriol M, Tranbaloc P. Vaillant JM. Adenoid cystic carcinoma of minor salivary glands. Analysis of 86 cases. Clinico-pathological, histo-enzymological and ultrastructural studies. *Virchows Archives A, Pathological Anatomy and Histopathology* 1982; **395:** 289–301.

55 Matsuba HM, Simpson JR, Mauney M, Thawley SE. Adenoid cystic salivary gland carcinoma: a clinicopathologic correlation. *Head and Neck Surgery* 1986; **8:** 200–4.

56 Nascimento AG, Amaral AL, Prado LA, Kligerman J, Silveira TR. Adenoid cystic carcinoma of salivary glands. A study of 61 cases with clinicopathologic correlation. *Cancer* 1986; **57:** 312–19.

57 Szanto PA, Luna MA, Tortoledo ME, White RA. Histologic grading of adenoid cystic carcinoma of the salivary glands. *Cancer* 1984; **54:** 1062–9.

58 Hamper K, Lazar F, Dietl M *et al.* Prognostic factors for adenoid cystic carcinoma of the head and neck: a retrospective evaluation of 96 cases. *Journal of Oral Pathology and Medicine* 1990; **19:** 101–7.

59 Aberle AM, Abrams AM, Bowe R, Melrose RJ, Handlers JP. Lobular (polymorphous low-grade) carcinoma of minor salivary glands. A clinicopathologic study of twenty cases. *Oral Surgery, Oral Medicine, Oral Pathology* 1985; **60:** 387–95.

60 Norberg LE, Burford-Mason AP, Dardick I. Cellular differentiation and morphologic heterogeneity in polymorphous low-grade adenocarcinoma of minor salivary gland. *Journal of Oral Pathology and Medicine* 1991; **20:** 373–9.

61 Freedman PD, Lumerman H. Lobular carcinoma of intraoral minor salivary gland origin. Report of twelve cases. *Oral Surgery, Oral Medicine, Oral Pathology* 1983; **56:** 157–66.

62 Batsakis JG, Pinkston GR, Luna MA, Byers RM, Sciubba JJ, Tillery GW. Adenocarcinomas of the oral cavity: a clinicopathologic study of terminal duct carcinomas. *Journal of Laryngology and Otology* 1983; **97:** 825–35.

63 Evans HL, Batsakis JG. Polymorphous low-grade adenocarcinoma of minor salivary glands. A study of 14 cases of a distinctive neoplasm. *Cancer* 1984; **53:** 935–42.

64 Miliauskas JR. Polymorphous low-grade (terminal duct) adenocarcinoma of the parotid gland. *Histopathology* 1991; **19:** 555–7.

65 Mitchell DA, Eveson JW, Ord RA. Polymorphous low-grade adenocarcinoma of minor salivary glands – a report of three cases. *British Journal of Oral and Maxillofacial Surgery* 1989; **27:** 494–500.

66 Batsakis JG, el Naggar AK. Terminal duct adenocarcinomas of salivary tissues. *Annals of Otology, Rhinology and Laryngology* 1991; **100:** 251–3.

67 Hamper K, Brugmann M, Koppermann R *et al.* Epithelial-myoepithelial duct carcinoma of salivary glands: a follow-up and cytophotometric study of 21 cases. *Journal of Oral Pathology and Medicine* 1989; **18:** 299–304.

68 Thackray AC, Sobin LH. *Histological typing of salivary gland tumours.* Geneva: World Health Organization, 1972.

69 Palmer RM. Epithelial-myoepithelial carcinoma: an immunocytochemical study. *Oral Surgery, Oral Medicine, Oral Pathology* 1985; **59:** 511–15.

70 Ellis GL, Wiscovitsh JG. Basal cell adenocarcinomas of the major salivary glands. *Oral Surgery, Oral Medicine, Oral Pathology* 1990; **69:** 461–9.

71 Takata T, Ogawa I, Nikai H. Sebaceous carcinoma of the parotid gland. An immunohistochemical and ultrastructural study. *Virchows Archives A, Pathological Anatomy and Histology* 1989; **414:** 459–64.

72 Peel RL, Gnepp DR. Diseases of salivary glands. In: Barnes L ed. *Surgical Pathology of the Head and Neck.* New York: Marcel Dekker, 1985: 612–15.

73 Mills SE, Garland TA, Allen MS Jr. Low-grade papillary adenocarcinoma of palatal salivary gland origin. *American Journal of Surgical Pathology* 1984; **8:** 367–74.

74 Goode RK, Corio RL. Oncocytic adenocarcinoma of salivary glands. *Oral Surgery, Oral Medicine, Oral Pathology* 1988; **65**: 61–6.

75 Luna MA, Batsakis JG, Ordonez NG, Mackay B, Tortoledo ME. Salivary gland adenocarcinomas: a clinicopathologic analysis of three distinctive types. *Seminars in Diagnostic Pathology* 1987; **4**: 117–35.

76 Afzelius LE, Cameron WR, Svensson C. Salivary duct carcinoma – a clinicopathologic study of 12 cases. *Head and Neck Surgery* 1987; **9**: 151–6.

77 Brandwein MS, Jagirdar J, Patil J, Biller H, Kaneko M. Salivary duct carcinoma (cribriform salivary carcinoma of excretory ducts). A clinicopathologic and immunohistochemical study of 12 cases. *Cancer* 1990; **65**: 2307–14.

78 Batsakis JG, El Naggar AK, Luna MA. 'Adenocarcinoma, not otherwise specified': a diminishing group of salivary carcinomas. *Annals of Otology, Rhinology and Laryngology* 1992; **101**: 102–4.

79 Singh R, Cawson RA. Malignant myoepithelial carcinoma (myoepithelioma) arising in a pleomorphic adenoma of the parotid gland. An immunohistochemical study and review of the literature. *Oral Surgery, Oral Medicine, Oral Pathology* 1988; **66**: 65–70.

80 di Palma S, Pilotti S, Rilke F. Malignant myoepithelioma of the parotid gland arising in a pleomorphic adenoma. *Histopathology* 1991; **19**: 273–5.

81 LiVolsi VA, Perzin KH. Malignant mixed tumors arising in salivary glands. I. Carcinomas arising in benign mixed tumors: a clinicopathologic study. *Cancer* 1977; **39**: 2209–30.

82 Takata T, Nikai H, Ogawa I, Ijuhin N. Ultrastructural and immunohistochemical observations of a true malignant mixed tumor (carcinosarcoma) of the tongue. *Journal of Oral Pathology and Medicine* 1990; **19**: 261–5.

83 Takeda Y. True malignant mixed tumor (carcinosarcoma) of palatal minor salivary gland origin. *Annals of Dentistry* 1991; **50**: 33–5.

84 Chen KT. Metastasizing pleomorphic adenoma of the salivary gland. *Cancer* 1978; **42**: 2407–11.

85 Batsakis JG. Primary squamous cell carcinomas of major salivary glands. *Annals of Otology, Rhinology and Laryngology* 1983; **92**: 97–8.

86 Gnepp DR, Corio RL, Brannon RB. Small cell carcinoma of the major salivary glands. *Cancer* 1986; **58**: 705–14.

87 Gnepp DR, Wick MR. Small cell carcinoma of the major salivary glands. An immunohistochemical study. *Cancer* 1990; **66**: 185–92.

88 Hui KK, Luna MA, Batsakis JG, Ordonez NG, Weber R. Undifferentiated carcinomas of the major salivary glands. *Oral Surgery, Oral Medicine, Oral Pathology* 1990; **69**: 76–83.

89 Chomette G, Auriol M, Vaillant JM, Kasai T, Okada Y, Mori M. Basaloid carcinoma of salivary glands, a variety of undifferentiated adenocarcinoma. Immunohistochemical study of intermediate filament proteins in 24 cases. *Journal of Pathology* 1991; **163**: 39–45.

90 Lanier AP, Clift SR, Bornkamm G, Henle W, Goepfert H, Raab Traub N. Epstein–Barr virus and malignant lymphoepithelial lesions of the salivary gland. *Arctic Medicine Research* 1991; **50**: 55–61.

91 Huang DP, Ng HK, Ho YH, Chan KM. Epstein–Barr virus (EBV)-associated undifferentiated carcinoma of the parotid gland. *Histopathology* 1988; **13**: 509–17.

15 Management of salivary gland tumours

JD Langdon and JM Henk

Introduction

Salivary gland tumours are relatively uncommon, accounting for approximately 3 per cent of all tumours.[1] In the UK the annual incidence is 1.1 per 100 000 population.[2] Of all salivary tumours, those of the minor glands comprise only a small proportion of the total. Thackray[3] reported that, in the UK, for every 100 parotid tumours there will be 10 submandibular tumours, 10 minor salivary gland tumours and one in the sublingual gland. Reports from the USA suggest a rather higher proportion. A literature review by Frable and Elzay[4] revealed that minor salivary gland tumours comprised 18 per cent of the total. Conley,[5] in a review of 200 patients, reported that tumours of the minor salivary glands were one-fifth as common as those of the parotids and not quite twice as common as those of the submandibular glands.

The mucosa of the oral cavity contains an abundance of minor salivary glands. Ranger *et al.*[6] showed that there were normally between 450 and 750 minor salivary glands within the oral cavity. They are distributed in the mucosa of the lips, cheeks, palate, floor of mouth and retromolar area. Similar structures are found in many other parts of the body; for example, the oropharynx, larynx and trachea. They all have a histological structure resembling that of the major salivary and lacrimal glands.

Salivary gland tumours, because of their varied histopathology, frequently complex anatomical relations and rarity continue to be a fertile area for discussion amongst surgeons and for re-evaluation of current management techniques.[7]

In the British Salivary Gland Tumour Panel (SGTP) series of 3000 unselected tumours, the peak age incidence for benign tumours was in the sixth decade and, for malignant tumours, the seventh.

Women are slightly more frequently affected, until the eighth and ninth decades when they are almost twice as commonly affected as men. This, however, must be related to female predominance of 2 to 1 at these ages in the general population.

Malignant tumours are more common as age advances and relatively more frequent in the minor salivary glands. In the third decade only 5 per cent of tumours are malignant, but by the seventh decade this has risen to 30 per cent. This incidence of malignant tumours in individual glands varies widely; the lowest incidence is in the parotid glands where they form only 20 per cent.[8] At the other extreme, virtually all sublingual tumours are malignant.

The distribution of histological types of tumour arising in the minor salivary glands differs from that of tumours arising in the major salivary glands.[9] Approximately 50 per cent of minor salivary gland tumours are malignant. Of the malignant tumours approximately half are of the adenoid cystic variety; the remainder are muco-epidermoid carcinomas, malignant pleomorphic adenomas and adenocarcinomas.

Over 70 per cent of all tumours arise in the parotid glands. Eleven per cent arise in the submandibular glands, and the remainder occur in the sublingual and minor salivary glands (Table 15.1).

Incidence and pathology

Pleomorphic adenoma

This is the most common type of salivary gland tumour and accounts for 63 per cent of all parotid tumours. Almost any age can be affected, but the

Table 15.1   Distribution of major salivary gland tumours

90% Parotid				10% Submandibular			
70% Benign		30% Malignant		50% Benign		50% Malignant	
Pleomorphic adenoma	75%	Adenocarcinoma	24%	Pleomorphic adenoma	56%	Adenoidcystic carcinoma	24%
Warthin's tumour	16%	Muco-epidermoid carcinoma	22%	Lymphangioma	9%	Adenocarcinoma	24%
Adenoma	4%	Squamous cell carcinoma	20%	Haemangioma	9%	Squamous cell carcinoma	24%
Haemangioma	3%	Anaplastic carcinoma	13%	Oncocytoma	4%	Mucoepidermoid carcinoma	14%
Lymphangioma	1%	Adenocystic carcinoma	7%	'Other'	22%	Malignant pleomorphic adenoma	5%
'Other'	1%	Malignant pleomorphic adenoma	7%			'Other'	9%
		'Other'	7%				

peak incidence is in the fourth and fifth decades. There is a slight female predominance.

Although in itself benign and slow growing, pleomorphic adenoma causes considerable problems, namely:

(1) Biopsy is not feasible except for the minor gland tumours, because the tumour can seed in the line of incision to produce multiple recurrences.
(2) Removal of pleomorphic adenomas from the parotid gland is technically difficult.
(3) Encapsulation is often incomplete.
(4) Pleomorphic adenomas are frequently mucinous in texture and can readily burst to produce multiple seedings if enucleation is attempted.
(5) Removal of recurrences, which are typically multifocal, becomes more difficult with each attempt and an unlucky patient can end up with innumerable nodules of tumour in the neck spreading far beyond the original site.[10]
(6) Rarely, a cytologically benign pleomorphic adenoma can show invasive behaviour.
(7) Pleomorphic adenoma is one of the few benign tumours which can undergo malignant change, particularly if allowed to persist for, or recur, over a long period.[11, 12]

Warthin's tumour (adenolymphoma)

This is the most common type of monomorphic adenoma, and probably only affects the parotid in which it accounts for 14 per cent of all tumours. Descriptions of adenolymphoma in other glands, particularly the submandibular gland, are open to question. The mean age affected is 62.5 years and the male to female ratio is currently thought to be 1.6 to 1.

Warthin's tumour usually presents as a soft painless swelling in the parotid. Although they are said to be slow growing, about 40 per cent of these tumours will have been present for 6 months or less, whilst occasionally the history is only a few weeks. In a few cases the tumour causes pain or, rarely, facial weakness. Sometimes fluctuation or rapid increase in size is noticed; this is almost certainly due to the partly cystic nature of most of these tumours.

The tumour is bilateral in about 5 per cent of cases, and in about 10 per cent of cases is multifocal within a single parotid. There is a suggestion that with the more widespread use of computed tomography (CT) and ultrasound for the investigation of parotid masses Warthin's tumour will be found to be frequently multifocal and bilateral.

Excision of adenolymphoma is usually curative, but incomplete excision leads to recurrence.[13]

Alternatively, recurrence may result from the tumour being multifocal.

Muco-epidermoid carcinoma

Although both benign and malignant varieties of the muco-epidermoid tumour are described, it is probably wise to regard all such tumours as having a malignant potential and therefore they should be classified as carcinomas.[14–17] The tumour presents a spectrum from benign to frankly malignant.[17–19]

The relative incidence of muco-epidermoid carcinomas in the intra-oral regions (10 per cent) is higher than in the major salivary glands (5 per cent).[20,21] Approximately 40 per cent occur in the palate, 20 per cent in the retromolar and tuberosity regions, and 20 per cent in the floor of the mouth. Almost any age can be affected but peak incidence is in the fifth decade.

The 'low grade' tumours behave like benign tumours, presenting as painless swellings with a normal overlying epithelium, whereas the 'high grade' tumours present as squamous cell carcinomas with pain and ulceration.

The prognosis depends on histological grade. Less than 10 per cent of patients with well differentiated (Stages I and II) tumours die of the disease, whereas the mortality from poorly differentiated (Stage III) tumours has been reported to be as high as 70 per cent.[22] Stage III tumours are prone to both local recurrence and lymph node metastases. Distant metastases are uncommon; when they occur they usually follow lymph node involvement.

Clinically, muco-epidermoid carcinomas are unlikely to be distinguishable from benign tumours. The chief problem with these tumours is that their behaviour is not reliably predictable from the histological appearances. It has to be accepted that even the most benign-looking of these tumours can metastasise. Thus all muco-epidermoid tumours should be regarded as potentially malignant and fully excised. The 5 and 10 year survival figures are 71 per cent and 50 per cent respectively.[23]

Acinic cell carcinomas

Acinic cell carcinomas form about 2.5 per cent of parotid tumours but are rarer in the submandibular glands. They are another difficult entity usually with a highly characteristic histological appearance. Despite their generally benign appearance they can behave unpredictably.

Acinic cell carcinomas are among the rarest tumours of the minor salivary glands. Fewer than 30 cases were reported in the world literature up to 1978.[24] They have been reported in all parts of the oral cavity, but mainly in the upper lip and cheek.

In view of the fact that even benign-appearing acinic cell carcinomas can occasionally metastasise, they should be treated in the same manner as muco-epidermoid carcinomas.[25] Hickman *et al.*[23] quote 5 and 10 year survival figures of 82 per cent and 68 per cent respectively.

Adenoid cystic carcinoma

This forms 2 per cent of parotid gland tumours, but is the commonest malignancy affecting the minor salivary glands. They occur most frequently in the palate and are sometimes also seen in the cheek or floor of the mouth. They present as a painless lump. The typical appearance is of a smooth dome-shaped swelling, cherry-red in colour. Typically there is no ulceration, but this may occur as a result of trauma to the lesion from opposing teeth or denture flanges. This lesion is painless initially, but at a late stage pain may result from invasion of adjacent nerves. The tumour is slow growing and most patients give a history of 1 year or more at presentation.

Adenoid cystic carcinomas characteristically grow slowly and relentlessly;[26] there is wide local spread due mainly to the propensity of the tumour for perineural invasion. They have, typically, an insidious and often inexorably infiltrative growth pattern.[26] Lymph node metastases are often late events,[27,28] occurring in 10–15 per cent of cases (see Chapter 13). By contrast, systemic metastases are common. Spiro *et al.*[27] found distant spread in 40 per cent of cases, although this was the cause of death in only 10 per cent. Metastases are found in the lungs, bones and brain.[29–31] The lungs are the commonest site of blood-borne metastases. Pulmonary deposits have a 'cannonball' appearance on chest X-ray; they often grow slowly and remain asymptomatic for many years.

The usual course of the disease is one of relentless progression with local invasion, and persistence or recurrence of tumour after repeated surgical excision, leading ultimately to death from local disease, although distant metastases may contribute. The persistence of the tumour despite radical excision is due to the locally infiltrative behaviour with proneness to follow the routes of the cranial nerves.[32] Conley and Dingman[28] reported a 50 per cent local recurrence rate. The common story is that of an apparently adequate excision followed 3–5 years later by repeated recurrences treated by even wider excisions over the following 10–15 years, before the patient ultimately dies of intracranial spread or chest infection. In the long term, the prognosis is very poor. Although the 5 year survival rate may be as high as 58 per cent, this falls to 30 per cent at 10 years and 13 per cent at 20 years.[1] An actuarial disease-free rate at 30 years of 8 per cent was calculated by Conley.[5] It is therefore never possible to say that any individual patient is cured of this disease, although survival for many years is not uncommon.

In view of the propensity for adenoid cystic carcinoma to spread widely along perineural spaces excision must also be wide and in the parotid gland sacrifice of branches of the facial nerve obviously involved is unavoidable.

The present consensus is that supraradical surgery is not indicated[33–36] even though this tumour is relentless. The best control is achieved by 'simple' radical excision followed by radiotherapy.[37]

Adenocarcinoma

This formed only 1 per cent of 651 parotid gland tumours reported by Thackray and Lucas[38] but 4.3 per cent of the slightly larger series of both Eneroth[1] and of Foote and Frazell.[7]

Only a relatively small proportion of minor salivary gland tumours fall into the group (reports are of between 7.5 per cent and 33 per cent).[20,39] Growth tends to be rapid, with a high rate of local recurrence. Metastases occur frequently to lymph nodes, and occasionally to distant sites.[27]

In the major salivary glands adenocarcinoma is often fixed and painful and may cause facial palsy, ultimately ulcerating through the overlying skin.

Many histological variants of salivary adenocarcinoma exist, with no clear difference in behaviour or prognosis. The terminal duct carcinoma shares clinical and pathological features with adenoid cystic carcinoma and can be deceptive histologically.[40]

Squamous cell carcinoma

This presents in salivary glands but is rare despite the relative frequency with which squamous metaplasia is seen in pleomorphic adenomas.[40] In the SGTP series of 2410 cases,[7] epidermoid carcinoma accounted for only 1.1 per cent. This is the same figure as found by Thackray and Lucas[38] but lower than the 3.4 per cent quoted by Foote and Frazell[8] in the USA.

These tumours occur in the elderly and the mean age affected is 70 years (range, 50 to 90 years). There is male predominance (2.3 to 1).

It is not clear whether or not squamous carcinomas occur in minor salivary glands in the mouth. If they do it is impossible to distinguish them from squamous carcinomas arising in the mucosa.

Macroscopically, epidermoid carcinomas do not seem to have any distinct features although they may be particularly hard upon palpation and readily ulcerate.

It is important to exclude the possibility that such carcinomas are not metastases from other organs as the prognosis under such circumstances is even poorer.

In view of the rarity of epidermoid carcinoma in salivary glands there are no reliable figures for survival rates to indicate the likely response to treatment. The latter is by radical excision and radiotherapy.

Undifferentiated carcinoma

This is an epithelial tumour that is too poorly differentiated to be categorised as any of the other types of carcinoma. It may even be difficult by light microscopy alone to distinguish such tumours from lymphomas but such problems have now largely been resolved by such means as the use of immunocytochemistry.

Undifferentiated carcinoma is rare, and in the SGTP series accounts for only 1.8 per cent of epithelial tumours and is not included as an entity by Foote and Frazell.[7] In the Thackray and Lucas series,[38] however, undifferentiated carcinoma accounted for 3.7 per cent of their cases.

Relatively speaking, undifferentiated carcinoma is more common in the sublingual and submandibular glands. Within the oral cavity, it is often difficult to be certain that an undifferentiated carcinoma is of salivary gland origin. Koss *et al.*[41] reported a group of 14 undifferentiated carcinomas of the head and neck, nine of which were in the oral cavity, and which had a histological structure resembling an oat-cell carcinoma of the bronchus. They arose beneath intact oral epithelium and contained remnants of normal salivary gland, and were therefore considered to be probably of salivary gland origin. There was a high incidence of lymph node metastases, and a poor prognosis with only four of the patients surviving 5 years.

Rapid spread of undifferentiated carcinomas is

to be expected, particularly to regional lymph nodes, and distant metastases are likely to be the chief cause of death.

Treatment should be by radical excision of the gland followed by radiotherapy. Thackray and Lucas[38] suggest that the 5 year survival rate may be up to 30 per cent.

Malignant change in benign tumours

Clinically, malignant change in a benign salivary gland tumour is suggested by a sudden increase in growth rate after years of gradual progress. Even more convincing, however, are the microscopic appearances where both pleomorphic adenoma and carcinoma can be seen adjacent in the same section. According to the stage of development of the malignant component it may form only a minute part of the tumour or so large a proportion of the mass that the original pleomorphic adenoma may be difficult to find.

The reported incidence of carcinoma in pleomorphic adenoma shows wide variation. In the SGTP series the overall incidence was 3.2 per cent, but Foote and Frazell[7] reported an incidence of 6.3 per cent. However, as Thackray and Lucas[38] point out, such figures must be looked at with due consideration of the length of time the tumour has been present. It has only rarely been reported to arise in the minor salivary glands. They further suggest that up to 25 per cent of pleomorphic adenomas might undergo malignant changes if left untreated for a sufficient number of years.

As might be expected, carcinoma in pleomorphic adenoma is a tumour of older persons with a mean age of 63 years (range, 25 to 83 years). There is little difference in the gender ratio. Malignant change in a pleomorphic adenoma is more common in long standing tumours (more than 12 years) or in multinodular recurrences in which one nodule is found to be malignant.

Carcinoma in pleomorphic adenoma must be expected to behave in the manner of the carcinomatous component with metastasis initially to regional lymph nodes and later to distant sites. Treatment is by radical excision in the first instance. The value of radiotherapy is unclear.

On the basis of analysis of 383 reported cases, the 5 year survival rate appears to be 56 per cent and the 10 year rate 31 per cent.[23]

Non-epithelial tumours and tumour-like lesions

Almost any variety of tumour can develop from the connective tissue stroma of salivary glands. Tumours can also develop in the associated lymphoid tissues and lymphomas are the most common non-epithelial tumours of salivary glands. Overall, however, no more than approximately 4 per cent of salivary gland tumours are of connective tissue or lymphoreticular origin.

The parotid swelling of lympho-epithelial lesions is typically smooth, firm and without fixation superficially or deeply. Pain may be present in up to 40 per cent of patients. Usually the history is of no more than 6 months or occasionally of a year or two.

Excision of the whole mass is desirable to allow full examination for possible lymphomatous change.

In addition, the patient should be investigated for possible Sjøgren's syndrome and prolonged follow up is essential because of the risk of salivary lymphoma. The term *benign* lymphoepithelial lesion (BLL) is misleading. In view of the inherent risk of lymphoma in BLL the hazard should not be increased by use of irradiation or cytotoxic/immunosuppressive drug treatment. The effects of BLL in itself may be only that of progressively decreased salivary function. If, however, lymphoma develops, the prognosis is that of the tumour. *Lymphomas* formed 41 per cent of the non-epithelial tumours in the SGTP material. In such cases, the lymphoma may have arisen in the salivary gland or in the latter may be the first clinical manifestation of more widespread disease.[42] This problem has to be resolved by CT scanning or other staging procedures.

Treatment will depend both on the histological subtype and on whether the tumour is systemic or localised to the salivary gland. Excision is likely to have been carried out in the first instance, but in addition, radiotherapy and/or chemotherapy will be necessary.[43]

Haemangioma of the parotid gland

Juvenile haemangioma of the parotids is said to be the most common mesenchymal tumour (or hamartoma) of salivary glands, and is certainly so in children.

Haemangioma of the parotid may be evident at

birth or early infancy, and forms a soft, sometimes bluish enlargement of the gland.

In view of the possibility of spontaneous regression of these haemangiomas, treatment should not be hasty. If, however, it cannot be avoided, excision appears to be curative.

Mesenchymal tumours are rare in salivary glands, and range from haemangiopericytomas to malignant fibrous histiocytoma or neurofibrosarcoma.

Clinical features

The majority of patients with tumours of the major salivary glands have painless swellings. (Fig. 15.1) For example, only 13 of 68 patients with parotid masses in a personal series experienced any pain. Eleven of the 50 patients with parotid gland tumours complained of a dull ache radiating deeply into the ear.[44] Of these 11 patients, only one had malignant disease and in three the symptoms were probably due to ascending infection. Although numbness, paraesthesia and lymphadenopathy or facial nerve paralysis are well recognised features of malignancy, in this series, of the 15 patients who presented with such symptoms, only three proved to have malignant tumours. Of 17 patients with malignant tumours, not one had any facial nerve weakness, one element of the triad of symptoms (with ear pain and sensory loss in the second and third divisions of the trigeminal nerve) that are occasionally associated with the condition.[45,46]

Growth of some adenomas can be exceedingly slow, and they may have been present for years before treatment is sought. There are no reliable indicators of malignancy but rapid growth, pain and lymphadenopathy are strongly suggestive.

All the histological types of minor salivary gland tumour tend to present initially with similar symptoms and signs, and cannot be distinguished from each other clinically. The first sign is a painless firm swelling beneath the mucosa, which is usually shiny on the surface and cherry-red in colour. Growth is characteristically slow, as the majority of such tumours are well differentiated. The lesion can reach a diameter of several centimetres before causing any other symptoms. The patient may then complain of difficulty in chewing, or of difficulty in swallowing owing to the bulk of the tumour, or of pain from pressure on bone or involvement of nerves. Ulceration does not normally occur until the tumour is large and is traumatised by teeth or dentures, except in the case of a poorly differentiated rapidly growing tumour which is more likely to ulcerate early and is therefore difficult to distinguish clinically from a squamous carcinoma of the mucosa.

Investigations

Although there are many possible causes of swelling in or around the parotid and submandibular glands, generally the pattern is sufficiently characteristic

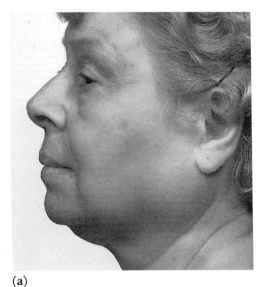

(a)

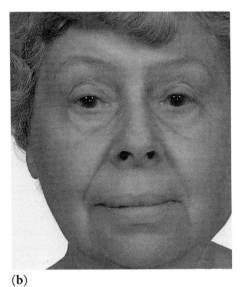

(b)

Fig. 15.1   (a) and (b) Typical appearance of a parotid tumour, in this case a benign pleomorphic adenoma.

to allow diagnosis. However, special investigations may be necessary to distinguish neoplastic from inflammatory disease.[47]

Biopsy

Because of the risk of seeding tumour cells into clean tissue planes and thus jeopardising the subsequent excision, major salivary gland tumours should not be biopsied before definitive surgery.[48] Indeed Conley[5] has called superficial parotidectomy 'The Grand Biopsy' and suggests that nothing less is acceptable as treatment for parotid tumours in the superficial lobe. An exception to this is in the obviously malignant tumour involving the overlying skin where there is nothing to be lost by performing a biopsy.

There have been suggestions that fine needle aspiration biopsy (FNAB) might be helpful in making a pre-operative diagnosis.[49–51] Further experience will show whether this is so. In view of the variations in the histological appearances within many salivary gland tumours, it seems highly unlikely that such a random sampling technique could be reliable. Indeed it is often only after viewing multiple sections taken throughout the tumour that the histopathologist is able to make a definitive diagnosis. A few cells aspirated through a needle give no indication of the architecture of the tumour. The present authors do not rely on FNAB in salivary gland disorders. Tru-cut biopsies are also unacceptable in the major salivary glands because of the risks of seeding the tumour.

Sialography

Sialography is the investigation of choice in chronic inflammatory disease, auto-immune disease and duct obstruction, and is often performed as part of the routine assessment of a salivary mass (Fig. 15.2). The best assessment of gland function is obtained from a post-stimulation emptying film. A mass may be confirmed by its displacement of ducts and adjacent glandular tissue, with deeper tumours typically giving a 'grasping hand' appearance.

However, this only shows that the gland is displaced by a mass, and contributes nothing more.

Most parotid tumours are benign, slow growing masses with readily palpable borders. Retrospective review shows that most sialograms are unnecessary and do not influence clinical decisions. At best they only reassure the surgeon of what he already knows, namely that there is a mass within the gland.[47]

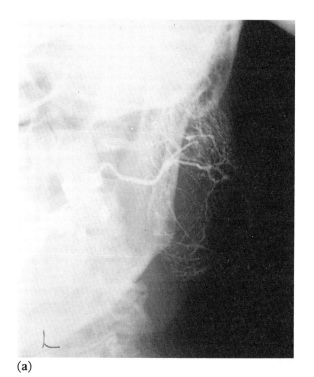

(a)

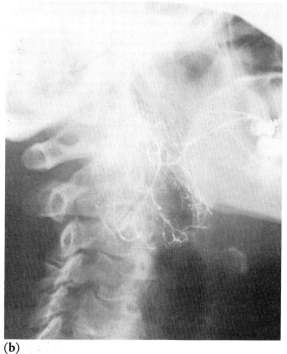

(b)

Fig. 15.2   (a) and (b) Sialogram showing an obvious space occupying lesion in the parotid gland.

Sialograms are often difficult to interpret, particularly with small or peripheral lesions. The technique cannot be relied upon to indicate malignancy or show spread beyond the gland capsule, or indeed to distinguish superficial and deep lobe masses. Clinical features, such as recent onset of rapid growth, fixation of the tumour to the skin, facial weakness or lymphadenopathy when present are more important in identifying malignant lesions but are all late and inconsistent signs.

Computed tomography scanning

CT demonstrates small differences in soft tissue X-ray attenuation and the distinction between gland and adjacent soft tissue is greatly improved (Fig 15.3). It also allows examination in the transverse plane. The density of the gland varies considerably but is always greater than that of fat but less than that of muscle. The parotid gland is divided into superficial and deep lobes joined by an isthmus, the facial nerve lying in a plane between the two lobes. When a mass occupies a position along the course of the nerve, CT may help to demonstrate the relation of the mass to the nerve. Such information is of pre-operative value to the surgeon, as removal of a lesion which distorts the anatomy at the stylomastoid foramen, or has a significant component deep to the nerve, is likely to be more time-consuming. Most parotid masses have a relatively low density similar to soft tissue and are easily demonstrated. Deep lobe tumours are as easy

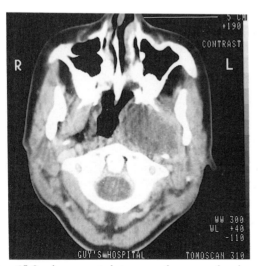

Fig. 15.3 A computed tomography scan showing a tumour arising in the deep lobe. The attenuated plane of parapharyngeal fat can be seen.

to visualise as superficial tumours, and the extent of a lesion is precisely demonstrated.

CT cannot reliably predict whether a lesion is benign or malignant, but most benign lesions have well defined, although occasionally lobulated, borders. However, on occasions, a malignant lesion or enlarged lymph node may give an identical picture. Aggressive lesions with irregular or indistinct margins suggest malignancy. Extension into the infratemporal fossa, base of skull or the presence of metastatic deposits confirm the diagnosis. Multiple lesions suggest malignant lymphoma, Warthin's or metastatic tumour.

CT scanning is of great value in distinguishing intrinsic and extrinsic salivary disease, and may help to distinguish deep lobe parotid from lateral pharyngeal tumours. Parapharyngeal tumours are usually separated from the gland by a layer of normal fat. If this layer is not seen between the mass and parotid gland, the lesion is probably a deep lobe parotid tumour, although very large lesions obliterate this plane and make diagnosis difficult.

The use of an intravenous contrast medium may be of value in demonstrating the relation of tumours of the major salivary glands to major vessels and vascular malformations. Glomus vagale tumours and arteriovenous malformations enhance dramatically after contrast. Both of these lesions may mimic deep lobe parotid tumours clinically.

In the past, CT sialography has been advocated. With modern scanners the resolution is such that there is nothing to be gained from injection of contrast medium into the gland.

Magnetic resonance imaging

Despite the advantage that magnetic resonance imaging (MRI) does not involve ionising radiation, it is an expensive investigation and is currently less readily available than CT. In terms of imaging of salivary gland tumours, it has little advantage over CT for the major glands as both modalities clearly distinguish tumour from normal structures. However, for minor gland tumours in the palate and for any tumours within the infratemporal fossa or around the base of the skull MRI is more effective in displaying early bone invasion.

Ultrasound

The role of ultrasound in parotid disease has yet to be established. The superficial portion of the gland, like the thyroid, is readily accessible to ultrasound examination. The deep part is, however, obscured by the mandible. Similarly, the superficial lobe of the submandibular gland is accessible.

The normal gland is homogenous and gives fine, medium-range echoes. Its borders, although not sharply delineated, are easily visualised. Useful adjacent landmarks are the mandible, which is linear and far more echogenic, and the masseter and sternomastoid muscles which are echo-poor compared with the parotid or submandibular glands. Ultrasound cannot characterise a focal lesion, but various ultrasonic characteristics may indicate the probable aetiology. Pleomorphic adenomas, for example, are echo-poor, fairly well defined, and may exhibit posterior acoustic enhancement. Warthin's tumours are often more echogenic. Enlarged lymph nodes appear as echo-poor areas, and again tend to show posterior acoustic enhancement. Chronic inflammation makes the gland appear less homogenous than normal, and it may be possible to distinguish dilated ducts in advanced cases. Stones can also be visualised as echo-bright regions with acoustic shadowing posteriorly, and this can be useful when sialography is contra-indicated in acute inflammation.

Although ultrasound requires further evaluation of its role in salivary imaging, it would appear to be useful in the detection of focal lesions, the echo-structure and margins sometimes giving indications between benign and malignant lesions.[52] The technique is non-invasive, inexpensive and relatively quick, and therefore might be considered as the first line of investigation of a salivary gland swelling.

Scintigraphy

In the past, technetium pertechnetate scintigraphy has been advocated.[7] Except for Warthin's tumour, which always appears as a hot spot, the results of scintigraphy are confusing. All other tumour types can be imaged variously as hot or cold spots within the gland, and therefore the investigation is of no help.

Scintigraphy to assess gland function can sometimes be useful. For example, occasionally patients complain of continuing symptoms following superficial lobectomy, and in this situation scintigraphy will reveal any persistent deep lobe activity.

Treatment

Surgery

Treatment of parotid tumours is surgical wherever possible by superficial parotidectomy (Fig. 15.4) for all benign tumours in the superficial lobe and total parotidectomy for all benign deep lobe and dumb-bell tumours.[44] Such tumours including large deep lobe tumours should never be approached from the pharyngeal aspect (Fig 15.5).[53,54] The facial nerve is preserved in all cases. Postoperative irradiation for benign tumours is not advocated.[11,55] Early authors claimed that it was impossible to remove the parotid gland and any associated disease without irreparably damaging the facial nerve. This was largely due to the ignorance of the anatomy of this region, as it was believed that the branches of the facial nerve were buried inextricably within the gland substance. The key to successful parotid surgery is the observation of two anatomical features:

(1) The parotid gland has two (superficial and deep) lobes united by an isthmus.
(2) The facial nerve and its branches are surrounded by these lobes, invested in loose connective tissue. The facial nerve, except when invaded by tumour, does not enter the substance of the parotid.[56]

The prognosis for *malignant parotid tumours* is poor, which makes a definitive surgical plan particularly important to minimise the difficulties of having to treat recurrences once anatomical land-

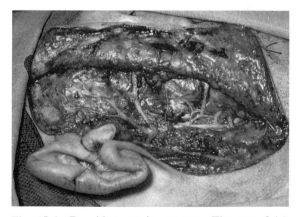

Fig. 15.4 Parotidectomy in progress. The superficial lobe containing the tumour has been excised. The branches of the facial nerve are seen overlying the deep lobe of the parotid and the mandibular ramus.

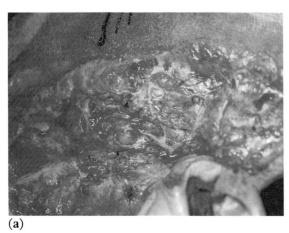
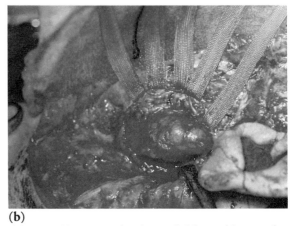

(a)   **(b)**

Fig. 15.5   (a) In this patient with a tumour in the deep lobe of the parotid a conventional superficial parotidectomy has been performed. (b) Following superficial parotidectomy the branches of the facial nerve are carefully mobilised to give access to the deep lobe together with the tumour.

marks have changed and scarring has occurred.[57] There is little evidence that radical parotidectomy, which includes sacrificing the entire facial nerve, adds significantly to the patient's chance of survival. It does, however, considerably increase the morbidity. For this reason, we advocate superficial or total parotidectomy depending on the site of the tumour with preservation of those branches of the facial nerve not macroscopically invaded by tumour, whilst bearing in mind that as true 'en bloc' resection of tumour and gland is not possible commensurate care must be taken not to invade tumour boundaries.[58] Whenever palpable nodes are present in the neck, a radical neck dissection is also performed in continuity with the parotidectomy. This is followed by radiotherapy.[59,60] For locally advanced tumours with skin involvement, a radical 'wipe out' procedure followed by appropriate reconstruction is necessary to achieve local control. Similarly, 'supraradical' surgery for adenoid cystic carcinoma is not advocated. This tumour, although probably always fatal in the long term, has an appreciable 10 year survival rate. It is difficult therefore to justify extensive mutilating surgery without offering a cure. Quite commonly, the natural history is one of limited local recurrences, each of which responds to local treatment, over the course of years. Our present policy for adenoid cystic carcinoma is radical resection with as wide a margin as is anatomically possible whilst being compatible with reasonable rehabilitation, followed by radiotherapy and careful follow up.

Surgery for submandibular tumours is not controversial. For patients presenting with a mass in the submandibular gland which is not fixed to adjacent structures, simple excision of the submandibular gland is advocated. For obviously malignant tumours, a supra-omohyoid clearance, if necessary including the inner table of the mandible, should be undertaken. If palpable nodes are present in the neck, a full radical neck dissection should be carried out. Obviously if there is overlying skin involvement, the area must be widely excised and reconstructed with appropriate flaps.

Malignant tumours of the minor salivary glands in the palate are treated by excision including a 1 cm margin and fenestration of the underlying bone. In the case of an adenoid cystic carcinoma, more radical surgery should be undertaken because of the risk of perineural spread. Maxillectomy based on the extent of the tumour as seen with CT or MRI is advocated followed by radical radiotherapy up to and including the base of the skull.

Malignant tumours arising in minor glands at other sites are treated by excision with wide margins followed by appropriate reconstruction. Whenever lymph node involvement is present, radical neck dissection should be undertaken.

Surgical technique of parotidectomy

Whenever the facility is available and the patient fit, we prefer to use hypotensive anaesthesia as this considerably reduces the oozing and thus makes it easier to trace the facial nerve branches. Nerve stimulators are misleading and are not advocated for routine use. Following a pre-auricular incision extending downwards to continue in a suitable skin crease in the neck, the skin flap is raised in the plane of the preparotid fascia, and then held forward by suturing the margins of the flap to the adjacent towels. By blunt dissection, the blood-free plane anterior to the external auditory meatus is opened up and leads the surgeon down to the base of the skull just superficial to the styloid process and stylomastoid foramen. This plane is then gently opened up in an inferior direction by blunt dissection until the trunk of the facial nerve is seen. With large posterior tumours this plane may be difficult to open up. In this situation it is helpful to identify the posterior belly of the digastric muscle in the cervical extension of the incision and trace this upwards and backwards to its insertion onto the mastoid which lies immediately below the stylomastoid foramen thus leading the operator to the facial nerve from below. Once the facial nerve trunk has been identified, the superficial lobe of the parotid can be 'exteriorised' by opening up the plane in which the branches of the facial nerve run between the two lobes by blunt dissection. Initially, as it leaves the stylomastoid foramen, the trunk of the facial nerve turns abruptly to become more superficial and also divides into the larger zygomatico-facial trunk and smaller cervicofacial trunk. The five main branches of the nerve are then followed peripherally through the parotid until the superficial lobe is completely freed.

If the tumour is within the deep lobe, the various branches of the facial nerve are mobilised and lifted on nylon tapes to enable the deep lobe to be freed around its margins and removed by dropping the mass downwards. As the parapharyngeal space is wedge-shaped with its apex superiorly, it is almost invariably possible to do this. Only very rarely is it necessary to perform a mandibulotomy (either vertical subsigmoid or angle) to gain access to the deep lobe. Very rarely – most often after recurrent infection and fibrosis – the trunk of the facial nerve cannot be confidently identified. In this situation, the peripheral branches of the nerve are identified at the anterior border of the parotid and traced centrally towards the stylomastoid foramen.

Following removal of the parotid gland, the blood pressure is returned to normal, all bleeding points are controlled, a vacuum drain placed and the wound closed in layers. A pressure dressing is then applied for 48 hours.

For malignant tumours with lymph node metastases, a radical neck dissection is undertaken in continuity with a total parotidectomy.

Permanent facial nerve paralysis following par-otidectomy should be rare (less than 1 per cent).[56] Transient disturbances of facial nerve function are observed following up to 30 per cent of parotidectomies but are usually of short duration.

According to Laage-Hellman,[61] Frey's syndrome is a regular sequel to parotidectomy while Morfit and Kramish[62] report a 54 per cent incidence and Glaister *et al*.[63] an incidence of 38 per cent. In the present author's series, Frey's syndrome developed in 13 per cent after an average delay in onset of 22 months and this long delay has been observed by many other authors.[56] Other rare complications, namely sialocele or salivary fistula occasionally follow parotid surgery.

Radiotherapy

Salivary tumours are often considered to be 'radioresistant'. This is not necessarily true; regression after radiotherapy is usually slow, but this reflects the slow cell turnover time of the majority of these tumours, rather than the inability of radiation to effect a cure. There are many reports of long term control of large inoperable tumours by radiotherapy.

Postoperative radiotherapy

The place of radiotherapy in the management of *pleomorphic adenoma* is controversial. Pleomorphic adenoma does not appear to respond when irradiated, in common with most benign neoplasms. However, the tumour cells sustain damage to DNA which may render them incapable of further growth, so that lack of tumour shrinkage does not necessarily indicate absence of a radiation effect. Experience of treatment of pleomorphic adenoma by 'enucleation' and radiotherapy many years ago strongly suggested that radiotherapy can prevent or delay regrowth of this tumour from microscopic residual disease.

It is now generally agreed that radiotherapy should not be a substitute for inadequate surgery, although a treatment policy of enucleation and radiotherapy still has its advocates.[64] In any case where tumour resection is thought to be incomplete, or where there has been spillage of tumour into the operative field, the risks of recurrence must be weighed against the risks of radiotherapy. The incidence of radiation-induced malignancy after irradiation of pleomorphic adenoma is uncertain. Tumours of tissue in the irradiated volume other than salivary gland have been reported but are rare, for example in the series reported by Dawson and

Orr,[65] one such tumour, a soft tissue sarcoma, occurred in over 300 patients followed for more than 10 years. Carcinomatous change in pleomorphic adenoma has been described more frequently after radiotherapy, but recurrences in patients who have not received radiotherapy occasionally show malignant change so the effect of radiation is difficult to assess. The authors' policy is to excise these tumours completely wherever possible. In the rare case of incomplete surgery or when a pleomorphic adenoma ruptures during surgery, we advocate radiotherapy.

Postoperative radiotherapy is probably advisable for nearly all cases of *malignant salivary tumours*. There have been no randomised studies, but many retrospective reviews have demonstrated a higher survival rate from combined surgery and radiotherapy than from surgery alone, despite the fact that in general combined treatment was used in more advanced tumours.[66–69]

Radiation fields should include the ipsilateral regional lymph nodes if the histological type is one with a high propensity for lymph node metastases, i.e. undifferentiated carcinoma, squamous cell carcinoma, adenocarcinoma and high grade mucoepidermoid carcinoma.[70] Lymph node irradiation is probably unnecessary for adenoid cystic carcinoma, but it is important to treat a wide volume including the base of the skull because of the extensive perineural spread characteristic of this tumour type.[71]

Radiotherapy as sole treatment

Treatment by radiotherapy alone should only be considered for inoperable malignant tumours, or when the patient is unfit for or refuses surgery. Some malignant salivary gland tumours may be cured solely by radiotherapy. Five year disease-free survival rates of 15 per cent have been reported for both major[65] and minor gland tumours.[72]

Adenoid cystic carcinoma has been reported to be the most consistently radioresponsive type. Cowie and Pointon[37] reported a five year local control rate of 40 per cent. However, this tumour may recur many years after treatment, and it is debatable whether or not it is ever truly radiocurable.

Technique

Parotid

A lateral photon field should not be used because the exit dose to the opposite parotid gland may be sufficient to cause severe permanent xerostomia. The choice lies between a lateral high energy electron field or oblique photon fields. The authors favour the latter technique (Fig. 8.2, p. 104). The patient is treated supine with the chin well up so that the plane of the superior border of the fields passes below the eyes. If it is necessary to irradiate the lymph nodes also, anterior and posterior neck fields can be matched to the lower border of the parotid volume (Fig. 13.6, p. 183).

Submandibular

The submandibular region is best irradiated by a pair of oblique fields. In the case of an adenoid cystic carcinoma the target volume should be extended posterosuperiorly to include the course of the mandibular nerve to the base of skull, to cover potential perineural spread.

Dose

For postoperative radiotherapy of pleomorphic adenoma a dose of 45 Gy in 20 fractions is adequate. Postoperative treatment of malignant tumours requires higher doses; for example 50 Gy in 20 fractions as used by Fitzpatrick *et al*.;[66] or the more conventional 60 Gy in 30 fractions.

Irradiation of inoperable tumours requires very high doses, to the maximum of normal tissue tolerance. Reported series such as that of Borthne *et al*.[67] and others have suggested that 70 Gy over 7 weeks is needed for best results. The authors have had some success using larger fraction sizes, giving 55 Gy in 15 fractions over 6 weeks. However, if large fractions are used great care must be exercised to avoid vulnerable structures such as the brain stem and optic nerve.

Neutron therapy

Improved results in treatment of inoperable tumours from the use of fast neutron therapy have been claimed by Catterall and Bewley[73] and others. A small prospective randomised study showed a significant improvement in local control.[74] However, severe late morbidity occuring 5 or more years after treatment has been recorded from neutron therapy in other head and neck sites, so longer follow up is needed before the relative merits of conventional high dose photon therapy and neutron therapy can be assessed. As Million *et al*.[75] have pointed out, the neutron results are no better than the best results of conventional therapy to date.

Side effects of radiotherapy

Acute effects include taste loss, mucositis in the oral cavity or oropharynx adjacent to the tumour bearing gland, and erythema of the skin. These all settle within a few weeks of radiotherapy. Late effects are rarely severe. If a very high dose is given to an inoperable parotid tumour fibrosis may occur causing trismus. Radiation complications may occur in the mandible after irradiation of a submandibular tumour (see Chapter 8). Parotid irradiation inevitably causes some degree of dryness of the skin of the external auditory meatus. Hard wax may become adherent and difficult to remove; it must be treated with great care, as trauma to the skin of the bony part of the canal can result in exposure of the bone with the risk of the rare but serious complication of temporal bone necrosis.

Chemotherapy

In general, there is little place for chemotherapy in the treatment of salivary gland tumours, and as yet it seems to be no more than a treatment of last resort. A possible exception is the patient with severe local symptoms such as pain, fungation or bleeding, in which case a non-toxic regime such as fluorouracil 1 gram intravenously once weekly is worth trying. Lymphoma presenting in the parotid region is, of course, an exception to this and responds well to radiotherapy and/or chemotherapy as does lymphoma at other sites.

There are very few reported cases of a complete response: Skibba *et al.*[76] reported a patient with an unusually rapidly growing adenoid cystic carcinoma of the parotid with metastases to the lungs and skull in whom complete regression was obtained with a combination of cyclophosphamide, adriamycin and vincristine. There was one complete response in a series of 19 patients treated with cisplatin based chemotherapy.[77]

Tannock and Sutherland[78] made the observation that an adenoid cystic carcinoma is a slow growing tumour with a doubling time of between 1.5 and 18 months, the mean being 12 months. They point out that with a slowly growing tumour, any response to chemotherapy is likely to be slow, so treatment must be given over a prolonged period. Accordingly, drugs with cumulative toxicity such as the anthracyclines, nitroso-ureas and bleomycin

are best avoided. They suggested fluorouracil to be the most promising single agent as it can be given once weekly intravenously for a prolonged period without cumulative toxicity. Of 12 patients so treated, four obtained partial response and two showed no further progression of disease for periods ranging from 4 to 24 months. This response rate is similar to other reports with many combinations of agents which have been tried, all of which were associated with some toxicity.

Adenocarcinomas and malignant mixed tumours are perhaps a little less insensitive to cytotoxic therapy than are adenoid cystic carcinomas. Rentschler *et al.*[79] found that doxorubicin was the best single agent. Alberts *et al.*[80] treated five cases with a combination of doxorubicin, cisplatinum and cyclophosphamide. There were two complete responses and three partial responses, with a median duration of 6 months.

References

1 Eneroth CM. Histological and clinical aspects of parotid tumours. *Acta Otolaryngologica Supplement* 1964; **191**: 1–99.
2 Evans RW, Cruickshank AH. Epithelial tumours of the salivary glands. In: Evans RW, Cruickshank AH eds. *Major Problems in Pathology*, Volume 1. Philadelphia, PA: WB Saunders, 1970.
3 Thackray AC. Salivary gland tumours. *Proceedings of the Royal Society of Medicine* 1968; **61**: 1089–92.
4 Frable WJ, Elzay RP. Tumours of minor salivary glands; a report of 73 cases. *Cancer* 1970; **25**: 932–41.
5 Conley, J. *Salivary Glands and the Facial Nerve.* Stuttgart: George Thieme, 1975.
6 Ranger D, Thackray AC, Lucas RB. Mucous gland tumours. *British Journal of Cancer* 1956; **10**: 1–16.
7 Foote FW, Frazell EL. Tumours of the major salivary glands. *Cancer* 1953; **6**: 1065–133.
8 Skolnik EM, Friedman M, Becker S, Sisson GA, Keyes GR. Tumours of the major salivary glands. *Laryngoscope* 1977; **87**: 843–61.
9 Batsakis JG. Neoplasms of the minor and lesser major salivary glands. *Surgery, Gynaecology and Obstetrics* 1972; **135**: 289–98.
10 Maran AGD, Mackenzie IJ, Stanley RE. Recurrent pleomorphic adenomas of the parotid gland. *Archives of Otolaryngology* 1984; **110**: 167–71.
11 Watkin GT, Hobsley M. Influence of local surgery and radiotherapy on the natural history of pleomorphic adenomas. *British Journal of Surgery* 1986; **73**: 74–6.
12 Stevens KL, Hobsley M. The treatment of pleomorphic adenomas by formal parotidectomy. *British Journal of Surgery* 1982; **69**: 1–3.

13 Ebbs SR, Webb AJ. Adenolymphoma of the parotid: aetiology, diagnosis and treatment. *British Journal of Surgery* 1986; **73**: 627–30.

14 Smith AG, Broadbent TR, Zaraletta AA. Tumours of oral mucous glands. *Cancer* 1954; **7**: 224–33.

15 Stewart FW, Foote FW, Becker WF. Muco-epidermoid tumours of the salivary glands. *Annals of Surgery* 1945; **122**: 820–44.

16 Woolner LB, Pettet JR, Kirklin JW. Muco-epidermoid tumours of the minor salivary glands. *American Journal of Clinical Pathology* 1954; **24**: 1350–62.

17 Bhaskar SN, Bernier JL. Muco-epidermoid tumours of major and minor salivary glands. Clinical features, histology, natural history and results of treatment in 144 cases. *Cancer* 1962; **15**: 801–17.

18 Lapp H. Uber den muco-epidermoidtumor, eine besondere. Art von speicheldrusengeswulst. *Deutsche Zahnärtliche Zeitschrift* 1958; **13**: 1006–19.

19 Weiss H. Zue pathogenese de Maligen mukoepidermoidtumors. *Zeitschrift für Laryngologie, Rhinologie, Otologie und ihre Grenzgebiete* 1964; **43**: 39–41.

20 Chaudhry AP, Vickers RA, Gorlin RJ. Intraoral minor salivary gland tumours; an analysis of 1414 cases. *Oral Surgery* 1961; **14**: 1194–226.

21 Epker BN, Henny FA. Clinical histopathologic and surgical aspects of intraoral minor salivary gland tumours: review of 90 cases. *Journal of Oral Surgery* 1970; **27**: 792–804.

22 Healy WV, Perzin KH, Smith L. Muco-epidermoid carcinomas of salivary gland origin – classification, clinicopathological correlation and results of treatment. *Cancer* 1970; **26**: 368–88.

23 Hickman RE, Cawson RA, Duffy SW. The prognosis of specific types of salivary gland tumours. *Cancer* 1984; **54**: 1620–4.

24 Chen SY, Brannon RB, Miller AS, White DK, Hooker SP. Acinic cell adenocarcinoma of minor salivary glands. *Cancer* 1978; **42**: 678.

25 Clemis JD, Bland J, Fung C. Acinic cell tumours of salivary gland origin. *Laryngoscope* 1977; **87**: 1500–8.

26 Cummings CW. Adenoid cystic carcinoma (cylindroma) of the parotid gland. *Annals of Otolaryngology* 1977; **86**: 280–92.

27 Spiro RJ, Koss LG, Hajdu SI, Strong EW. Tumours of minor salivary origin. A clinicopathologic study of 492 cases. *Cancer* 1973; **31**: 117–29.

28 Conley J, Dingman DL. Adenoid cystic carcinoma in the head and neck (cylindroma). *Archives of Otolaryngology* 1974; **100**: 81–90.

29 Stuteville OH, Corley RD. Surgical management of tumours of the intraoral minor salivary glands: report of 80 cases. *Cancer* 1967; **20**: 1578–86.

30 Moran JJ, Becker SM, Brady LW, Rambo VB. Adenoid cystic carcinoma: clinico pathological study. *Cancer* 1961; **14**: 1235–50.

31 Kleinsasser O. Einleitung, morphologie und verhalten der epithelialen speicheldrusentumoren. *HNO* 1969; **17**: 197–211.

32 Thackray AC, Lucas RB. The histology of cylindroma of mucous gland origin. *British Journal of Cancer* 1960; **14**: 612–20.

33 Harrison DFN. Conservation surgery in the management of adenoidcystic carcinoma of the head and neck. *Bulletin of the New York Academy of Medicine* 1986; **62**: 828–33.

34 Stell PM, Cruikshank AH, Stoney PJ, Canter R, McCormick MS. Adenoid cystic carcinoma: the results of radical surgery. *Clinical Otolaryngology* 1985; **10**: 205–8.

35 Matsuba HM, Thawley SE, Simpson JR, Levine LA, Mauney M. Adenoidcystic carcinoma of the major and minor salivary gland origin. *Laryngoscope* 1984; **94**: 1316–18.

36 Matsuba HM, Spector GJ, Thawley SE, Simpson JR, Mauney M, Pikul FJ. Adenoid cystic salivary gland carcinoma. *Cancer* 1986; **57**: 519–24.

37 Cowie VJ, Pointon RCS. Adenoid cystic carcinoma of the salivary glands. *Clinical Radiology* 1984; **35**: 331–3.

38 Thackray AL, Lucas RB. *Tumours of the Major Salivary Glands*. Washington DC: Armed Forces Institute of Pathology, 1974.

39 Isaacson G, Shear M. Intraoral salivary gland tumours; a retrospective study of 201 cases. *Journal of Oral Pathology* 1983; **12**: 57–62.

40 Batsakis JG. Primary squamous cell carcinomas of major salivary glands. *Annals of Otolaryngology, Rhinology and Laryngology* 1983; **92**: 97–8.

41 Koss LG, Spiro RH, Hajdu SI. Small cell (oat cell) carcinoma of minor salivary gland origin. *Cancer* 1972; **30**: 737–41.

42 Batsakis JG. Primary lymphomas of the major salivary glands. *Annals of Otolaryngology, Rhinology and Laryngology* 1986; **95**: 107–8.

43 Gleeson MJ, Bennett MH, Cawson RA. Lymphomas of salivary glands. *Cancer* 1986; **58**: 699–704.

44 Langdon JD. Tumours of the salivary glands: clinical analysis of 68 cases. *Journal of Oral and Maxillofacial Surgery* 1985; **43**: 688–92.

45 Broderick JP, Auger RG, de Santo LW. Facial paralysis and occult parotid cancer – a characteristic syndrome. *Archives of Otolaryngology – Head and Neck Surgery* 1988; **114**: 195–7.

46 Byers RM, Piorkowski R, Luna MA. Malignant parotid tumours in patients under 20 years of age. *Archives of Otolaryngology* 1984; **110**: 232–5.

47 Partridge M, Langdon JD, Borthwick-Clarke A, Rankin S. Diagnostic techniques for parotid disease. *British Journal of Oral and Maxillofacial Surgery* 1986; **24**: 311–22.

48 Olsen KD. The parotid lump – don't biopsy it! *Postgraduate Medicine* 1987; **81**: 225–34.

49 Berg HM, Jacobs JB, Kaufman D, Reede DL. Correlation of fine needle aspiration and CT scanning of

parotid masses. *Laryngoscope* 1986; **96**: 1357–62.

50 Cohen MB, Ljung B, Boles R. Salivary gland tumours, fine needle aspiration vs frozen section diagnosis. *Archives of Otolaryngology – Head and Neck Surgery* 1986; **112**: 867–9.

51 Qizilbash AH, Sianos J, Young JEM, Archibald SD. Fine needle aspiration biopsy cytology and cytopathology of major salivary glands. *Journal of Clinical Cytology* 1985; **29**: 503–12.

52 Ballerini G, Mantero M, Sbrocca M. Ultrasonic patterns of parotid masses. *Journal of Clinical Ultrasound* 1984; **12**: 273–7.

53 Baker DC, Conley J. Treatment of massive deep lobe parotid tumours. *American Journal of Surgery* 1979; **138**: 572–5.

54 Patey DH, Thackray AC. The pathological anatomy and treatment of parotid tumours with retropharyngeal extension (dumb-bell tumours). *British Journal of Surgery* 1956; **44**: 352–8.

55 Watkin GT, Hobsley M. Should radiotherapy be used routinely in the management of parotid tumours? *British Journal of Surgery* 1986; **73**: 601–3.

56 Langdon JD. Complications of parotid gland surgery. *Journal of Maxillo-Facial Surgery* 1984; **12**: 193–238.

57 Hanna DC, Dickason WL, Richardson GS, Gaisford JC. Management of recurrent salivary gland tumours. *American Journal of Surgery* 1976; **132**: 453–8.

58 Donovan DT, Conley JJ. Capsular significance in parotid tumour surgery: reality and myths of lateral lobectomy. *Laryngoscope* 1984; **94**: 324–9.

59 Rafla S. Malignant parotid tumours: natural history and treatment. *Cancer* 1977; **40**: 136–44.

60 Imperato JP, Weichselbaum RR, Ervin TJ. The role of post-operative radiation therapy in the treatment of malignant tumours of the parotid gland. *Journal of Surgical Oncology* 1984; **27**: 163–7.

61 Laage-Hellman JE. Treatment of gustatory sweating and flushing. *Acta Odontologica* 1958; **49**: 132–6.

62 Morfit, HM, Kramish D. Auriculotemporal syndrome (Frey's syndrome) following surgery of parotid tumours. *American Journal of Surgery* 1961; **102**: 777–80.

63 Glaister DH, Hearnshaw JR, Heffran PF, Peck AW. The mechanism of post-parotidectomy gustatory sweating (auriculotemporal syndrome). *British Medical Journal* 1958; **2**: 942–6.

64 Armistead PR, Smiddy FG, Frank HG. Simple enucleation and radiotherapy in the treatment of pleomorphic salivary adenoma of the parotid gland. *British Journal of Surgery* 1979; **66**: 716–17.

65 Dawson AK, Orr JA. Long-term results of local excision and radiotherapy in pleomorphic adenoma of the parotid. *International Journal of Radiation Oncology, Biology, Physics* 1985; **11**: 451–5.

66 Fitzpatrick PJ, Theriault C. Malignant salivary gland tumours. *International Journal of Radiation Oncology, Biology, Physics* 1986; **12**: 1743–7.

67 Borthne A, Kjellevold K, Kaalhus O, Vermund H. Salivary gland malignant neoplasms: treatment and prognosis. *International Journal of Radiation Oncology, Biology, Physics* 1986; **12**: 747–54.

68 North CA, Lee DJ, Piantadosi S. Carcinoma of the major salivary glands treated by surgery or surgery plus post-operative radiotherapy. *International Journal of Radiation Oncology, Biology, Physics* 1990; **118**: 1319–26.

69 Simpson JR, Matsuba HM, Thawley SE, Mauney M. Improved treatment of salivary adenocarcinomas: planned combined surgery and irradiation. *Laryngoscope* 1986; **96**: 904–7.

70 McNaney D, McNeese MD, Guillamondegui OM, Fletcher GH, Oswald MJ. Post-operative irradiation in malignant epithelial tumours of the parotid. *International Journal of Radiation Oncology, Biology, Physics* 1983; **9**: 1289–95.

71 Vikram B, Strong EW, Shah JP, Spiro RH. Radiation therapy in adenoid-cystic carcinoma. *International Journal of Radiation Oncology, Biology, Physics* 1984; **10**: 221–3.

72 Ellis ER, Million RR, Mendenhall WM, Parsons JT, Cassisi NJ. The use of radiation therapy in the management of minor salivary gland tumours. *International Journal of Radiation Oncology, Biology, Physics* 1988; **15**: 613–17.

73 Catterall M, Bewley DK. *Fast Neutrons in the Treatment of Cancer.* London: Academic Press, 1979.

74 Griffin TW, Pajak TF, Laramore GE. Neutron vs photon irradiation of inoperable salivary gland tumours: results of an RTOG-MRC co-operative randomised study. *International Journal of Radiation Oncology, Biology, Physics* 1988; **15**: 1085–90.

75 Million RR, Cassisi NJ, Wittes ES. Minor salivary glands. In: de Vita VT, Hellman S, Roseberge SA eds. *Cancer Principles and Practice of Oncology.* Philadelphia, PA: JB Lippincott, 1982.

76 Skibba JL, Hurley JD, Ravelo HV. Complete response of metastatic adenoid cystic carcinoma of the parotid gland to chemotherapy. *Cancer* 1981; **47**: 2543–8.

77 Dick de Haan L, de Mulder PHM, Vermorken JB *et al.* Cisplatin-based chemotherapy in advanced adenoid cystic carcinoma of the head and neck. *Head and Neck* 1992; **14**: 273–7.

78 Tannock IF, Sutherland DJ. Chemotherapy for adenocystic carcinoma. *Cancer* 1980; **46**: 452.

79 Rentschler R, Burgess MA, Byers R. Chemotherapy of major salivary neoplasms: a twenty-five year review of M.D. Anderson Hospital experience. *Cancer* 1977; **40**: 612–19.

80 Alberts DS, Manning MR, Coulthard SW, Koopman CF, Herman TS. Adriamycin/cisplatinum/cyclophosphamide combination chemotherapy for advanced carcinoma of the parotid gland. *Cancer* 1981; **47**: 645–8.

16 Primary tumours of the jaws

D Archer and JD Langdon

It is not always possible to be certain whether some tumours of the jaws have arisen from osseous or odontogenic tissues, but such a distinction is usually of little practical significance. Many of these tumours are rare in the jaws but are more common in other parts of the skeleton.[1-5]

(1) *Tumours of osseous tissues*
Ossifing fibroma
Osteoma, exostoses and tori
Osteoid osteoma
Osteoblastoma
Giant cell tumours and granulomas
Osteosarcoma
Chondroma and chondrosarcoma
Chondromyxoid fibroma
Chondroblastoma
Desmoblastic fibroma
Fibrosarcoma
(2) *Miscellaneous primary tumours of the jaws*
Ewing's sarcoma
Haemangioma and angiosarcoma
Lymphoma
(3) *Multifocal and secondary bone tumours*
Carcinomas
Myeloma, multiple or solitary
Histiocytosis X
Others
(4) *Odontogenic tumours*
Ameloblastoma
Adenomatoid odontogenic tumour
Calcifying epithelial odontogenic tumour
Cementomas and cemental dysplasias
Myxoma of the jaws
Other odontogenic tumours and odontomes

Assessment of tumours of the jaws

The histological features alone are sometimes insufficient to categorise a jaw tumour correctly and in most cases it is necessary to take into account also the history and clinical features and the radiographic findings.[6]

In the absence of adequate information of this sort it may not be possible to decide whether or not a bone tumour is malignant and unnecessarily extensive surgery may be carried out. By contrast, to attempt to distinguish between odontogenic tumours and their osseous counterparts may be little more than an academic exercise if their management and outcome are going to be the same.

Ossifying fibroma

This uncommon tumour is seen in young adults, but almost any age can be affected. This tumour when in the tooth bearing areas is not necessarily distinguishable, microscopically, from a cementifying fibroma. To try to do so seems to be little more than academic as their behaviour and treatment is the same.[7]

It is important however to differentiate this lesion from fibrous dysplasia.

Osteoma and other bony overgrowths

Tumours consisting of bone, either compact or cancellous, are occasionally seen; localised overgrowths of bone (exostoses) are more common. Small exostoses may form irregularly on the surface of the alveolar processes and on the palate (torus palatinus) or mandible (torus mandibularis). Exostoses consist of lamellae of compact bone, but exceptionally large specimens may have a core of cancellous bone.

Torus palatinus

This may start to develop in early adult life, but is not usually noticed until middle age. The common site is towards the posterior of the mid-line of the hard palate and the swelling is rounded and symmetrical, sometimes with a mid-line groove. If the swelling is large enough to interfere with the fitting of a denture or otherwise gets in the way, it should be removed.

Tori mandibularis

These form on the lingual aspect of the mandible opposite the mental foramen. They are typically bilateral, forming hard, rounded swellings. Local excision is necessary if the torus is troublesome.

Compact and cancellous osteoma

The compact osteoma consists of dense bone containing occasional vascular spaces, and is of very slow growth. The cancellous osteoma consists of trabeculae of bone, between which are marrow spaces, surrounded by a lamellated cortex.

Osteomas should be excised only if they become large enough to cause symptoms or make the fitting of a denture difficult.

Gardner's syndrome

Gardner's syndrome comprises multiple osteomas of the jaws and long bones, *Polyposis coli* with a high malignant potential, and often other features such as dental defects and epidermal cysts. It is inherited as an autosomal dominant trait.[8]

The osteomas of the jaws are typically multiple and may be ranged along the alveolar ridge, along the borders of the mandible or form endosteal radiopacities.

The chief importance of this syndrome is that most of those affected die of bowel cancer by the age of 50, but some members of the family can have multiple osteomas without *Polyposis coli*.

Osteochondroma

This is a bony overgrowth growing by ossification beneath a cartilagenous cap. Clinically, the mandible is more commonly affected than any other part of the head and neck region, and approximately 95 per cent of cases arise from the region of the coronoid or condylar process.[9] The lesion forms a hard bony protruberance like that of an osteoma.

It can interfere with temporomandibular joint function and limit opening of the mouth. The cartilagenous cap may not be visible in radiographs. Almost any age can be affected.

There is doubt as to whether osteochondromas are true neoplasms or developmental anomalies; usually, growth of the tumour ceases with skeletal maturation. In any case they are benign and complete excision together with the overlying periosteum is curative.

Osteoid osteoma and osteoblastoma

These tumours are not histologically distinguishable, but though it is not universally agreed that they are separate entities, they appear to have different clinical and radiographic features.[10] They are both rare in the jaws and more common in other bones such as the femur. Most patients are below the age of 30 and males are affected twice as often as females.

Osteoid osteoma

The mandible is affected approximately twice as frequently as the maxilla: the typical complaint is of pain which is characteristically worse at night but variable in nature and severity.[11] The pain is also characteristically relieved by adequate doses of aspirin, and can occasionally precede radiologically detectable changes. Osteoid osteomas are less than 2 cm in diameter, and appear to have limited growth potential.

Radiographically, osteoid osteoma is considerably more frequently cortical than medullary in site and typically shows a central nidus of radiolucency surrounded by a zone of densely sclerotic bone. In a minority the nidus becomes calcified.

Osteoblastoma

Osteoblastomas are even more rare than osteoid osteomas, particularly in the head and neck region. In this area the mandible is also the most frequently affected site. As with osteoid osteoma osteoblastoma occurs below the age of 30, and males predominate in the ratio of 2 to 1. The chief complaint is of dull aching pain, but this is not usually nocturnal, and frequently does not respond to aspirin. More important however, osteoblastomas have a potential for progressive growth, can produce swelling of the jaw and may cause loosening of teeth.[12]

Radiographically, an osteoblastoma appears as a rounded area of radiolucency, usually in the medulla and containing variable amounts of mineralisation. Unlike osteoid osteoma, there is no nidus, perilesional sclerosis is usually slight and the mass can be larger (2 to 10 cm in diameter). However, the radiographic features are variable and can mimic osteosarcoma or other malignant tumours in up to 25 per cent of cases and show a sun-ray appearance or Codman's triangles.

The osteoblastoma is benign and responds to conservative excision, but recurrence is likely if this is incomplete.[13] There have been isolated reports of malignant change in osteoblastoma, but such lesions may have been low grade osteosarcomas from the start. However, even 'malignant osteoblastomas' appear only to be locally aggressive and, unlike osteosarcoma, appear to have little or no potential for metastasis.

Cementoblastoma is also histologically similar to, and can be regarded as a counterpart of, osteoblastoma. If the lesion is originating from and surrounding the root of a tooth, it seems reasonable to regard it as a cementoblastoma, if the microscopic findings are consistent with this diagnosis. Like osteoblastoma an aggressive variant of cementoblastoma has been reported.[14]

Giant cell granuloma of the jaw

Central giant cell lesions affecting the jaws are, in most cases, hyperplastic lesions and can be clearly distinguished from neoplasms by their behaviour.

The giant cell tumour (osteoclastoma) is an aggressive neoplasm that chiefly affects the limbs. Osteoclastomas occasionally form in such bones as the temporal or sphenoid, but it is questionable how many of the few reported cases of these neoplasms in the jaws can be authenticated; a report in 1981 of a primary malignant giant cell tumour of the jaw was claimed to be the first documented case. This tumour metastasised to lungs and a lymph node.

Although the giant cell granuloma is the main type of giant cell lesion affecting the jaw, it is uncommon. Its important and characteristic feature is that although it may grow rapidly and simulate a neoplasm clinically, wide excision is unnecessary and regression follows mere curettage.

It is probable that this lesion is a developmental disorder and similar collections of giant cells can be seen in fibrous dysplasia and related conditions. Previously the lesion was referred to as the giant cell *reparative* granuloma, but there is no evidence to suggest a role for 'repair' in these tumours.[15]

Clinical features

Central giant cell granuloma is usually seen in young people under 20, and females are twice as frequently affected as males. The mandible is the usual site, and the great majority of lesions are anterior to the first molars, where the teeth have had deciduous predecessors. There is frequently only a painless swelling, but growth is sometimes rapid, and there may occasionally be pain or paraesthesia of the lower lip. Radiographs show a rounded cyst-like area of radiolucency often with a suggestion of loculation or a soap bubble appearance. The roots of related teeth can be displaced, or less frequently may be resorbed, and the mass can occasionally break through the bone, particularly of the alveolar ridge, to produce a soft tissue swelling. Biopsy is necessary to make the diagnosis but this should be supplemented by blood chemistry to exclude hyperparathyroidism.

There are no changes in blood chemistry, but the histological features are indistinguishable from hyperparathyroidism. These giant cells have been shown by Flanagan *et al.*,[16] in their response to calcitonin, their activity in tissue culture and by osteoclast-specific monoclonal antibodies, to have all the properties of and to be indistinguishable from osteoclasts.

Differential diagnosis of giant cell granuloma

(1) Hyperparathyroidism. The histological appearances are identical. Blood chemistry should be undertaken and a raised serum, calcium and bony alkaline phosphatase indicate hyperparathyroidism. Skeletal radiographs may also show other affected bones. No treatment is needed for the bone lesions which normally heal after the removal of the parathyroid tumour.

(2) Fibrous dysplasia. A limited biopsy may show foci of giant cells but the radiographic and histological features, and behaviour are distinctive.

(3) Cherubism. The microscopic features may be indistinguishable from giant cell granuloma, but typically there are symmetrical lesions, par-

ticularly near the angle of the mandible and sometimes in the maxilla also.

(4) Giant cell tumour (osteoclastoma) as mentioned earlier affects long bones, but may not be distinguishable with certainty by microscopy alone from a giant cell granuloma. Aggressive behaviour and recurrence after surgery would be confirmatory.

(5) Aneurysmal bone cysts may contain many giant cells but their other histological features and in particular the multiple blood-filled spaces, should enable the distinction to be readily made.

Treatment

Curettage of giant cell granulomas is adequate and wide excision is unnecessary; small fragments that may be left behind seem to cause little trouble, rarely require further treatment and appear to resolve spontaneously. Rarely, recurrence follows incomplete removal and a further limited operation becomes necessary. Harris[17] has recently reported a series of central giant cell granulomas of the jaws which regressed with calcitonin therapy.

Osteosarcoma

This highly malignant tumour is the most common primary neoplasm of bone, but overall is rare, especially in the jaws. According to Garrington *et al.*,[18] the annual incidence of osteosarcoma of the jaws in the USA is 1 per 1.5 million persons.

Most cases of osteosarcoma have no identifiable aetiological factors apart from the few which have followed irradiation. Osteosarcoma is also a recognised complication of Paget's disease of bone but hardly ever in the jaws.

Clinical features

Osteosarcoma of the jaws characteristically affects patients considerably later than in the long bones, namely at a mean age of 30 to 39. Rarely it may develop even later as a result of irradiation many years previously. Males are slightly more frequently affected than females. The mandible, in particular the body, is more frequently affected than the maxilla.

A characteristic picture is that of a firm swelling, which grows in a few months and becomes painful. The teeth may be loosened and there may be par-

aesthesia or loss of sensation in the mental nerve area. Metastases to the lungs may develop early. The radiological features are variable but irregular bone destruction usually predominates over bone formation in most cases. A soft tissue mass may be associated and bone formation in such a mass is highly characteristic of osteosarcoma. A sun-ray appearance at the surface or Codman's triangles at the margins due to elevation of the periosteum and new bone formation may be seen on appropriate radiographs in only a minority of cases and are not specific to osteosarcoma. The extent of the tumour can be shown by computed tomography (CT) scanning.

Diagnosis depends on biopsy, which may need to be repeated if there is any doubt. Radiographs of the chest should also be taken as secondary deposits may be present when the patient is first seen. Serum alkaline phosphatase levels are raised in about 50 per cent of cases and particularly with those tumours where new bone formation predominates.

Behaviour and management

Osteosarcoma of the jaws is a rapidly invasive tumour but metastases to the lungs are usually later events than in the case of osteosarcoma of long bones. Nevertheless local recurrence within a year of initial treatment is seen in approximately 50 per cent of cases and the prognosis then deteriorates sharply. Rarely there may be metastases to the regional lymph nodes.

The treatment of osteosarcoma is early radical excision.[19] This involves mandibulectomy or maxillectomy together with wide excision of any soft tissue extensions of the tumour. This is often combined with external beam, interstital or stereotactically guided radiotherapy followed immediately by surgery.[20] The value of adjuvant chemotherapy cannot be said as yet to be established and immunotherapy has proved to be disappointing; possibly because of the small numbers in any recorded series.

The prognosis depends mainly on the extent of the tumour at operation and deteriorates with spread to the soft tissues, to lymph nodes or to the base of the skull. McKenna *et al.*[21] in an analysis of 552 osteogenic sarcomas found that the 5 year survival rate ranged from 40 per cent for tumours less than 5 cm in diameter to zero for tumours over 15 cm. However, osteosarcomas of the jaws appear to have a significantly better prognosis than those in the long bones.

Juxtacortical osteosarcoma

Juxtacortical osteosarcoma is a rare variant which, like endosteal osteosarcoma, mainly affects the limbs, but can occasionally involve the jaws. Its chief importance is its better prognosis.

Clinically, juxtacortical osteosarcoma typically affects the mandible, and the average age of patients is about 35 years. Females are said to be more commonly affected, but this is not apparent in the small numbers of reported jaw tumours of this type.

Juxtacortical osteosarcoma forms a slow growing mass which may cause dull aching pain on the surface of the bone or in the adjacent parosteal tissues. The mass is typically rounded with a broad base.

Radiographically, juxtacortical osteosarcoma characteristically has a radiopaque base and is more radiolucent superficially. The pattern of and amount of opacity and radiolucency however varies widely between individual cases.

Management and prognosis

It is obviously essential to establish the diagnosis firmly and an adequate biopsy of the superficial radiolucent areas is most likely to provide an accurate answer.

Wide excision, including underlying bone, is desirable, although treatment in some reported cases has been limited to curettage. Recurrence is then likely and may happen after excision; it has also happened even after hemimandibulectomy. Too little information is available on the behaviour of juxtacortical osteosarcoma of the jaws, but with those affecting long bones the overall 5 year survival rate is about 80 per cent. With high grade, poorly differentiated tumours, however, there may eventually be spread to the lungs in nearly 70 per cent of cases.[22]

Chondroma and chondrosarcoma

Chondroma

The chondroma is a particularly rare tumour of the jaws. It is more frequently found in the nose or nasal sinuses and hence can occasionally be found in the maxilla rather than the mandible. Clinically, true chondromas are small and likely to be no more than chance findings. However, it has been reported that 20 per cent of chondrosarcomas in the maxillo-facial area were originally thought to be chondromas.

Microscopically, chondromas consist of hyaline cartilage, but the cells are irregular in size and distribution. Calcification or ossification may develop within the cartilage.

Behaviour and management

The treatment is by wide excision, including an adequate margin of normal tissue all round, because of the difficulty in distinguishing benign from malignant tumours and the fact that chondrosarcomas in the maxillofacial region are considerably more common than chondromas.[23]

Chondrosarcoma (Figs 16.1 and 16.2)

Chondrosarcomas of the jaws affect adults at an average age of about 45. The maxilla is affected in

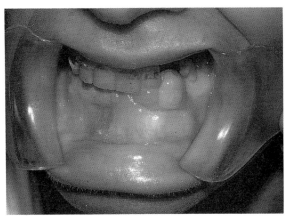

Fig. 16.1 Chondrosarcoma arising in the lower canine region of a male patient aged 44 years.

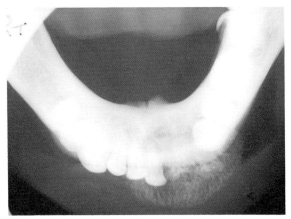

Fig. 16.2 Radiograph of patient shown in Fig. 16.1. The sun-ray appearance of this expansile lesion is clearly seen.

60 per cent of cases, most frequently in the anterior alveolar region, and the mandible in 40 per cent but with no special site of predilection.

Pain, swelling or loosening of teeth associated with an area of greater or lesser radiolucency are typical features. Radiographically, chondrosarcoma of the jaws can be well or poorly circumscribed, or may appear multilocular. Although radiolucency is typical, calcifications are frequently present and may be widespread and dense.

Behaviour and management

Chondrosarcomas of the maxillofacial region are aggressive and the main cause of death is local recurrence or persistent tumour. Fewer than 10 per cent of these tumours metastasise; the lungs or other bones are the usual sites of distant spread.

Chondrosarcomas must therefore be widely excised as early as possible. The first operation is critical as inadequate excision is likely to lead to recurrences beyond the original area of operation with inevitable problems of management. Chondrosarcomas only occasionally respond to radiotherapy and chemotherapy appears to be of little value.

The prognosis of chondrosarcomas of the maxillofacial region is generally worse than for other sites because of the difficulties of adequate excision in this area.[3] The 5 year survival rate ranges from 40 to 60 per cent and depends on the tumour stage and grade, and on the extent of the original excision.

Mesenchymal chondrosarcoma

Mesenchymal chondrosarcoma is considerably more uncommon than chondrosarcoma but a relatively high proportion (15 to 35 per cent) occur in the craniofacial region. A minority form in the soft tissues.

Clinical features

Mesenchymal chondrosarcoma has a wide age distribution and presents no specific signs or symptoms. Rapidly developing pain and swelling, sometimes with loosening of teeth, are however typical.

Radiographically there is an area of radiolucency, usually speckled with calcifications. There is only partial circumscription and no peripheral sclerosis. This is a highly cellular tumour in which only small foci of tissue can be recognised as poorly formed cartilage.

Behaviour and prognosis

Mesenchymal chondrosarcoma is highly malignant and the frequency of metastases is high. Spread is usually to the lungs but can be to lymph nodes and frequently follows local recurrences.

Early radical surgery followed by combined chemotherapy is therefore the treatment of choice. However, its value is as yet uncertain and either local recurrences or metastases can appear 10 or more years after treatment.[24] There are no reliable microscopic indicators of value in assessing prognosis.

Chondromyxoid fibroma (fibromyxoid chondroma)

This rare tumour has occasionally been reported in the mandible. Fewer than 20 cases have been reported in the head and neck region and the chief importance of this tumour is that it is benign but can be mistaken microscopically for a chondrosarcoma.

Clinical features

Most patients are below the age of 30. Chondromyxoid fibroma has been reported sometimes to behave like a malignant tumour and can cause pain, swelling of the jaw or loosening of teeth. There is relatively little information on the radiographic features of these tumours in the jaws but they are likely to appear as radiolucent areas with irregular but, typically, sclerotic margins or an appearance suggesting loculation. Opacities are rarely seen in the tumour area.

Behaviour and management

Chondromyxoid fibroma is benign but can recur if excision is inadequate and, like other chondroid tumours can grow in the soft tissues as a result of seeding of tumour cells at operation.[25] Moreover sarcomatous change has rarely been reported. Excision of the tumour with as wide as possible a margin of normal tissue is therefore desirable.

Chondroblastoma

Chondroblastoma is a benign tumour that slightly more commonly affects the long bones than chondromyxoid fibroma but involves the maxillofacial region even more rarely and has considerably more frequently been found in the temporal bone than in the jaws.

Clinical features

The median age of presentation of this tumour in the head and neck region is approximately 40; males are affected twice as frequently as females. However, data on tumours in this region are scanty. Characteristic radiographic appearances in the long bones are a rounded area of radiolucency with a thin sclerotic border which may sometimes show a scalloped pattern and varying amounts of calcification. These appearances may however be less well defined in the jaws.

Behaviour and management

As indicated earlier, information about chondroblastomas of the jaws is scanty. They are, in general, benign and curettage (followed if necessary by bone grafting) has been reported to be successful, though with recurrences in 5 to 35 per cent of cases.[26] If however aneurysmal bone cyst is associated, curettage alone is inadequate and its combination with cryosurgery is probably more effective. There is in either case a good response to radiotherapy for otherwise uncontrollable or surgically inaccessible lesions.

Ewing's sarcoma

Ewing's sarcoma is rare and predominantly affects the legs or pelvis, but of the few that affect the head and neck region, there is a strong predilection for the body of the mandible.

The histogenesis of Ewing's sarcoma has long been controversial but immunocytochemistry has shown that the cells stain for neural markers. Moreover the tumour cells may form rosette-like patterns as seen in neuroblastoma and retinoblastoma.

Clinical features

The usual age group affected is from 5 to 30 years, and the typical symptoms are bone swelling and often pain, progressing over a period of months. Teeth may become loosened by bone destruction, and the overlying mucosa may become ulcerated. Fever, leukocytosis, raised erythrocyte sedimen-

tation rate (ESR) and anaemia may be associated features and indicate a poor prognosis.

Behaviour and management

The most common sites for metastases are the lungs and other bones. Since Ewing's sarcoma is so rare as a primary tumour in the jaws, the possibility that such a tumour is a metastasis from another bone should always be investigated by means of a skeletal survey. Lymph nodes are involved in 10 to 20 per cent of cases.

Currently the initial treatment of choice is probably wide excision including radical neck dissection or megavoltage irradiation when excision is not possible. In addition, multi-agent chemotherapy should be given, and this combination treatment appears to have improved the 5 year survival rate from about 10 to 60 per cent or more by reducing the incidence of subsequent metastases.[27]

Desmoplastic fibroma (Fig. 16.3)

The terminology of these and related tumours is confusing. Desmoplastic fibroma is histologically indistinguishable from the periosteal desmoid. 'Desmoid' means band- or ligament-like and is

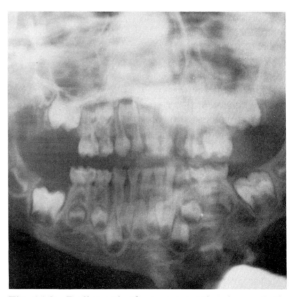

Fig. 16.3 Radiograph of a very extensive desmoplastic fibroma involving the soft tissues of the left neck and lower border of the mandible in a 4 year old boy. This tumour underwent spontaneous regression over a 2 year period following surgical debulking.

not a helpful term in this context as it derives from the fibrous masses which arise in muscle sheaths particularly of the abdominal wall. The abdominal desmoid is a form of fibromatosis, a term that describes tumour-like fibrous proliferations which infiltrate the surrounding tissues like a fibrosarcoma, but never metastasise. The rare desmoplastic fibroma of the jaws has the same salient features.

Clinical features

The majority of patients (75 per cent) are below the age of 30 and 50 per cent are between the ages of 10 and 20. The mandible is the most common site in the head and neck region.[28] The majority of these lesions are at the junction between the ramus and the body of the mandible.

The main symptom is a gradually enlarging swelling but occasionally there is aching pain. Radiographically, desmoplastic fibroma gives rise to a well circumscribed area of lucency which has a honeycomb or trabeculated appearance, and in most cases has some sclerosis around its margins. Roots of related teeth may be resorbed, and rarely the margins suggest infiltration of the surrounding bone.

Behaviour and management

Desmoplastic fibroma is a progressive lesion, but as mentioned earlier, it does not metastasise. Because of its infiltrative character however, curettage or local excision are followed by recurrence in up to 30 per cent of cases.[28] Excision with an adequate margin of normal bone is therefore required and wider excision still is necessary for lesions that have extended into the soft tissues. However, mutilating surgery is not justified as any recurrences are purely local and can be controlled when they appear. Malignant change has been reported after radiotherapy which is therefore contra-indicated. Rarely, desmoplastic fibromas have been reported to undergo spontaneous regression particularly in infancy.[29]

Fibrous histiocytoma (Fig. 16.4)

Fibrous histiocytomas range in behaviour from benign to malignant. These tumours are predominantly soft tissue tumours but a minority are intra-osseous. In an analysis of 88 reports of these tumours involving the head and neck region, Barnes[30] found that 7 per cent were in the man-

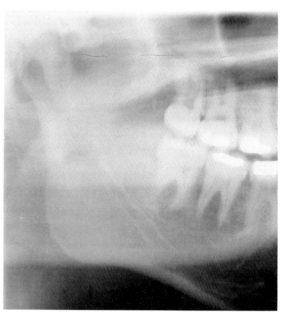

Fig. 16.4 Radiograph of a malignant fibrous histiocytoma arising in the third molar region of the mandible in a 19 year old male. Malignant resorption of the roots of the molar teeth can be seen.

dible, which was considerably more frequently involved than the maxilla or the oral and peri-oral soft tissues.

Clinical features

Malignant fibrous histiocytomas of the jaws do not show any specific features to distinguish them from other sarcomas. Pain, swelling and loosening of teeth are typical effects.

Treatment

Fibrous histiocytomas, even if histologically benign should be widely excised. The possibility of lymph node involvement should be considered and neck dissection carried out if necessary.

Haemangioma of bone (Fig. 16.5)

Solitary haemangiomas form less than 1 per cent of tumours of bone, but a high proportion are in the head and neck region. Of these, about 30 per cent are in the jaws, the mandible being involved twice

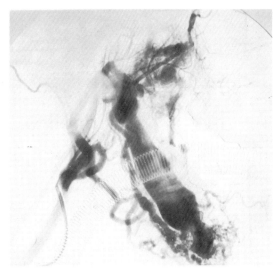

Fig. 16.5 Superselective subtraction carotid angiogram of an arteriovenous haemangioma occupying the entire left mandible of a 28 year old female.

as often as the maxilla. Women are twice as frequently affected as men, but the tumour can be seen at virtually any age.

Clinical features

A haemangioma of the jaw gives rise to progressive painless swelling. When the overlying bone becomes sufficiently thinned, the swelling may become pulsatile, teeth may be loosened and there may be profuse bleeding particularly from the gingival margins involved by the tumour. Some behave aggressively with rapid erosion of surrounding bone. Growth and extension may be periodic, with periods of apparent quiescence of many years followed by rapid spontaneous growth.

Radiographic features

A haemangioma appears as a generally rounded or pseudoloculated area of radiolucency with ill defined margins and often a soap bubble appearance.

Superselective angiography, however, indicates when haemangiomas are venous (cavernous) capillary or arteriovenous. The last (fast flow angiomas) have one or more large feeder arteries, and are likely to be the most rapidly expanding and most likely to bleed severely, if opened.

Diagnosis and management

The chief problem is that of haemorrhage at operation, but in view of the overall rarity of such tumours, the possibility of an intra-osseous haemangioma may be unsuspected, particularly if there has been no history of bleeding or superficial signs suggestive of a vascular lesion. Theoretically, however, haemangioma should be considered in the differential diagnosis of any cyst-like lesion of the jaws, particularly those having radiographic features such as those described above. It is clearly not feasible to carry out angiography on all such lesions, but it is certainly an argument for aspiration of cyst-like lesions where the diagnosis is uncertain. Another warning sign is that at operation elevation of the overlying periosteum may reveal a bluish swelling.

Opening a haemangioma or extracting a related tooth can give rise to torrential bleeding – losses of 3.5 litres of blood have not uncommonly been reported – but by no means all haemangiomas bleed as freely as might be expected from their histological picture.

Once the diagnosis has been made, wide en bloc resection is the only practical method of dealing with the problem. Radiotherapy has been tried, but has considerable disadvantages. When there are identifiable feeder vessels, selective arterial embolisation makes any subsequent resection very much easier and safer. Surgery should follow embolisation as soon as possible, and certainly within 3 days. The haemodynamics of these lesions are such that soon after embolisation further channels open up due to a 'steal' effect. When arteriography reveals identifiable feeder vessels it is often possible to tie off these vessels, or even the external carotid artery on that side, and then radically curette the affected area retaining the cortex and periosteum. The ensuing defect is then packed with bone mush harvested from the iliac crest and once healing is completed the bone becomes reconstituted. When a haemangioma expands to include the skull base treatment may become impossible.

Secondary neoplasms – carcinoma
(see Chapter 17)

Primary growth is usually in the bronchus, breast or prostate, and cancer cells reach the jaws by the bloodstream.[31] These are common tumours and are the most common carcinomas to cause bony metastases. Other important sites of primary growth are the thyroid and kidney, but adenocarcinomas from almost any primary site can metastasise to the jaws.

Symptoms from a malignant deposit in the jaw are, on rare occasions, the first sign of the disease and can lead to diagnosis of the primary. In other cases the jaw is the first apparent site of secondary deposits from a growth treated a year or more previously. Although the jaw is much less frequently involved than other bones, secondary carcinoma is an important malignant tumour.

Patients are usually middle-aged or elderly. The common symptoms are pain, which is often severe, or swelling of the jaw. Paraesthesia (numbness or tingling) of the lip may be caused by involvement of a nerve trunk.

Radiological examination

This usually shows an area of radiolucency with a hazy outline which sometimes simulates an infected cyst or may be quite irregular and simulate osteomyelitis. A typical site is at the base of the condylar neck. Sometimes the entire mandible may have a moth-eaten appearance. Areas of new bone formation may rarely be the main feature.

The secondary deposits are usually adenocarcinomas or less often squamous cell carcinoma, according to the nature of the primary growth. Bone destruction by osteoclasts near the periphery of the deposit is the most common effect, but bone sclerosis can result particularly from metastases from the prostate.

A careful history, especially of previous operations, and general examination are necessary. A technetium bone scan of the rest of the skeleton will show whether there are other deposits, and blood examination is necessary in case widespread metastases are replacing the marrow, causing anaemia. Biopsy of the jaw should be carried out to confirm the diagnosis.

Treatment

The primary growth should be treated if this is still feasible, and in the case of the breast and prostate, hormone therapy may cause secondary deposits to regress for a time. In most cases bony metastases are a sign of blood-borne spread of the disease and palliative treatment is usually all that can be achieved. Irradiation may make the patient more comfortable and make the lesion in the jaw regress for a time. Should the deposit fungate into the oral cavity or face, cryosurgery may be helpful in controlling pain and haemorrhage, and reducing bulk.

Multiple myeloma and solitary plasmacytoma

Multiple myeloma

Multiple myeloma is by far the most common neoplasm of plasma cells, and solitary plasmacytomas, whether endosteal or soft tissue, usually progress after a variable period to multiple myeloma.[32]

The initial symptoms of multiple myeloma may occasionally result from a jaw lesion or one of the complications of myeloma, in particular amyloidosis, which may be the main clinical feature. More rarely solitary plasmacytoma of the jaw or of oral or peri-oral soft tissues may be seen.

Multiple myeloma is unusual among lymphoreticular neoplasms in producing bone-destructive lesions, which are usually the main cause of symptoms, namely, bone pain and tenderness. Skeletal radiographs typically show multiple punched-out areas of radiolucency, particularly in the vault of the skull.

As a result of the proliferation of myeloma cells in the marrow, there is frequently anaemia and sometimes thrombocytopenia. Depressed production of other immunoglobulins may lead to increased susceptibility to infection.

Cases such as these represent fully developed disease, which is only rarely detected early in its asymptomatic phase by the chance finding of a monoclonal gammopathy as a result of a routine blood examination.

Investigation

Serological findings which may suggest the diagnosis of multiple myeloma are a greatly raised ESR, rouleaux formation of red cells in a blood sample and raised plasma protein levels, all of which result from the increased immunoglobulin production, but are also seen in related conditions such as Waldenstrom's macroglobulinaemia.

Bone marrow biopsy is usually diagnostic. Immunocytochemical demonstration of monoclonal production of immunoglobulin (Ig) or immunoglobulin fragments provides confirmation and serum electrophoresis shows a monoclonal spike.

The majority of myelomas are IgG-producing, but about 20 per cent are IgA-producing. Other immunoglobin types are rare. Light chain overproduction, demonstrable by serum electrophoresis, is common. If sufficiently sensitive techniques are used, Bence–Jones proteinuria (also due to light chain overproduction) may be detectable in about 75 per cent of patients.

Management

Although there is frequently an initial response to treatment with combination chemotherapy, the median survival for multiple myeloma is about 2 years, and fewer than 20 per cent of patients survive for 5 or more years.

Surgical treatment of patients with myeloma may be complicated by anaemia, haemorrhagic tendences or increased susceptibility to infection.

Solitary plasmacytoma of bone

This rare tumour occasionally develops in the jaw. Clinical features are bone pain, tenderness or a swelling and a sharply defined area of radiolucency or, rarely, a soap bubble appearance are typical features.

Microscopically, the cellular features are the same as those of multiple myeloma, which should be excluded as described above. However, a small rise in serum or urine monoclonal immunoglobulin, which disappears with treatment, is detectable in a minority of patients with solitary endosteal plasmacytoma. Persistence of a monoclonal peak in the serum is indicative of inadequate treatment or of dissemination of the disease.

The treatment of choice is localised radiotherapy. Over sixty-five per cent of patients survive for ten or more years, but the majority eventually develop multiple myeloma, occasionally even after several decades.

Langerhans cell histiocytosis (histiocytosis X) (Fig. 16.6)

This term is given to a rare, predominantly osteolytic disease, where there is thought to be malignant proliferation of histiocyte-like Langerhans cells. The latter are dendritic intra-epithelial cells with many of the functions of macrophages. They are recognisable by the presence of the surface markers of macrophages and, at the ultrastructural level, of rod-shaped Birbeck granules.[33]

Three main forms of Langerhans cell histiocytosis, in order of severity, are recognised, namely:

(1) Solitary eosinophilic granuloma
(2) Multifocal eosinophilic granuloma (including Hand–Schuller–Christian disease)
(3) Letterer–Siwe syndrome

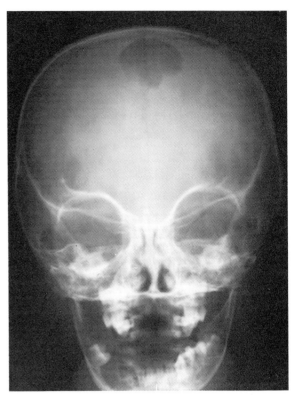

Fig. 16.6 Multifocal eosinophilic granuloma involving the skull and right mandible of a child of 5 years of age.

Solitary eosinophilic granuloma

Solitary eosinophilic granuloma predominantly affects adults, and when involving the jaws, usually affects the mandible, to produce a localised area of bone destruction with swelling and often pain. A typical radiographic appearance is a rounded area of radiolucency with margins somewhat less sharply defined than those of a cyst, and frequently extending to the alveolar ridge. An appearance of teeth 'floating in air' is typical. Occasionally, gross periodontal destruction with exposure of the roots of the teeth is a feature.

Multifocal eosinophilic granuloma

In addition to the mandible, other sites of predilection are the skull, axial skeleton and femora.

Almost any of the viscera (hepatosplenomegally) or the skin (seborrhoeic dermatitis) may be involved in multifocal disease, but rarely without osseous lesions. Such disease may be referred to as Hand–Schuller–Christian disease, but the classical triad of exophthalmos, diabetes insipidus and lytic skull lesions is present only in a minority.

The natural history of Langerhans cell histiocytosis ranges from isolated lesions with spontaneous regression, to widespread disease and a rapidly fatal outcome despite treatment.[34,35] Although the behaviour of this disease is unpredictable, the very young have the worst prognosis with a mortality rate of about 50 per cent. In those over 2 years, the mortality is reported to be about 15 per cent. In general, the greater the number of organ systems affected, the poorer the prognosis. Monocytosis or thrombocytopenia are also associated with a high mortality. Pulmonary involvement, producing large cystic lesions, may after successful treatment, usually involving multi-agent chemotherapy, require the consideration of heart/lung transplantation.

Management
In addition to biopsy of the oral lesions, physical examination, skeletal survey and blood picture will give an indication of any dissemination and its degree.

For a localised jaw lesion, curettage followed if necessary by corticosteroid or cytotoxic chemotherapy, or irradiation, usually suffices, but, as mentioned earlier, the course of the disease is so unpredictable that prolonged careful follow up, and sometimes further treatment, is necessary. For multisystem disease, a combination of cytotoxic agents (often vinca alkaloids), corticosteroids and irradiation of active bone lesions is required.[36]

Letterer–Siwe disease

Letterer–Siwe disease differs from the other types of Langerhans cell histiocytosis in that infants, or less often young children, are affected and the disease may be rapidly fatal. Both soft tissues and bone are commonly involved and rashes may be the earliest manifestation. Other features can include lymphadenopathy and splenomegaly, fever, anaemia and thrombocytopenia, and infections such as otitis media. Many organs can become involved and become enlarged as a result of histiocytic infiltration.

Radiographically the bone lesions do not differ from those in other types of Langerhans cell histiocytosis.

Vigorous chemotherapy is said to have greatly improved the prognosis.[36]

Odontogenic tumours

The odontogenic tissues, both ectodermal and mesenchymal, can give rise to true neoplasms.[2,5,37] These tissues act in a highly integrated fashion in the process of tooth formation and it is not surprising that this process can occasionally become disturbed or that when tumours develop several of these tissues are included. The ameloblastoma is the most important of the odontogenic tumours but all of them are uncommon and many, particularly their malignant counterparts, are very rare indeed. As a consequence only the most important will be discussed.

Odontomes

The odontogenic tissues can occasionally produce malformations known as odontomes. An odontome consists of dental tissues in normal relation to one another but in more or less irregular form. Like a tooth an odontome usually calcifies, ceases to grow once it has reached maturity and ultimately erupts. Intermediate forms also exist where it is uncertain whether the lesion is an odontome or a neoplasm. The lesion's behaviour is then the ultimate indicator of its nature.

Odonotogenic tumours are all rare, but the ameloblastoma is the least uncommon.

Ameloblastoma (Fig. 16.7)
The ameloblastoma is a tumour of odontogenic ephithelium and found only in the jaws. The most striking histological feature is the ameloblast-like cells. The most typical radiological appearance is that of a multilocular cyst. The ameloblastoma is slowly invasive locally but otherwise benign.

Clinical features
Most tumours are first recognised in patients aged 40 or 50. They are rare in children and old people except in Africa where young adults are commonly affected. Eighty per cent form in the mandible; of these 70 per cent develop in the molar region and often involve the ramus.[38,39] They are symptomless until the swelling becomes large enough to be noticed. If neglected the tumour can break through

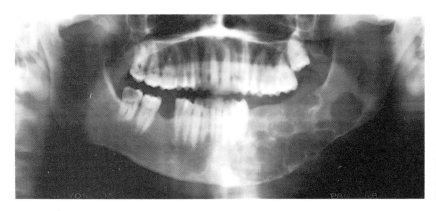

16.7 Radiograph of an ameloblastoma showing the classical multilocular radiolucency in the left mandible.

the bone and, ultimately, spread into the soft tissues. Lingual expansion is common and was once considered to be pathognomonic of ameloblastoma but this is not absolutely true.

Radiological features

These tumours resemble cysts, that is, a rounded well defined radiolucent area with well defined margins. The most readily recognised pattern is that of a multilocular cyst, particularly a few large radiolucent areas with small daughter cysts near their margins.

Other variants are a honeycomb pattern of radiolucency, or a single well defined cavity indistinguishable from a simple cyst.

Management

The diagnosis must be confirmed by biopsy. Treatment is by wide excision, preferably taking up to 2 cm of apparently normal bone around the margin. Complete excision will produce a cure but anything less is followed by recurrence.

Complete excision of a large ameloblastoma may mean total resection of the jaw and bone grafting. It is preferable therefore to avoid so extensive an operation whenever possible by leaving the lower border of the jaw intact and extending the resection subperiosteally provided the tumour has not penetrated the cortex. Bony repair can then take place and a good deal of the jaw reforms. The tumour penetrates cancellous bone more readily than compact and the lower border may be uninvolved. If tumour is left behind recurrence follows but this may take several years and regular radiographic follow up should be carried out. A further limited operation can then be carried out to remove the recurrence. This approach is generally less unpleasant for the patient, who must be warned of

the necessity of regular follow up and, possibly, of a further operation.

Adenomatoid odontogenic tumour

This rare lesion (at one time known as adeno-ameloblastoma) is completely benign and is probably a hamartoma. It has little in common with the ameloblastoma in behaviour and also has no glandular component.

Clinical features

This lesion affects young people, either in late adolescence or as young adults, and is rare in older persons.[40] Women are more often affected than men. The tumour forms a very slow growing swelling and may be noticed incidentally on a radiograph. A dental or dentigerous cyst may be simulated and its nature unsuspected until removed at operation and found to be solid.

Treatment and prognosis

These lesions shell out readily and enucleation seems to be adequate.

Calcifying epithelial odontogenic tumour

This rare and bizarre tumour is often also referred to, for simplicity, as a Pindborg tumour after the first author to describe it.[41] Although exceedingly rare, this tumour is important, partly because of its unusual structure, and particularly because it is occasionally mistaken for a poorly differentiated carcinoma.

These tumours are not encapsulated, are locally invasive and their behaviour seems to be similar to that of the ameloblastoma.

Clinical features

Adults are mainly affected at an average age of about 40. The typical site is the posterior body of the mandible.

Symptoms are usually lacking until a swelling becomes apparent.

Radiographs show a translucent area with a poorly defined margin and, according to the maturity of, and the amount of calcification within the tumour, areas of radiopacity.

Management

Diagnosis depends on histological examination.

It is particularly important to distinguish the highly pleomorphic epithelium from a poorly differentiated carcinoma, as the treatment and prognosis are widely different.

Adequate excision of the tumour with a border of normal bone appears to be effective. If excision is inadequate recurrence follows.[42]

It must be emphasised that this tumour is so rare that there is little information about its long-term behaviour.

Cementomas and cemental dysplasias

Cementum being a bone-like tissue or a modified form of bone might be expected to be subject to changes comparable to the dysplasias of bone or to neoplastic change. Cementomas or cemental dysplasias are a group of lesions characterised by continued proliferation of cementum, but they form a difficult group with poorly defined characteristics.[2] Four main types are usually described, but many cases do not fit precisely into any of these categories. They are all rare.

Benign cementoblastoma

This is regarded as a benign neoplasm and is characterised by the formation of a mass of cementum-like tissue which forms an irregular or rounded mass attached to the root of a tooth.

Clinically the benign cementoblastoma is mainly seen in young adults, usually below the age of 25. Men are predominantly affected. The lesion is usually attached to a mandibular molar or premolar tooth. Rarely they produce bony expansion and the majority are symptom-free.

The radiographic features are a radiopaque mass with a radiolucent periphery. The mass may be densely radiopaque or mottled and is usually rounded but may be more irregular in shape. Immature lesions are predominantly radiolucent and as they mature they become increasingly radiopaque from the centre outwards. Resorption of the roots of the tooth to which the mass is attached is common. Occasionally growth of a benign cementoblastoma may be very rapid.[14]

The cementoblastoma is readily enucleated and shows little or no tendency to recur.

Cementifying fibroma

This lesion is characterised by a rounded area of connective tissue which forms within the jaw and contains spherical or lobulated, heavily calcified nodules of cementum-like tissue.

The lesion is seen mostly in patients of about middle age and the mandibular premolar or molar region is usually affected.[43] Once fully calcified the lesion does not seem to progress and is probably therefore not a true neoplasm. Female Afro-Caribbeans are predominantly affected. Bony expansion is rare and unless infected there are no symptoms; the diagnosis is made on incidental radiographic findings.

However, if a tooth in the region is extracted the densely calcified masses frequently become infected resulting in a chronic osteomyelitis which only resolves when the entire lesion is removed surgically.

Peri-apical cemental dysplasia (peri-apical fibrous dysplasia)

This lesion is similar in structure to the cementifying fibroma.

The lesion mostly affects women past middle age and is most often seen in the mandibular incisor region.[44] On radiographs a rounded radiolucent area may be seen in the early stages related to the apices of the teeth, and may simulate a peri-apical granuloma. The related teeth are however vital. Later there is increasing radiopacity until the mass becomes densely radiopaque, but usually retains a peripheral radiolucent margin. No treatment is necessary.

Gigantiform cementoma

This lesion consists of masses apparently formed by the fusion of rounded nodules of cementum-like tissue, to produce a lobulated form. Afro-Caribbean women of middle age are mostly affected and the lesions are both multiple and often bilaterally symmetrical, suggesting that the lesion is dysplastic. The masses may grow until there is expansion of the jaw. Radiologically the gigantiform cementoma appears as radiopaque, often lobulated masses without a radiolucent border. Resection may be required to restore facial contour.

Myxoma of the jaws (Figs 16.8 and 16.9)

This tumour appears to be peculiar to the jaws and can fairly be regarded as being of odontogenic origin.[45]

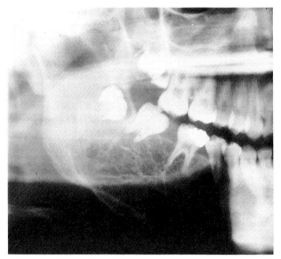

Fig. 16.8 Radiograph of an odontogenic myxoma in the mandible of a 16 year old girl. The classical soap bubble appearance can be seen.

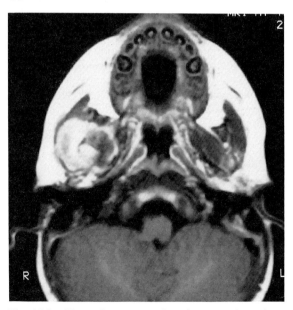

Fig. 16.9 Magnetic resonance imaging scan of an odontogenic myxoma arising in the vertical ramus of the mandible in a 2 year old boy.

Tumours consisting of myxomatous tissue with varying amounts of fibrous tissue may be found elsewhere in the skeleton. These are probably fibromas in which an unusually large amount of connective tissue mucoid has formed. Those in the jaws, however, appear to be a different entity. Myxomas of the jaws usually develop in young persons in the maxilla, a tooth is usually absent and in addition these tumours show a close structural resemblance to dental mesenchyme.

Young people are predominantly affected and the tumour produces a fusiform swelling of the jaw. Radiologically the appearance is an area of radiolucency with soap bubble pattern which may be indistinguishable from an ameloblastoma.

Myxoma of the jaws is usually slow growing, but it is infiltrative and recurrence after excision is common. Apart from this locally invasive character, the tumour is otherwise benign.

Wide excision is therefore desirable in the hope of preventing recurrence, but is not always successful.[46] In spite of vigorous treatment some tumours persist and recurrences have been described over 30 years after the original operations. By this time the tumour appears inactive however and is symptomless.

Other odontogenic tumours
(Figs 16.10 and 16.11)

Ameloblastic fibroma

This tumour, though rare, is important in the differential diagnosis of ameloblastoma and because it may be a true mixed tumour.

The ameloblastic fibroma usually affects young adults, that is an earlier age group than does the ameloblastoma.[47]

Histologically the tumour comprises an epithelial and a connective tissue component. The epithelium consists of ameloblast-like or more cuboid cells surrounding others resembling stellate reticulum. The epithelium is within a highly cellular connective tissue matrix which forms little collagen and resembles the immature dentine papilla.

It is widely believed that both the epithelial and mesenchymal components are neoplastic.

The radiological appearances may be identical to that of ameloblastoma.

The ameloblastic fibroma appears to be benign. It shows little tendency to recur following local resection.

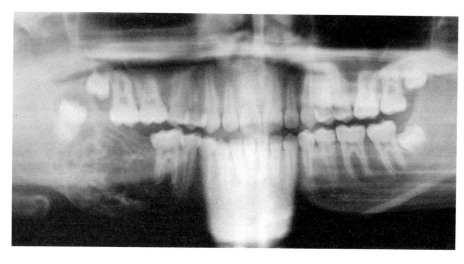

16.10 Radiograph of an ameloblastic fibroma in the mandible of a 15 year old male.

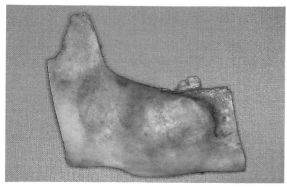

Fig. 16.11 Resection specimen of the tumour seen in Fig. 16.10. Gross expansion of the mandible is clearly visible.

Malignant odontogenic tumours

Malignant counterparts of many odontogenic tumours have been occasionally described, but are so rare as to be of little more than academic interest. Ameloblastoma is not a malignant tumour, in that apart from slow local invasion there is no true metastasis and the tumour's behaviour is benign overall. Implantation into the lungs following aspiration of fragments of a fungating ameloblastoma has been described. Malignant odontogenic tumours will not therefore be discussed further here.

Odontomes

The term 'odontome' has been used in the past to include virtually any abnormal structure arising from dental tissues. The term odontome should however be used only for malformations of dental tissues of developmental origin. They are *not* neoplasms and, like teeth, once fully calcified do not develop further. Odontomes are therefore hamartomas of dental tissues and even when the morphology is grossly distorted (as in complex composite odontomes) the pulp, dentine, enamel and cementum are formed in correct anatomical relation with one another. Furthermore, odontomes also tend to erupt and once they have become exposed to the saliva usually become infected. This is the usual cause of symptoms from odontomes. Nevertheless as discussed earlier intermediate forms exist and are difficult to classify.

Odontomes contain all the dental tissues and are in effect composite in nature; odontoblasts become differentiated only under the inductive stimulus of enamel epithelium: enamel forms only after dentine has been deposited, and cementum only forms in relation to other dental hard tissues. Odontomes are named according to the predominant tissue.

References

1 Dockerty MB, Parkhill EM, Dahlin DC, Woolnert LB, Soule EH, Harrison EG. *Tumours of the Oral Cavity and Pharynx. Atlas of Tumour Pathology*, Section IV, Fascicle 10b. Washington DC: Armed Forces Institute of Pathology, 1968.
2 Pindborg JJ, Kramer IRH, Torlori H. *Histological Typing of Odontogenic Tumours, Jaw Cysts and Allied Lesions. International Histological Classification of Tumours, No. 5*. Geneva: World Health Organization, 1971.

3 Spjut HJ, Dorfman HD, Fechner RE, Ackerman LV. *Tumours of Bone and Cartilage. Atlas of Tumour Pathology*, Series II, Fascicle 5. Washington DC: Armed Forces Institute of Pathology, 1971.

4 Schajowicz F, Ackerman LV, Sissons HA, Sobins LH, Torloni H. *Histological Typing of Bone Tumours. International Histological Classification of Tumours*, No. 6. Geneva: World Health Organization, 1972.

5 Lucas RB. *Pathology of Tumours of the Oral Tissues*. 3rd edn. Edinburgh: Churchill Livingstone, 1977.

6 Batsakis JG. *Tumours of the Head and Neck*, 2nd edn. Baltimore, MD: Williams & Wilkins, 1979.

7 Smith AG, Zaraleta A. Osteoma, ossifying fibroma, fibrous dysplasia of facial and cranial bones. *Archives of Pathology* 1952; **54**: 507–27.

8 Rayne J. Gardner's syndrome. *British Journal of Oral Surgery* 1986; **6**: 11–17.

9 Thoma KH. Tumours of the condyle and temporo-mandibular joint. *Oral Surgery* 1954; **7**: 1091–107.

10 Schajowicz F, Lemos C. Osteoid osteoma and osteoblastoma – closely related entities of osteoblastic derivation. *Acta Orthopaedica Scandinavica* 1970; **41**: 272–91.

11 Prabhakar B, Reddy DR, Dayananada B, Rao GR. Osteoid osteoma of the skull. *Journal of Bone and Joint Surgery* 1972; **54b**: 146–7.

12 Brady CL, Browne RM. Benign osteoblastoma of the mandible. *Cancer* 1972; **30**: 329–33.

13 Marsh BW, Bonfiglio M, Brady LP, Enneking WF. Benign osteoblastoma: range of manifestations. *Journal of Bone and Joint Surgery* 1975; **57a**: 1–9.

14 Langdon JD. The benign cementoblastoma – just how benign? *British Journal of Oral Surgery* 1976; **13**: 239–49.

15 Waldron CA, Shafer WG. The central giant cell reparative granuloma of the jaws. An analysis of 38 cases. *American Journal of Clinical Pathology* 1966; **45**: 437–47.

16 Flanagan AM, Tinkler SMB, Horton MA, Williams DM, Chambers TJ. The multinucleate cells in giant cell granulomas of the jaw are osteoclasts. *Cancer* 1988; **62**: 1139–43.

17 Harris M. Central giant cell granulomas of the jaws regress with calcitonin therapy. *British Journal of Oral and Maxillofacial Surgery* 1933; **31**: 89–94.

18 Garrington GE, Scofield HH, Cornyn J, Hooker SP. Osteosarcoma of the jaws. Analysis of 56 cases. *Cancer* 1967; **20**: 377–91.

19 Pease GL, Maisel RH, Cantrell RW. Surgical management of osteogenic sarcoma of the mandible. *Archives of Otolaryngology* 1975; **101**: 761–2.

20 Chambers RG, Mahoney WD. Osteogenic sarcoma of the mandible: current management. *American Journal of Surgery* 1970; **36**: 463–71.

21 McKenna RJ, Schwinn CP, Soong KY, Higinbotham NL. Sarcomata of the osteogenic series. An analysis of 552 cases. *Journal of Bone and Joint Surgery* 1966; **48a**: 1–26.

22 Bras JM, Donner R, van der Kwast WAM, Snow GB, van der Wall I. Juxtacortical osteogenic sarcoma of the jaws. Review of the literature and report of a case. *Oral Surgery* 1980; **50**: 535–44.

23 Chawdhry AP, Robinovitch MR, Mitchell DR, Vickers RA. Chondrogenic tumours of the jaws. *American Journal of Surgery* 1961; **102**: 403–11.

24 Dahlin DC, Henderson ED. Mesenchymal chondrosarcoma: further observations on a new entity. *Cancer* 1962; **15**: 410–17.

25 Kyriakos M. Soft tissue implantation of chondromyxoid fibroma. *American Journal of Surgical Pathology* 1979; **3**: 363–72.

26 Dahlin DC, Ivins JC. Benign chondroblastoma. A study of 125 cases. *Cancer* 1972; **30**: 401–13.

27 Rosen G, Caparros B, Nirenberg A *et al*. Ewing's sarcoma: ten-year experience with adjuvant chemotherapy. *Cancer* 1981; **47**: 2204–13.

28 Freedman PD, Cardo VA, Kerpel SM, Lumerman H. Desmoplastic fibroma (fibromatosis) of the jaw bones: report of a case and review of the literature. *Oral Surgery* 1978; **46**: 386–95.

29 Carr RJ, Zaki GA, Leader MB, Langdon JD. Infantile fibromatosis with involvement of the mandible. *British Journal of Oral and Maxillofacial Surgery* 1992; **30**: 257–62.

30 Barnes L. Tumours and tumour-like lesions of the soft tissues. In: Barnes L ed. *Surgical Pathology of the Head and Neck*. New York: Marcel Dekker, 1985: 801–6.

31 Zachariades N. Neoplasms metastatic to the mouth, jaws and surrounding tissues. *Journal of Cranio-Maxillofacial Surgery* 1989; **17**: 283–90.

32 Osserman EF, Fahey JL. Plasma cell dyscrasias. Current clinical and biochemical concepts. *American Journal of Medicine* 1968; **44**: 256–9.

33 Hartman KS. Histiocytosis X: a review of 114 cases with oral involvement. *Oral Surgery* 1980; **49**: 38–54.

34 Fitzpatrick R, Rapaport MJ, Silva DG. Histiocytosis X. *Archives of Dermatology* 1981; **117**: 253–7.

35 Groopman JE, Golde DW. The histiocytic disorders: a pathophysiologic analysis. *Annals of Internal Medicine* 1981; **94**: 95–107.

36 Starling LA, Donaldson MH, Haggard ME, Vietti TJ, Sutow WW. Therapy of histiocytosis X with vincistine, vinblastine and cyclophosphamide. The Southwest Cancer Chemotherapy study group. *American Journal of Diseases of Childhood* 1972; **123**: 105–10.

37 Pindborg JJ. *Pathology of the Dental Hard Tissues*. Copenhagen: Munksgaard, 1970.

38 Small IA, Waldron CA. Ameloblastomas of the jaws. *Oral Surgery* 1955; **8**: 281–97.

39 Mehlisch DR, Dahlin DC, Masson JK. Ameloblastoma: a clinicopathologic report. *Journal of Oral Surgery* 1972; **30**: 9–22.

40 Smith RRL, Olsen JL, Hutchins GM, Crawley WA, Levin SL. Adenomatoid odontogenic tumour – ultra-

structural demonstration of two cell types and amyloid. *Cancer* 1979; **43**: 505–11.

41 Pindborg JJ. Calcifying epithelial odontogenic tumours. *Acta Pathologica Microbiologica Scandinavica Supplement* 1956; **111**: 71.

42 Vickers RA, Dahlin DC, Gorlin RJ. Amyloid-containing odontogenic tumours. *Oral Surgery* 1965; **20**: 476–80.

43 Langdon JD, Rapidis AD, Patel MF. Ossifying fibroma – one disease or six: an analysis of 39 fibro-osseous lesions of the jaws. *British Journal of Oral Surgery* 1976; **14**: 1–11.

44 Hamner JE, Scofield HH, Cornyn J. Benign fibro-osseous jaw lesions of periodontal membrane origin. An analysis of 249 cases. *Cancer* 1968; **22**: 861–78.

45 Stout AP. Myxoma, the tumour of primitive mesenchyme. *Annals of Surgery* 1948; **127**: 706–19.

46 Kangue TT, Dahlin CC, Turlington EG. Myxomatous tumours of the jaws. *Journal of Oral Surgery* 1975; **33**: 523–8.

47 Trodahl JN. Ameloblastic fibroma. A survey of cases from the Armed Forces Institute of Pathology. *Oral Surgery*, 1972; **33**: 547–58.

17 Rare tumours and metastases to the mouth, jaws and surrounding tissues

JD Langdon and JM Henk

A wide variety of malignant tumours can arise in this region. Most are so rare as to merit isolated case reports only and these will not be discussed here. Two tumours are however of significant importance, melanoma and granular cell tumour.

Malignant melanoma

Melanoma rarely arises in the oral cavity. Less than 10 per cent of head and neck melanoma are mucosal, of which 50 per cent arise in the oral cavity.[1] Oral cavity melanoma has a peak incidence between the ages of 40 and 60 years. Fifty per cent arise on the hard palate and 25 per cent on the upper gingiva. Approximately a third arise from pre-existing pigmented lesions (Fig. 17.1).

Usually the melanoma is pigmented and appears black or brown, but about 15 per cent are amelanotic with a red appearance. These tumours are often very rapidly growing and therefore often extensive at presentation. They are usually raised or nodular and are asymptomatic until they eventually become ulcerated and bleed.

Pathology

Oral melanomas are usually nodular with malignant melanocytes invading both the epithelium and connective tissue. The cells are round or spindle-shaped. There may be pseudo-epitheliomatous hyperplasia. Superficial spreading melanomas and lentigo maligna are very rarely seen in the mouth.[2]

Prognosis

The prognosis is very poor, with a 5 year survival rate of about 5 per cent.[3] The poorer prognosis of oral compared with cutaneous melanomas is probably due to their late detection and the rarity of the more favourable variants, superficial spreading melanoma and lentigo maligna. The Breslow thickness measured from the granular cell layer to the deepest identifiable melanocyte is the best guide to prognosis in cutaneous melanoma, but is difficult to apply to mucosal tumours. Large size, rapid growth, and especially association with bone destruction are poor prognostic factors. Other indicators of a poor prognosis are malignant cells within blood vessels and multiple atypical mitoses.

Treatment

The diagnosis must be established by biopsy. Once the diagnosis is confirmed the patient must be screened for the presence of metastatic disease;

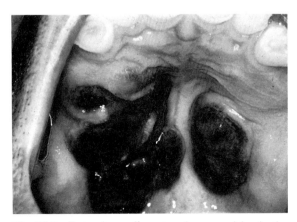

Fig. 17.1 Extensive malignant melanoma arising in the hard palate of a patient aged 51 years.

metastases are especially frequent in regional lymph nodes, lungs and liver.

If the disease is localised the only chance of cure is with radical excision. The value of elective neck dissection in node negative disease is not established, but there is no doubt that this operation should be performed if regional lymph nodes are involved. There is some suggestion that post-operative radiotherapy reduces the incidence of local recurrence in mucosal melanomas generally,[4] although there is insufficient data on the oral cavity *per se*. It has been claimed that prophylactic chemotherapy may prevent or delay the incidence of subsequent metastatic disease but its value is unproven. The natural history of metastatic disease is variable, with the occasional patient surviving for several years but the majority growing rapidly with survival of only a few months. In general response rates to a variety of chemotherapy schedules have been disappointing. Fit patients with locally recurrent or metastatic disease may be considered for trials of chemotherapy within a specialist unit.

Granular cell tumour

Granular cell tumours are rare lesions which can occur in all parts of the body, but have a predilection for head and neck sites. The tongue is the commonest site; this tumour has also been reported in the larynx, trachea, cheek, pharyngeal muscles and orbit. Multiple tumours of this type are occasionally seen. The cell of origin in not known for certain. It was formerly believed to be skeletal muscle, hence the old term 'myoblastoma' which is almost certainly a misnomer. Ultrastructural studies suggest an origin either from Schwann or undifferentiated mesenchymal cells; the latter is now favoured.[5]

Pathology

Granular cell tumours consist of nests of round or oval cells with small central nuclei. The cytoplasm contains periodic acid-Schiff (PAS) positive granules. In the tongue the overlying mucosa is frequently hyperkeratotic and may show pseudo-epitheliomatous hyperplasia, which consequently may be misdiagnosed as squamous cell carcinoma. Some of these tumours may infiltrate surrounding tissues, but the true incidence of malignancy is difficult to assess. Metastases to regional lymph nodes have been reported but are exceedingly rare.

Clinical features

The commonest presentation is as a smooth firm non-ulcerated swelling, immediately below the mucosa of the tongue, most often on the dorsum near the mid-line. There are no features to distinguish granular cell tumours from other benign tumours.

Treatment

The treatment is wide local excision. The recurrence rate is about 5 per cent, so follow up is advisable.

Metastatic disease

Incidence

The oral cavity is occasionally the site for distant metastases from primary malignant tumours below the clavicle. It has been estimated that 1 per cent of all malignant neoplasms metastasise to the jaws and oral cavity, and that 1 per cent of all malignancies found in these sites are in fact metastatic foci from elsewhere.[6]

The figures quoted for the incidence of oral metastases may be falsely low due to the fact that the standard skeletal survey does not include detailed examination of the jaws, and postmortem examination does not routinely encompass the peri-oral area (Fig. 17.2).

Site

The jaws are by far the most frequent site for metastatic disease in this region (Fig. 17.3). In 1989 Zachariades[6] reviewed the literature and found reports of 422 metastatic lesions in the mouth, jaws and surrounding tissues in 365 patients. Of these patients 56.5 per cent were over 50 years of age. Of these metastases 58.5 per cent were to the mandible, 11 per cent to the maxilla, 25.8 per cent to the oral soft tissues and 4.7 per cent to the major salivary glands (Table 17.1). Most metastases which involve the soft tissues of the oral cavity do so by secondary spread from an initial deposit in the underlying bone.

The gingivae are the most common sites for metastases confined to the oral soft tissues.[6]

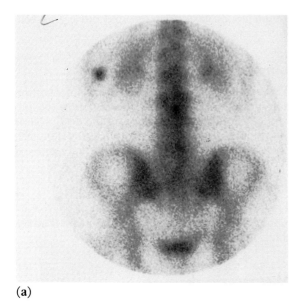

(a)

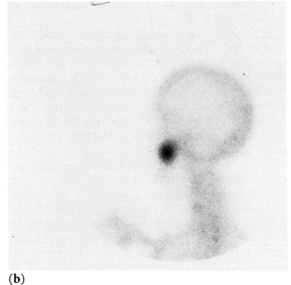

(b)

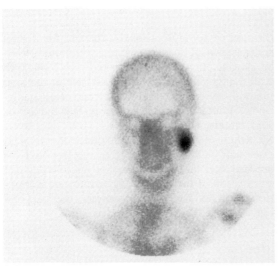

(c)

Fig. 17.2 Bone scan of a patient with breast cancer revealing an asymptomatic metastasis in the ramus of the mandible.

Needleman and Salah,[7] when reporting a patient with multiple gingival metastases arising from carcinoma of the breast, reviewed the literature and emphasised that many of these lesions are initially diagnosed as pregnancy epulis, pyogenic granuloma, peripheral giant cell granuloma, gingival fibroma or primary gingival neoplasm.

Metastases to the parotid glands are reported from time to time.[8,9] When they occur, the primary tumours are usually in the head and neck and it is often argued that they are lymphatic metastases to intraparotid lymph nodes. However, Goldberg and Georgiade[9] when reviewing the literature found

60 cases of parotid metastases from distant sites; these were, in order of frequency, bronchus, kidney, breast, colon, prostate, stomach and uterine sarcoma.

Origin

The most common sites for primary lesions metastasising to this region are lungs, breast, kidney and adrenal glands (Fig. 17.4).[6] Many authors have reported bronchogenic tumours which have metastasised to the gingivae; Kaugars and Svirsky[10] analysed the English language literature and identi-

Table 17.1 Sites of metastases to the mouth, jaws and salivary glands

	No. of cases
Mandible	203
Maxilla	47
Condyle	24
Upper gingiva	40
Lower gingiva	25
Tongue	34
Palate	8
Upper and lower jaw	6
Cheek	4
Pulp (dental)	3
Lower lip	3
Buccal mucosa	3
Other mucosa	2
Parotid	10
Submandibular	2

Source: Zachariades.[6]

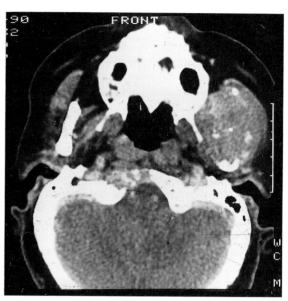

Fig. 17.4 A computed tomography scan demonstrating a very large metastatic deposit destroying the ramus of the mandible. The primary tumour was in the breast.

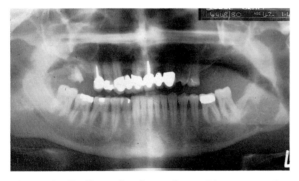

Fig. 17.3 Radiograph of a patient with an extensive metastasis from a melanoma in the angle of the left mandible.

fied 37 cases of lung tumours metastatic to the oral cavity and jaws. They added one further case. In their series there were 34 men and only four females. The average age at presentation was 54 years. Twenty-one of the metastases were associated with the mandible; the maxilla was involved in seven. One case was in the floor of the mouth. Nine cases appeared to be primarily soft tissue metastases, eight being in the tongue and one in the lip. In 18 of the 38 cases, the oral metastasis predated the diagnosis of the primary lesion. Eleven cases within the series gave a history of tooth extraction followed by the appearance of metastatic tumour at the healing socket.

The route by which carcinomas of the lung metastasise to the mouth is a subject of controversy. According to classic theory tumour spread occurs by direct extension, blood and lymph channels or by transcoelomic spread. Blood-borne metastases seem a likely explanation for metastatic disease appearing in the oral soft tissues.

The mechanism of metastatic spread of tumour to the head and neck was investigated by Batson.[11] He injected radiopaque dye into the dorsal vein of the penis in cadavers and monkeys, and demonstrated an extensive interconnecting system of veins up and down the spine which are subject to frequent reversals of flow.

This venous system explains how cranial metastases are so frequent in lung cancer. When the patient coughs, blood containing malignant emboli flows from the bronchial vein into the spinal veins and up to the head and neck rather than into the pulmonary veins and into the right heart. Another common source of metastases to the mouth, jaws and surrounding tissues is renal tumour, which can also spread via the vertebral venous plexus and so reach the head and neck.[12]

Of particular interest is the repeated finding of metastasis to the jaws and gingivae of hepatocellular carcinoma.[13] The present author has in fact seen a gingival metastasis in a patient who had successfully undergone a hepatic transplant for a primary hepatoma.

The probable explanation for the occasional appearance of metastases at the site of a healing tooth socket following dental extraction is that the tissue in which the tumour cells have become embedded were traumatised at the time of extraction. The local vasculature would have had a reduced blood flow and increased vascular permeability, allowing malignant cells to settle and seed.

Arguing against operative trauma as a factor in site selection for blood-borne metastases, MacGregor and Lewis[14] pointed out that a much higher incidence of postextraction metastases would be expected on this basis than actually occurs. Kaugars and Svirsky[10] raised the possibility that the teeth were extracted initially owing to symptoms of an already present underlying metastasis, and that this metastasis subsequently proliferated through the sockets.

The equivalent to transcoelomic spread from the lung is dissemination of malignant cells in the mucous secretions, which eventually are expectorated into the mouth. It is well recognised that tuberculosis may be disseminated via the sputum, and it seems reasonable that the same should happen with bronchial carcinoma. This hypothesis is supported by O'Niel,[15] MacGregor and Lewis[14] and Donoff et al.[16] Barnard[17] reported a case of metastatic carcinoma of bronchus appearing in the cheek adjacent to an upper molar which had previously been extracted under local anaesthesia. He postulated that malignant cells in the sputum might have been implanted in the cheek by the local anaesthetic needle.

Many other tumours have been reported on rare occasions to metastasise to this region, e.g. lymphangiosarcomas,[18] carcinomas of the ovary,[19] chorio-epithelioma,[20] carcinoma of the thyroid,[21] carcinoma of the pancreas,[22] carcinoma of the rectum,[23] melanoma,[24] retinoblastoma,[25] carcinoma of the prostate,[26] cholangiocarcinoma[27] and angiosarcomas.[28]

Clinical features and diagnosis

Initial symptoms of metastases which have been described include swelling, pain, paraesthesia, trismus, loosening of teeth, and poor healing following dental extractions. These metastatic tumours are often misdiagnosed as they may mimic dental pathology such as gingivitis, pericoronitis, periodontal abscess, pyogenic granuloma, various epulides, and in particular infected tooth sockets following dental extractions (Table 17.2). Biopsy is necessary to establish the diagnosis.

Symptoms from a malignant deposit in the jaws are, on rare occasions, the first sign of the disease and can lead to diagnosis of the primary. In other cases the jaw is the first apparent site of secondary deposits from a growth treated a year or more previously. Although the jaw is much less frequently involved than other bones, secondary carcinoma is an important malignant tumour.

The common symptoms are pain, which is often severe, or swelling of the jaw. Paraesthesia (numbness or tingling) of the lip may be caused by involvement of a nerve trunk.

Radiological examination usually shows an area of radiolucency with a hazy outline which sometimes simulates an infected cyst, or maybe quite irregular and simulate osteomyelitis. Areas of new bone formation may rarely be the main feature. In the case of metastases from carcinoma of the prostate the predominant sign may be increased bone density.

Diagnosis requires a careful history, especially of previous operations, and a general physical examination. Radiographs or bone scans of the rest of the skeleton will show whether there are other deposits and blood examination may show evidence of marrow involvement, e.g. leuko-erythroblastic anaemia. Biopsy of the lesion is necessary to confirm the diagnosis except in a patient with obvious widespread malignancy from a primary elsewhere.

Table 17.2 Provisional diagnosis of metastases

	No. of cases
Metastasis	52
'Epulis'	20
Abscess	18
Sarcoma	12
'Other'	12 – includes osteomyelitis, cyst, pulpitis, temporomandibular joint dysfunction, trigeminal neuralgia

Source: Zachariades.[6]

Treatment

In general a patient presenting with metastatic disease in the oral cavity will have widespread malignant disease and so radical treatment is not indicated. Just occasionally a single oral metastasis may be the presenting sign of an as yet undetected but treatable primary; such patients should be investigated by appropriate means in order to discover the primary. Often this will be suggested by the histology of the oral lesion, but in anaplastic tumours it may be more difficult. Some malignant conditions are treatable even in the presence of bone or soft tissue metastases, for example breast carcinoma and prostatic carcinoma by hormone therapy, and testicular teratoma and small cell carcinoma of the lung by cytotoxic chemotherapy. Rarely a solitary metastasis from a renal primary may be found, in which case early excision may prolong survival or even effect a cure.

Otherwise, most oral metastases indicate widespread dissemination of disease which can only be managed by palliative treatment. If the lesion is bulky, painful or haemorrhagic, local surgical excision, cryosurgery or local external beam radiotherapy will relieve symptoms. Bony metastases often respond well to palliative radiotherapy which can relieve pain and bring about temporary regression of the lesion.

References

1 Conley J, Pack GT. Melanoma of the mucous membranes of the head and neck. *Archives of Otolaryngology* 1974; **99**: 315–19.
2 Batsakis JG, Regezi JA, Soloman AR, Rice DH. The pathology of head and neck tumours: mucosal melanomas. *Head and Neck Surgery* 1982; **4**: 404–18.
3 Gaze MN, Kerr GR, Smyth JF. Mucosal melanoma of the head and neck: The Scottish experience. *Clinical Oncology* 1990; **2**: 277–83.
4 Lund V. Malignant melanoma of the nasal cavity and para-nasal sinuses. *Journal of Laryngology and Otology* 1982; **96**: 347–55.
5 Regezi JA, Batsakis JG, Courtney RM. Granular cell tumours of the head and neck. *Journal of Oral Surgery* 1979; **37**: 402–6.
6 Zachariades N. Neoplasma metastatic to the mouth, jaws and surrounding tissues. *Journal of Cranio-Maxillo-Facial Surgery* 1989; **17**: 283–90.
7 Needleman IG, Salah MW. Metastatic breast carcinoma presenting with multiple gingival epulides. *British Dental Journal* 1992; **172**: 448–50.
8 Kukan JO, Frank DH, Robson MC. Tumours metastatic to the parotid gland. *British Journal of Plastic Surgery* 1981; **34**: 299–302.
9 Goldberg JA, Georgiade GS. Accessory parotid glands as a site of metastases from outside the head and neck: case report. *Head and Neck* 1990; **12**: 421–5.
10 Kaugars GE, Svirsky JA. Lung malignancies metastatic to the oral cavity. *Oral Surgery* 1981; **51**: 179–86.
11 Batson OV. The function of the vertebral veins and their role in the spread of metastases. *Annals of Surgery* 1940; **112**: 138.
12 Batsakis JG. *Tumours of the Head and Neck*, 2nd edn. Baltimore, MD: Williams & Wilkins, 1979: 240.
13 Wedgewood D, Rusen D, Balk S. Gingival metastasis from parimary hepatocellular carcinoma. *Oral Surgery* 1979; **47**: 263–6.
14 MacGregor AJ, Lewis DA. Metastasis of carcinoma of the lung by implantation in tooth sockets. *British Journal of Oral Surgery* 1972; **9**: 195–9.
15 O'Neil R. Bronchial adenocarcinoma presenting as an epulis. *British Journal of Oral Surgery* 1964; **2**: 148–51.
16 Donoff RB, Albert R, Olson DJ, Guralnick W. Metastatic bronchogenic carcinoma to the mandible. *Journal of Oral Surgery* 1976; **34**: 1007–11.
17 Barnard JDW. Primary clinical manifestation of bronchial carcinoma as a buccal metastasis. *British Dental Journal* 1975; **138**: 174–6.
18 Wertheimer FW, Crayle LJ. Lymphangiosarcoma of the gingiva. *International Journal of Oral Surgery* 1973; **2**: 159–61.
19 Brown JB, Keefe CD. Sarcoma of the ovary with unusual oral metastasis. *Annals of Surgery* 1928; **87**: 467–8.
20 Bakeen G, Hiyarat AM, Al-Ubaidy SS. Chorioepithelioma presenting as a bleeding gingival mass. *Oral Surgery* 1976; **41**: 467–71.
21 Al-Ani S. Metastatic tumours to the mouth: report of two cases. *Journal of Oral Surgery* 1973; **31**: 120–2.
22 Schofield JJ. Oral metastatic deposit from carcinoma of the head of the pancreas. *British Dental Journal* 1974; **137**: 355–6.
23 Moffat DA. Metastatic adenocarcinoma of the rectum presenting as an epulis. *British Journal of Oral Surgery* 1976; **14**: 90–2.
24 Pilskin ME, Mastrangelo MJ, Brown AM, Custer RP. Metastatic melanoma of the maxilla presenting as a gingival swelling. *Oral Surgery* 1976; **41**: 101–3.
25 Perriman AO, Figuris KH. Metastatic retinoblastoma of the mandible. *Oral Surgery* 1978; **45**: 741–8.
26 Wolujewicz MA. Condylar metastasis from a carcinoma of the prostate gland. *British Journal of Oral Surgery* 1980; **18**: 175–82.
27 Watts PG. Secondary cholangiocarcinoma in the mandible. *British Dental Journal* 1979; **146**: 385.
28 Toth BB, Fleming TJ, Lomba JA, Martin JW. Angiosarcoma metastatic to the maxillary tuberosity region. *Oral Surgery* 1981; **52**: 71–4.

18 Malignant neoplasms of the oral cavity in HIV disease

C Scully and M Spittle

One in six persons with the acquired immuno-deficiency syndrome (AIDS) in Europe and USA has cancer.[1] A decade since the first recognition of AIDS and the identification of the responsible retroviruses – the human immunodeficiency viruses (HIV) – there is now an appreciation of the various malignant tumours affecting persons with HIV disease, and the fact that these not infrequently affect the oral tissues.[2–4] Throughout this decade however, there has been a change in pattern of risk groups for HIV, a changing pattern of disease and the introduction of antiretroviral treatments such as zidovudine. The resulting longer survival of infected persons, and therefore duration of immuno-deficiency, may influence the frequency and progression of tumours over the next few years. The size of these problems is already a cause of quite some concern with an expected annual increase in the USA of up to about 8000 cases of Kaposi's sarcoma and up to about 3000 cases of lymphomas related to HIV disease.[5] Nevertheless, it is important to remember that such tumours can also be seen in those without HIV infection, particularly in other immunocompromised persons.

The most common malignant tumours in HIV disease are Kaposi's sarcoma (KS; sometimes termed epidemic KS or EKS), which currently affects up to 40 per cent of those with AIDS, and lymphomas, which affect up to 10 per cent or more.[6] The incidence of KS continues to be higher in homosexual men (about 1 in 5) than other high risk groups (about 1 in 30 of those with non-sexually acquired AIDS) although it is diminishing among homosexual men in the USA[7–9] and in Europe,[10] including in the UK,[11] possibly due to changed sexual behaviour or other habits.[12] However, more patients are developing extensive vis-ceral KS and dying because of widespread dissemination. Currently 15 to 23 per cent of homosexual HIV-infected males present with KS.[9,10]

HIV-associated lymphomas are increasingly re-cognised.[13] Approximately 3 per cent of persons with AIDS have non-Hodgkin's lymphoma (NHL) at the onset of AIDS, and projections indicate that many will later develop NHL.[14] Indeed, one autopsy study showed NHL in 20 per cent of HIV-infected persons.[15] Most are high grade B cell malignancies, particularly diffuse large cell lymphomas and immunoblastic lymphomas, but primary lymphomas of the brain and especially Burkitt's lymphoma are also common.[16,17] Burkitt's lymphoma is one of the earliest NHL to manifest.[18] Epstein–Barr virus (EBV) is associated with about one-half of NHL in HIV disease.[19] Lymphomas have also emerged as an increasingly common cause of death.[11] Compared with lymphomas in non-HIV-infected persons they often present at an advanced stage with extranodal involvement and respond poorly to chemotherapy.[17,20]

Thus, two main neoplasms are known to be as-sociated with HIV disease and both are possibly infectious in origin. A variety of other malig-nancies, including oral squamous cell carcinoma, have been noted in clinical reports and there is con-cern that there may be increases in a range of other tumours – particularly those with an infectious basis.[16] Nevertheless, demographic evidence from the epidemic thus far records no increase in inci-dence of neoplasms other than KS and lymphomas, at least from studies of young males from both coasts of the USA.[5,21] However, the incidence of such tumours may well be underestimated because they are not diagnostic of HIV disease.

Indeed, when groups of known HIV-infected

persons have been studied, a range of malignant tumours have been noted.[22,23] Furthermore, while KS and lymphomas often appear in other immuno-compromised persons at about 1 year after onset of the immune defect, other neoplasms tend to appear only after about 2 years.[24] It may be premature, therefore, to suggest that there is no increased predilection to these other tumours in HIV disease. This chapter however, will concentrate on discussion of oral KS and lymphomas in HIV disease.

Management of patients with neoplasms in HIV disease is an evolving science, not least because of the increasing use of zidovudine (azidothymidine), dideoxyinosine and other antiviral agents. The aggressive course of the tumours, together with concurrent leukopenia and infections also make treatment difficult. Management of oral lesions must only be carried out after consultation with the AIDS physician and other involved colleagues.

Kaposi's sarcoma

KS in western countries is now found mainly in HIV-infected homosexual or bisexual men[9] but is also occasionally seen in such sexually active groups who are not infected with HIV.[25-32] KS has been regarded as an endothelial cell multicentric malignant neoplasm characterised by increased capillary growth and prominent spindle-shaped cells with surprisingly few mitoses, extravasation of erythrocytes and the appearance of haemosiderin (Fig. 18.1).[33] The proliferating cells are ultrastructurally similar to endothelial cells[34] and even clinically normal oral mucosa from HIV-positive persons may show vascular changes histologically similar to

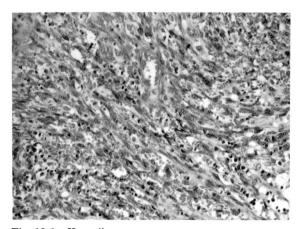

Fig. 18.1 Kaposi's sarcoma.

those seen in early KS.[35] Indeed there is now a body of opinion that suggests that KS is a multifocal vascular proliferative disorder and not a true neoplasm. The endothelial proliferation may be related to various angiogenic or other factors[36,37] released by CD4 lymphocytes.[38,39]

AIDS KS cells have been maintained in culture by a soluble factor which is produced by HIV-infected cells and which may be oncostatin M.[40] The growth of these cultured cells is promoted by the *tat* gene of HIV but no HIV sequences have been seen in the cells either of KS or of NHL – the other AIDS related malignancy.[41]

The findings of positive cytomegalovirus (CMV) serology and CMV-DNA, CMV-RNA, and CMV antigens in biopsy specimens suggested an association of CMV with KS.[42-46] Oral KS also appears to contain CMV-DNA,[47] but CMV can however be latent in endothelium even in non-HIV-infected persons. Epidemiologic data – particularly cases of KS in homosexuals who were non-HIV antibody positive after 8 to 10 years – suggests that KS in HIV disease may be associated with a transmissible agent other than HIV.[9,28,29,32] CMV may be an opportunistic infection within the KS tissue: a mycoplasma or other agent may be responsible for KS.[48,49]

The prevalence of KS in AIDS has been decreasing during the recent past,[50] and it is now perhaps a less common oral manifestation than, for example, oral candidiasis and hairy leukoplakia.

KS is usually characterised by multifocal, widespread lesions at the onset of illness. These lesions may involve the skin, oral mucosa, lymph nodes and visceral organs such as the gastro-intestinal tract, lung, liver and spleen. Lesions from KS have been observed at autopsy in all organs including brain, pancreas, heart and major vessels. These lesions remain generally asymptomatic, although in some cases patients present with headache or bowel obstruction. Visceral involvement, particularly in the gastro-intestinal tract, affects nearly half of the reported cases.

KS is oral or peri-oral in 50 per cent or more of patients with mucocutaneous KS and is often an early manifestation of severe HIV disease.[51-59] KS may also present as a cervical lymph node enlargement or in the salivary glands.[60-62]

The clinical appearance of oral KS is variable. Early lesions typically present in the palate as pigmented macules (Fig. 18.2) but later become nodular.[59] Palatal and alveolar margin involvement is common and may denote more widespread gastro-intestinal involvement. (Fig. 18.3) Sometimes the tongue, gingiva or elsewhere are affected and KS may present as red, bluish or purple patches or nodules, sometimes ulcerated (Fig. 18.4). Reports of non-discoloured oral KS are now appearing[63–66] and therefore a high index of suspicion is required in order not to overlook such early lesions. Biopsy may well be indicated.

The overall prognosis for survival in patients with KS appears to depend on the severity of immune suppression and HIV infection, rather than

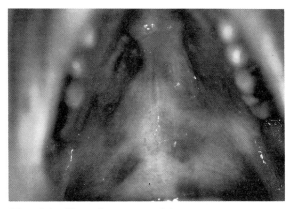

Fig. 18.2   Kaposi's sarcoma of the palate.

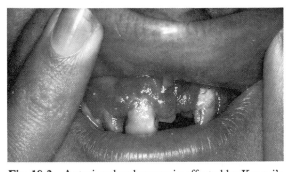

Fig. 18.3   Anterior alveolar margin affected by Kaposi's sarcoma with loosening of teeth.

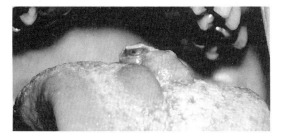

Fig. 18.4   Nodular Kaposi's sarcoma.

on the neoplastic proliferation and tumour load.[67] At 2 years, survival is more than 80 per cent in patients without opportunistic infections and less than 20 per cent in patients with opportunistic infections.

No universally accepted classification exists for this type of KS. The most widely used staging classifications are those of Krigel and Friedman-Kien[68] and Mitsuyasu (Table 18.1).[69] The staging system of Krown[70] offers uniform and precise criteria for disease evaluation, and prognosis since it incorporates measures of extent of disease, severity of immunodeficiency and presence of systemic symptoms (Table 18.2). Clinical staging is carried out as per Table 18.3.

Lymphomas

Lymphomas are fairly common in HIV-infected persons. High grade non-Hodgkin's B cell lymphomas occur most frequently.[71] The incidence of Hodgkin's disease appears not to be increased in New York men at risk of HIV,[21] but HIV-infected intravenous drug abusers in Italy do have some increase in Hodgkin's disease.[17,22] In one-third of cases the onset of lymphomas in HIV disease is preceded by persistent generalised lymphadenopathy (PGL). Enlargement of pre-existent palpable lymph nodes is always an indication for a biopsy to exclude malignant lymphoma. At initial presentation the lymphoma is typically widely disseminated, with extranodal sites reported to be involved in 65 per cent to 98 per cent of patients. Lymphoma is also found in unusual sites such as the myocardium, adrenals, earlobes, maxillae, gall bladder and rectum. Aside from these unusual sites of disease, there is also bone marrow involvement in 20–46 per cent of cases. Gastro-intestinal tract involvement is seen in 7–45 per cent of cases. The central nervous system is commonly involved, either as leptomeningeal lymphoma associated with systemic disease, or as the primary site[13,72]

Oral lymphoma, almost exclusively of the NHL type is now a recognised but uncommon complication of HIV (Fig. 18.5), typically presenting as a rapidly growing mass in the fauces or elsewhere, an ulcer or tooth mobility.[17,72–84] HIV-related Burkitt's lymphoma may also present orally[85] and there is also an increase in salivary gland lymphomas in HIV disease.[86–88]

Lymphomas in HIV disease may be associated with EBV; this also applies to oral lymphomas.[78]

Table 18.1 Staging systems for Kaposi's sarcoma

STAGE	STAGING SYSTEMS	
	Krigel	*Mitsuyasu*
I	Cutaneous, locally indolent	Limited cutaneous (<10 lesions or one anatomical area)
II	Cutaneous, locally aggressive, no lymph node involvement	Disseminated cutaneous (>10 lesions or more than one anatomical area)
III	Generalised* cutaneous and/or lymph node involvement	Visceral only (GI, LN)
IV	Visceral	Cutaneous and visceral, or pulmonary
Subtypes		
A	No systemic symptoms	No systemic symptoms
B	Systemic symptoms: weight loss (10%) or fever (>37.8°C, unrelated to an identifiable source of infection lasting 2 weeks)	Fever >37.8°C unrelated to identifiable infection for 2 weeks or weight loss (10%)

*Generalised includes minimal gastro-intestinal tracts (GI) disease. LN, lymph nodes.
Source: Errante *et al.*[67]

Table 18.2 Krown staging classification of Kaposi's sarcoma (KS)

	Good risk (0) *(all of the following)*	*Poor risk (1)* *(any of the following)*
Tumour (T)	Confined to skin and/or lymph nodes and/or minimal oral disease*	Tumour-associated oedema or ulceration Extensive oral KS Gastrointestinal KS KS in other non-nodal viscera
Immune system	CD4 cells >200/μl	CD4 cells <200/μl
Systemic illness	No history of OI or thrush No B symptoms Performance status >70 (Karnofsky)	History of OI and/or thrush B symptoms present Other HIV-related illness (e.g. neurological disease, lymphoma)

*Minimal oral disease is non-nodular KS confined to the palate; B, symptoms are unexplained fever, night sweats, >10% involuntary weight loss or diarrhoea persisting more than 2 weeks; OI, opportunistic infections; HIV, human immunodeficiency virus.
Source: Krown *et al.*[70]

Table 18.3 Staging of Kaposi's sarcoma

Physical examination (including oral and rectal examination)
Biopsy of lesions and/or lymph nodes
Chest radiograph (bronchoscopy*)
Gastroscopy and colonendoscopy
CT scan of abdomen
Laboratory studies: complete blood count, HIV serology, CD4 and CD8 lymphocyte count

*In patients with abnormal chest radiograph. CT, computed tomography; HIV, human immunodeficiency virus.
Source: Errante *et al.*[67]

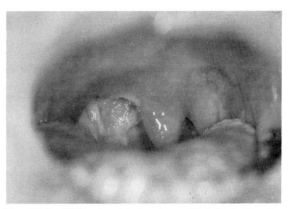

Fig. 18.5 HIV-related isolated non-Hodgkin's lymphoma of the tonsil.

Lymphomatoid granulomatosis

Lymphomatoid granulomatosis is an unusual entity characterised by a mixed mononuclear cell infiltrate and areas of necrosis with atypical lymphoreticular cells. EBV infection has been implicated in HIV-related lymphomatoid granulomatosis.[89] Some 20 to 50 per cent of cases progress to malignant lymphoma[90] and several cases of lymphomatoid granulomatosis presenting with oral ulcers have now been reported in AIDS.[91,92]

Some cases of lymphomatoid granulomatosis have responded to corticosteroids and cyclophosphamide, others to ranitidine and zidovudine, and yet others to α-interferon.

Other neoplasms

Early in the AIDS epidemic, oral carcinoma was reported in one male homosexual partner of a person with KS, and a small group of similar patients was subsequently reported by the same group of workers.[52,93] One oral carcinoma was found in an Italian study of HIV disease.[23] One recent study of head and neck carcinomas in HIV-infected patients failed to show an increased prevalence of oral carcinoma.[94] Other studies have shown increasing incidence of oral squamous carcinoma in younger males in the USA and UK and elsewhere, although there is no evidence that HIV disease has contributed.[95]

It is clearly encumbent on the professions to keep an open mind on the possibility that tumours other than KS and lymphomas will appear in HIV-infected persons, and it will be interesting to watch the progress of oral carcinoma – particularly in view of the suggested link of neoplasm with infective agents such as herpes simplex and human papillomaviruses.[96]

Management

The HIV epidemic has many implications for the oncologist. The development of malignancies in the head and neck area are a special challenge. Patients must be managed in the overall context of their disease in a multidisciplinary manner since the occurrence and treatment of the malignancy will affect the development and behaviour of other problems and therapies.

Kaposi's sarcoma

Neither local nor systemic treatment of KS have been shown to alter the ultimate course of the disease but they may cause a disappearance or reduction in size of lesions and thereby alleviate discomfort.[97] Because the natural course of KS disease progression is highly variable, evaluating the long term efficacy of systemic treatment has been difficult: no data show that treatment improves survival.

Radiation

Early lesions of KS may be a cosmetic nuisance particularly when they occur on the face. Localised patches may be covered with camouflaging make-up or may be treated with local radiotherapy. The radiotherapy may be given in a single dose of 8 Gy at 100 keV or may be fractionated giving 4 Gy in each of three treatments.[98] The violet indurated plaques will stop increasing in size and flatten. Lesions become paler and may disappear. Although there may be a circular area of post inflammatory pigmentation following the radiotherapy, this will gradually resolve. Most patients are pleased with the cosmetic result, especially when small nodules are treated. Should the lesion recur it may be retreated with the same dose at a later date. When irradiating KS on the face it must be remembered that temporary epilation (e.g. in the moustache area) will occur following this dose. Lesions occurring on the lower eyelid may be treated by radiation following the insertion of an eye shield.

Localised palatal lesions are extremely common, and these and involved areas on the alveolar margin respond very well to radiation, preventing pain, loss of dentition and bleeding. However, a mucositis has been noted which occurs following radiotherapy at doses very much lower that seen in the non-AIDS setting. This acute sensitivity of the mucosa of some patients has not been explained but may be due to altered endogenous interferon or glutathione levels and is seen most frequently in patients with low CD4 counts.[99] Radiotherapy to the palate, given by opposing supervoltage fields, is planned using the simulator and is given in a fractionated manner in an attempt to ameliorate this mucositis. A treatment of 3 Gy × 5 given on alternate days will give an excellent response and could be repeated if necessary after several months (Fig. 18.6).

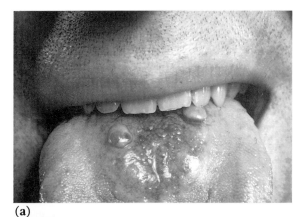

(a)

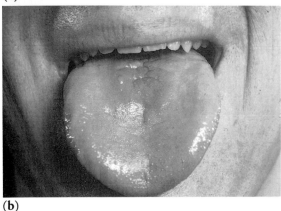

(b)

Fig. 18.6 Kaposi's sarcoma of tongue (a) before and (b) after irradiation.

Interferon

If KS becomes troublesome, but not life-threatening, and the patient has a CD4 count above 200, α-interferon may be given with success, commencing with 3 mega units subcutaneously three times a week. The dose is escalated in an attempt to achieve 30 mega units or above. There seems to be a dose-related response of KS but most patients find the side effects of high doses, namely fever, flu-like symptoms and headaches, intolerable. The ultimate dose achieved is therefore restricted by toxicity.[100] Interferon treatment is expensive and, in view of this and the side effects, assessment after 2–3 months enables a decision to be made about continuing therapy. Many patients are attracted by the concept of treatment that does not appear to be immunosuppressive. Success is related to the duration and size of the lesions. Response in 30–40 per cent, with complete regression in some, has been seen.[100–102] Interferon has also been used intralesionally.[103]

Chemotherapy

Without reversing the immunodeficiency there appears to be no cure for advanced KS. Where systemic treatment is thought clinically appropriate for patients with a CD4 count below 200, or where disease becomes life-threatening, the choice must be between moderate chemotherapy such as intravenous bleomycin and vincristine[104] or oral etoposide,[105,106] and more aggressive regimes including doxorubicin.[107] Doxorubicin and etoposide will cause epilation, which may affect the patient's opinion of appropriate agents. Bleomycin and vincristine can be given every 3 weeks with or without doxorubicin.[107] KS will respond to chemotherapy in 30 to 80 per cent of patients. However, when the chemotherapy is discontinued the lesions rapidly progress. Studies are in progress comparing these regimes with the use of liposomally encapsulated cytotoxics which are said to target the Kaposi's lesions which may have less toxicity.[108] Intralesional vinblastine has been successfully used in isolated skin and palatal lesions but produces pain for 1–3 days requiring moderate analgesia[109] and has little to offer over fractionated radiation.

Most patients with AIDS continue antiviral therapy such as zidovudine and this itself has occasionally been shown to improve KS lesions. However, if myelotoxicity occurs there is a choice between reducing the antiviral agent or reducing the chemotherapy. Although blood transfusions and the use of colony-stimulating factors may support the haemoglobin and leucocyte level, the dose-limiting toxicity of many agents used to treat AIDS patients is thrombocytopenia so the relative importance of continuing chemotherapy, for example in the presence of CMV retinitis, must be assessed.

Oedema commonly accompanies KS and widespread oedema of the face, boxer-short area and lower legs can be seen. Treatment of gross facial oedema with steroids, non-steroidal anti-inflammatory drugs, radiation and chemotherapy is often only minimally successful, and this oedema is often seen as a serious prognostic event.

Lymphoma

Clinical progression

The progression and clinical manifestations of the AIDS-related B cell lymphoma are unusual. The presentation is more frequently extranodal in nature. Lymphomatous involvement of the skin, gastro-intestinal tract, bone marrow, and head and neck is frequently seen (Figs 18.7 and 18.8). In 50 per cent of patients the lymphoma is the presenting sign of AIDS and is the one which indicates the least favourable progress. Survival is about 6 months with approximately half the patients dying of persistent lymphoma and others of opportunist infections.[110] The stage of disease at presentation surprisingly seems not to be associated with prognosis.[111] The disease is frequently disseminated (Stage IV) at presentation; B symptoms of fever and weight loss are usually present although it may be difficult to be sure these are caused by the lymphoma. Involvement of the head and neck is common and malignant lymphoma in the mouth,[4,74] particularly the tonsil, has been seen both as a Stage 1e isolated presentation and as part of disseminated disease. Involvement of the paranasal sinuses is also seen. In the USA, HIV NHL represent 3 per cent of all AIDS defining diagnoses.

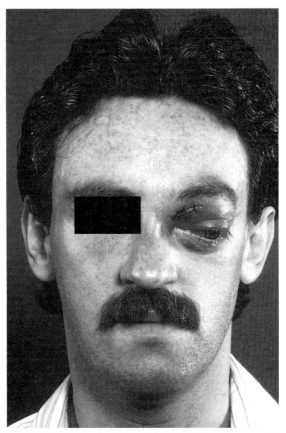

Fig. 18.8 HIV-related non-Hodgkin's lymphoma of the ethmoid.

Management

Since patients who are HIV positive manifest many pathological processes at the same time it is important to differentiate lymphoma from the other space occupying lesions or causes of lymphadenopathy from which they may be suffering. Staging procedures in HIV-related lymphomas ideally include bone marrow biopsy, chest radiograph, computed tomography scan of thorax and abdomen, gastrointestinal radiography, mouth, ear, nose and throat examination and lumbar puncture.[71] Although localised extranodal lymphoma may occur in the skin and isolated tonsillar involvement can be seen, the disease even when it first appears in the head and neck is usually part of a disseminated process and therefore localised radiotherapy, although helpful in treating bulk lesions, will only produce local remissions. When treating AIDS patients, management must always be problem-orientated even though the lymphoma is histologically aggressive. Several centres have shown that treating

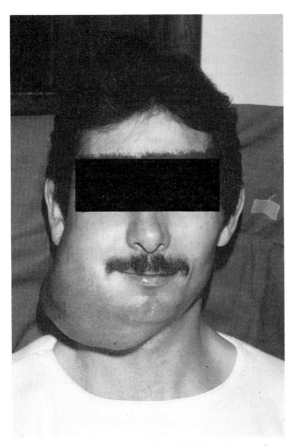

Fig. 18.7 HIV-related non-Hodgkin's lymphoma of cervical lymph nodes.

AIDS lymphoma patients with chemotherapy appropriate in the non-AIDS setting leads to an increased number of deaths from opportunist infections.[112] The three risk factors associated with a poorer prognosis in AIDS NHL are poor initial performance status, a previous AIDS defining diagnosis, and the presence of a CD4 count of less than 100. In patients with all adverse risk factors minimal treatment with steroids and vincristine or local radiotherapy is all that may be necessary. However, patients with a relatively good prognosis and only one risk factor may be treated more aggressively with CHOP (cyclophosphidamide, doxorubicin, vincristine and prednisolone) or other multi-agent chemotherapy,[112,113] but these are generally less effective than in lymphoma unassociated with HIV. Combinations of cytotoxic drugs with antiviral agents and marrow-protective colony-stimulating factors are under investigation.[114] International collaborative studies attempting to define the appropriate chemotherapy for individual risk groups and associated with the possibility of continuing other antiviral and antibacterial prophylaxis have been established.

Note added in proof: This chapter was completed in 1992.

References

1 Beral V, Jaffe H, Weiss R. Cancer surveys: cancer, HIV and AIDS. *European Journal of Cancer* 1991; **27**: 1057–8.

2 Scully C, Laskaris G, Pindborg J, Porter SR, Reichart P. Oral manifestations of HIV infection and their management. More common lesions. *Oral Surgery* 1991; **71**: 158–66.

3 Scully C, Laskaris G, Pindborg J, Porter SR, Reichart P. Oral manifestations of HIV infection and their management. Less common lesions. *Oral Surgery* 1991; **71**: 167–71.

4 Epstein JB, Scully C. Malignancies in the head and neck of patients with HIV disease. *International Journal of Oral and Maxillofacial Surgery* 1992; **2**: 219–26.

5 Rabkin CS, Biggar RJ, Horm JW. Increasing incidence of cancers associated with the human immunodeficiency virus epidemic. *International Journal of Cancer* 1991; **47**: 692–6.

6 Hiddemann W. What's new in malignant tumors in acquired immunodeficiency disorders? *Pathology, Research and Practice* 1989; **185**: 930–4.

7 Selik RM, Starcher ET, Curran JW. Opportunistic diseases reported in AIDS patients: frequencies, associations and trends. *AIDS* 1987; **1**: 175–82.

8 Rutherford GW, Schwarcz SK, Lemp GF *et al*. The epidemiology of AIDS-related Kaposi sarcoma in San Francisco. *Journal of Infectious Diseases* 1989; **159**: 567–71.

9 Beral V, Peterman TA, Berkelman RL, Jaffe HW. Kaposi's sarcoma among persons with AIDS: a sexually transmitted infection. *Lancet* 1990; **335**: 123–8.

10 Carabona J, Melbye M, Biggar RJ *et al*. Kaposi's sarcoma and non-Hodgkin's lymphoma in European AIDS cases. No excess risk of Kaposi's sarcoma in Mediterranean countries. *International Journal of Cancer* 1991; **47**: 49–53.

11 Peters BS, Beck EJ, Coleman DG *et al*. Changing disease patterns in patients with AIDS in a referral centre in the United Kingdom: the changing face of AIDS. *British Medical Journal* 1991; **302**: 203–7.

12 Haverkos HW, Friedman-Kien AE, Drotman DP, Morgan WM. The changing incidence of Kaposi's sarcoma among patients with AIDS. *Journal of the American Academy of Dermatology* 1990; **22**: 1250–3.

13 Karp JE, Broder S. Acquired immunodeficiency syndrome and non-Hodgkin's lymphomas. *Cancer Research* 1991; **51**: 4743–56.

14 Gail MH, Pluda JM, Rabkin CS *et al*. Projections of the incidence of non-Hodgkin's lymphoma related to acquired immunodeficiency syndrome. *Journal of the National Cancer Institute* 1991; **83**: 695–701.

15 Wilkes M, Fortin AH, Felix JC *et al*. Value of necropsy in acquired immunodeficiency syndrome. *Lancet* 1988; **2**: 85–8.

16 Beral V, Peterman T, Berkelman R, Jaffe H. AIDS-associated non-Hodgkin's lymphoma. *Lancet* 1991; **337**: 805–9.

17 Carbone A, Tirelli U, Vaccher E *et al*. A clinico-pathologic study of lymphoid neoplasias associated with human immunodeficiency virus infection in Italy. *Cancer* 1991; **68**: 842–52.

18 Roithmann S, Tourani JM, Andrieu JM *et al*. AIDS-associated non-Hodgkin lymphoma. *Lancet* 1991; **338**: 884–5.

19 Lenoir GM, Delecluse HJ. Lymphoma and immunocomprised host. In: Revilland JP, Wierzbicki N eds. *Immune Disorders and Opportunistic Infections*. Paris: Suresness Foundation Franco-Allemande, 1989: 173–83.

20 Myskowski PL, Straus DJ, Safai B. Lymphoma and other HIV-associated malignancies. *Journal of the American Academy of Dermatology* 1990; **22**: 1253–60.

21 Biggar RJ, Burnett W, Mikl J, Nasca P. Cancer among New York men at risk of acquired immunodeficiency syndrome. *International Journal of Cancer* 1989; **43**: 979–85.

22 Tirelli U, Carbone A, Monfardini S *et al*. Malignant tumours in patients with human immunodeficiency virus infection: a report of 580 cases. *Journal of Clinical Oncology* 1989; **7**: 1582–8.

23 Monfardini S, Vaccher E, Pizzocaro G *et al*. Unusual

malignant tumours in 49 patients with HIV infection. *AIDS* 1989; **3**: 449–52.

24 Hoover R. Effect of drugs-immunosuppression. In: Hiatt HH, Watson JD eds. *Origins of Human Cancer.* New York: Cold Spring Harbor Laboratory, 1977: 369–79.

25 Marquart KH, Oehschlaegel G, Engst R. Disseminated Kaposi's sarcoma that is not associated with the acquired immunodeficiency syndrome in bisexual men. *Archives of Pathology and Laboratory Medicine* 1986; **110**: 346–7.

26 Blayney DW, Ito JI, Jensen FC. Spontaneous remission of Kaposi's sarcoma in an HTVL-III negative homosexual man. *Cancer* 1986; **58**: 1583–4.

27 Afrasiabi R, Mitsuyasu RT, Nishanian P, Schwartz K, Fahey JL. Characterization of a distinct subgroup of high-risk persons with Kaposi's sarcoma and good prognosis who present with normal T4 cell number and T4:T8 ratio and negative HTLV-III/LAV serologic test results. *American Journal of Medicine* 1986; **81**: 969–73.

28 Archer CB, Spittle MF, Smith NP. Kaposi's sarcoma in a homosexual – 10 years on. *Clinical and Experimental Dermatology* 1989; **14**: 233–6.

29 Friedman-Kien AE, Saltzman BR, Cao Y *et al.* Kaposi's sarcoma in HIV-negative homosexual men. *Lancet* 1990; **335**: 168–9.

30 Kitchen VS, French MAH, Dawkins RL. Transmissible agent of Kaposi's sarcoma. *Lancet* 1990; **335**: 797–8.

31 Garcia Muret MP, Soriano V, Pujol RM, Hewlett I, Clotet B, de Morgas JM. AIDS and Kaposi's sarcoma pre-1979. *Lancet* 1990; **335**: 969–70.

32 Marquart KH, Engst R, Oehlschlaegel G. An 8-year history of Kaposi's sarcoma in an HIV-negative bisexual man. *AIDS* 1991; **5**: 346–7.

33 Green TL, Beckstead JH, Lozada-Nur F, Silverman S, Hansen LS. Histopathologic spectrum of oral Kaposi's sarcoma. *Oral Surgery* 1984; **58**: 306–14.

34 Kuntz AA, Gelderblom HK, Winkel T, Reichart PA. Ultrastructural findings in oral Kaposi's sarcoma (AIDS). *Journal of Oral Pathology* 1987; **16**: 372–9.

35 Zhang X, Langford A, Gelderblom H, Reichart P. Ultrastructural findings in clinically uninvolved oral mucosa of patients with HIV infection. *Journal of Oral Pathology and Medicine* 1989; **18**: 35–41.

36 Bovi PD, Curatola AM, Kern PG, Creco A, Ittmann M, Basilico C. An oncogene isolated by transfection of Kaposi's sarcoma DNA encodes a growth factor that is a member of the PSF family. *Cell* 1987; **50**: 729–37.

37 Ensoli B, Biberfeld P, Nakamura S, Salahuddin SZ, Wong-Staal F, Gallo RC. Possible role of growth factors and cytokines in the pathogenesis of Kaposi's sarcoma. IV International Conference on AIDS, 1988; Stockholm Abstract 2647.

38 Bayley AC, Lucas SB. Kaposi's sarcoma or Kaposi's disease? In: Fletcher CDM, McKee PH eds. *Patho-*

biology of Soft Tissue Tumours. London: Churchill Livingstone, 1990.

39 Nakamura S, Salahuddin SZ, Biberfeld P *et al.* Kaposi's sarcoma cells: long term culture with growth factor from retrovirus-infected CD4 + T cells. *Science* 1983; **24**: 426–30.

40 Nair BC, de Vico AL, Nakamura S, Copeland TD, Chen Y, Patel A. O'Neil T, Orozlan S, Gallo RC, Sarngadharan MG. Identification of a major growth factor for AIDS–Kaposi's sarcoma cells as oncostatin M. *Science* 1992; **255**: 1430–2.

41 Knowles DM, Chamulak G, Subar M *et al.* Clinicopathologic immunophenotypic and molecular genetic analysis of AIDS-associated lymphoid neoplasia. Clinical and biologic implications. *Pathology Annual* 1988; **23**: 33–69.

42 Giraldo G, Beth E, Haguenau F. Herpes type virus particles in tissue culture of Kaposi's sarcoma from different geographic regions. *Journal of the National Cancer Institute* 1972; **49**: 1509–26.

43 Giraldo G, Beth E, Henle W. Antibody patterns to herpes viruses in Kaposi's sarcoma with cytomegalovirus. *International Journal of Cancer* 1978; **22**: 126–31.

44 Drew WL, Miner RC, Ziegler JL *et al.* Cytomegalovirus and Kaposi's sarcoma in young homosexual men. *Lancet* 1982; **ii**: 125–7.

45 Civantos J, Penneys N, Ziegels-Weisman J. Kaposi's sarcoma: immunoperoxidase staining for cytomegalovirus. *AIDS Research* 1984; **1**: 121–5.

46 Boldogh I, Beth E, Huang E-S, Kyalwazi SK, Giraldo G. Kaposi's sarcoma. IV. Detection of CMV-DNA and CMV-RNA in tumor biopsies. *International Journal of Cancer* 1981; **28**: 469–74.

47 Newland JR, Adler-Storthz K. Cytomegalovirus in intraoral Kaposi's sarcoma. *Oral Surgery* 1989; **67**: 296–300.

48 Marquart KH, Oehlschlaegel G. Mycoplasma-like structures in a Kaposi's sarcoma not associated with AIDS. *European Journal of Clinical Microbiology* 1985; **4**: 73–4.

49 Lo SC, Shih JWK, Newton PB III *et al.* Virus-like infectious agent 9VLIA is a novel pathogenic mycoplasma: *Mycoplasma incognitus. American Journal of Tropical Medicine and Hygiene* 1989; **41**: 586–600.

50 DesJarlais DC, Stoneburner R, Thomas P. Declines in proportion of Kaposi's sarcoma among cases of AIDS in multiple risk groups in New York City. *Lancet* 1987; **ii**: 1024–5.

51 Abemayor E, Calceterra TC. Kaposi's sarcoma and community acquired immune deficiency syndrome. *Archives of Otolaryngology* 1983; **109**: 536–42.

52 Lozada F, Silverman S, Conant M. New outbreak of oral tumours, malignancies and infectious disease strikes young male homosexuals. *California Dental Association Journal* 1982; **10**: 39–42.

53 Lozada F, Silverman S, Migliorati CA, Conant MA, Volberding PA. Oral manifestations of tumours and

opportunistic infections in the acquired immuno-deficiency syndrome (AIDS) findings in 53 homo-sexual men with Kaposi's sarcoma. *Oral Surgery* 1983; **56**: 491–4.

54 Eversole LR, Leider AS, Jacobsen PC, Shaber EP. Oral Kaposi's sarcoma associated with acquired immunodeficiency syndrome among homosexual males. *Journal of the American Dental Association* 1983; **107**: 248–53.

55 Ficarra G, Berson AM, Silverman S *et al.* Kaposi's sarcoma of the oral cavity: a study of 134 patients with a review of the pathogenesis, epidemiology, clinical aspects and treatment. *Oral Surgery* 1988; **66**: 543–50.

56 Lummerman H, Freedman PD, Kerpel SM, Phelan JA. Oral Kaposi's sarcoma: a clinicopathologic study of 23 homosexual and bisexual men from the New York metropolitan area. *Oral Surgery* 1988; **65**: 711–16.

57 Keeney K, Abaza NA, Tidwel O, Quinn P. Oral Kaposi's sarcoma in acquired immune deficiency syndrome. *Journal of Oral Maxillofacial Surgery* 1987; **45**: 815–21.

58 Scully C, Epstein JB, Porter SR, Luker J. Recognition of oral lesions of HIV infection. *British Dental Journal* 1990; **169**: 295–6; 332–3; and 370–2.

59 Epstein JB, Scully C. HIV infection: clinical oral features and management in 33 homosexual males referred with Kaposi's sarcoma. *Oral Surgery* 1991; **71**: 38–41.

60 Patow CA, Steis R, Longo DL. Kaposi's sarcoma in the head and neck in the acquired immune deficiency syndrome. *Otolaryngology – Head and Neck Surgery* 1983; **92**: 255–60.

61 Finfer MD, Schinella RA, Rothstein SG, Persky MS. Cystic parotid lesions in patients at risk for acquired immunodeficiency syndrome. *Archives of Otolaryngology – Head and Neck Surgery* 1988; **11**: 1290–4.

62 Yeh CK, Fox PC, Fox CH, Travis WD, Lane HC, Baum BJ. Kaposi's sarcoma of the parotid gland in acquired immunodeficiency syndrome. *Oral Surgery* 1989; **67**: 308–12.

63 Greenspan D, Greenspan JS. Oral mucosal manifestations of AIDS. *Dermatologic Clinics* 1987; **5**: 733–7.

64 Barrett AP, Bilous AM, Buckley DJ, Kefford RF, Packham DR. Clinicopathological presentation of oral Kaposi's sarcoma in AIDS. *Australian Dental Journal* 1988; **33**: 395–9.

65 Daly CG, Allan BP. Bhagwandeen SB, Sutherland DC. Kaposi's sarcoma of the palate in a patient with AIDS: an unusual presentation. *Australian Dental Journal* 1989; **34**: 101–5.

66 Reichart PA, Schiodt M. Non-pigmented oral Kaposi's sarcoma (AIDS). Report of two cases. *International Journal of Oral and Maxillofacial Surgery* 1989; **18**: 197–9.

67 Errante D, Vaccher E, Tirelli U, Tumulo S, Monfardini S. Management of AIDS and its neoplastic complications. *European Journal of Cancer* 1991; **27**: 380–9.

68 Krigel RL, Friedman-Kien AE. Kaposi's sarcoma in AIDS: diagnosis and treatment. In: de Vita V, Hellman S, Rosenberg SA eds. *AIDS Etiology, Diagnosis, Treatment and Prevention*, 2nd edn. Philadelphia, PA: JB Lippincott, 1988: 245–61.

69 Mitsuyasu RT. Clinical variants and staging of Kaposi's sarcoma. *Seminars in Oncology* 1987; **14** (suppl. 3): 13–18.

70 Krown S, Metroka C, Wernz JC. Kaposi's sarcoma in the acquired immunodeficiency syndrome: a proposal for uniform evaluation, response and staging criteria. *Journal of Clinical Oncology* 1989; **7**: 1201–7.

71 Ioachim HL, Dorset B, Cronin W *et al.* Acquired immunodeficiency syndrome associated lymphomas: clinical, pathologic, immunologic and viral characteristics of 111 cases. *Human Pathology* 1991; **22**: 659–73.

72 Ziegler JL, Beckstead JA, Volbergind PA *et al.* Non-Hodgkin's lymphoma in 90 homosexual men. Relation to generalised lymphadenopathy and the acquired immunodeficiency syndrome. *New England Journal of Medicine* 1984; **311**: 565–70.

73 Lozada-Nur F *et al.* The diagnosis of AIDS and AIDS-related complex in the dental office: findings in 171 homosexual males. *California Dental Association Journal* 1984; **12**: 21–5.

74 Leess FR, Kessler DJ, Mickel RA. Non-Hodgkin's lymphoma of the head and neck in patients with AIDS. *Archives of Otolaryngology – Head and Neck Surgery* 1987; **113**: 1104–6.

75 Hommel DJ, Brown ML, Kinzie JJ. Response to radiotherapy of head and neck tumors in AIDS patients. *American Journal of Surgery* 1987; **154**: 443–6.

76 Brahim JS, Katz RW, Roberts MW. Non-Hodgkin's lymphoma of the hard palate mucosa and buccal gingiva associated with AIDS. *Journal of Oral and Maxillofacial Surgery* 1988; **46**: 328–30.

77 Kaugars GE, Burns JC. Non-Hodgkin's lymphoma of the oral cavity associated with AIDS. *Oral Surgery* 1989; **67**: 433–6.

78 Green TL, Eversole LR. Oral lymphomas in HIV-infected patients: associated with Epstein–Barr virus DNA. *Oral Surgery* 1989; **67**: 437–42.

79 Rubin MM, Gatta CA, Cozzi GM. Non-Hodgkin's lymphoma of the buccal gingiva as the initial manifestation of AIDS. *Journal of Oral and Maxillofacial Surgery* 1989; **47**: 1311–13.

80 Groot RH, van Merkesteyn JPR, Bras J. Oral manifestations of non-Hodgkin's lymphoma in HIV-infected patients. *International Journal of Oral and Maxillofacial Surgery* 1990; **19**: 194–6.

81 Soderholm AL, Lindquiet C, Heikinheimo K, For-

sell K, Happonen RP. Non-Hodgkin's lymphomas presenting through oral symptoms. *International Journal of Oral and Maxillofacial Surgery* 1990; **19**: 131–4.

82 Colmenero C, Gamallo G, Pintado V, Patron M, Sierra J, Valencia E. AIDS-related lymphoma of the oral cavity. *International Journal of Oral and Maxillofacial Surgery* 1991; **20**: 2–6.

83 Langford A, Dienemann D, Schuman D *et al.* Oral manifestations of AIDS-associated non-Hodgkin's lymphomas. *International Journal of Oral and Maxillofacial Surgery* 1991; **20**: 136–41.

84 Donkor P, Punnia-Moorthy A, Painter DM. A case of AIDS presenting as intra-oral malignant lymphoma. *Australian Dental Journal* 1991; **36**: 22–8.

85 Vallejo GH, Garcia MD, Lopez A, Mendieta C, Moskow BS. Unusual periodontal findings in an AIDS patient with Burkitt's lymphoma. *Journal of Periodontology* 1989; **60**: 723–7.

86 Shaha A, Thelmo W, Jaffe BM. Is parotid lymphadenopathy a new disease or part of AIDS? *American Journal of Surgery* 1988; **156**: 297–300.

87 Ioachim HL, Ryan JR, Blaugrund SM. Salivary gland lymphadenopathies and lymphomas associated with human immunodeficiency virus infection. *Archives of Pathology and Laboratory Medicine* 1988; **112**: 1224–8.

88 Poletti A, Manconi R, Volpe R, Carbone A. A study of AIDS-related lymphadenopathy in the intraparotid and perisubmaxillary gland lymph nodes. *Journal of Oral Pathology* 1988; **17**: 164–7.

89 Mittal K, Neri A, Feiner H, Schinella R, Alfonso F. Lymphomatoid granulomatosis in the acquired immunodeficiency syndrome. *Cancer* 1990; **63**: 1345–9.

90 Katzenstein ALA, Carrington CRB, Liebow AA. Lymphomatoid granulomatosis: a clinical study of 152 cases. *Cancer* 1979; **43**: 360–73.

91 Montilla P, Dronda F, Moreno S, Expeleta C, Bellas C, Buzon L. Lymphomatoid granulomatosis and the acquired immunodeficiency syndrome. *Annals of Internal Medicine* 1987; **106**: 166–7.

92 Lin-Greenberg A, Villacin A, Moussa G. Lymphomatoid granulomatosis presenting as ulcerodestructive gastrointestinal tract lesions in patients with human immunodeficiency virus infection. *Archives of Internal Medicine* 1990; **150**: 2581–3.

93 Conant MA, Volberding P, Fletcher V, Lozada FI, Silverman S. Squamous cell carcinoma in a sexual partner of a Kaposi's sarcoma patient. *Lancet* 1982; **i**: 286.

94 Roland JJ, Rothstein SG, Mittal KR, Perksy MS. Squamous carcinoma in HIV-positive patients under age 45. *Laryngoscope* 1993; **103**: 39–51.

95 Boyle P, Zheng T, Macfarlane GJ *et al.* Recent advances in etiology and epidemiology of head and neck cancer. *Current Opinion in Oncology* 1990; **2**: 539–45.

96 Scully C, Prime SS, Cox MF, Maitland NJ. Evidence for infective agents in the aetiology of oral cancer. In: Johnson NJ ed. *Risk Markers for Oral Diseases. 2 Oral Cancer. Detection of Patients and Lesions at Risk.* Cambridge: Cambridge University Press, 1991: 96–113.

97 Chachova A, Krigel R, Lafleur F *et al.* Prognostic factors and staging classification of patients with epidemic Kaposi's sarcoma. *Journal of Clinical Oncology* 1989; **7**: 774–80.

98 Hughes-Davies L, Spittle M. Cancer and HIV infection. *British Medical Journal* 1991; **302**: 673–4.

99 Hughes-Davies L, Young T, Spittle M. Radiosensitivity in AIDS patients. *Lancet* 1991; **337**: 1616.

100 Fishi MA, Uttamchandani RB, Resnick L *et al.* A phase 1 study of recombinant human interferon-alpha 2a or human lymphoblastoid interferon-alpha n 1 and concomitant zidovudine in patients with AIDS-related Kaposi's sarcoma. *Journal of Acquired Immune Deficiency Syndromes* 1991; **4**: 1–10.

101 Volberding PA, Mitsuyasu RT, Golando JP, Spiegel RJ. Treatment of Kaposi's sarcoma with interferon alpha-2b (Intron A). *Cancer* 1987; **59**: 620–5.

102 Groopman JE, Scadden DT. Interferon therapy for Kaposi's sarcoma associated with the Acquired Immunodeficiency Syndrome (AIDS). *Annals of Internal Medicine* 1989; **110**: 335–7.

103 Sulis E, Floris C, Sulis ML *et al.* Interferon administered intralesionally in skin and oral cavity lesions in heterosexual drug-addicted patients with AIDS-related Kaposi's sarcoma. *European Journal of Cancer and Clinical Oncology* 1989; **25**: 759–61.

104 Rarick MU, Gill PS, Montgomery T, Bernstein Singer M, Jones B, Levine AM. Treatment of epidemic Kaposi's sarcoma with combination chemotherapy (vincristine and bleomycin) and zidovudine. *Annals of Oncology* 1990; **1**: 147–9.

105 Laubenstein LJ, Krigel RL, Odajuk CM. Treatment of epidemic Kaposi's sarcoma with etoposide or a combination of doxorubicin and vinblastine. *Journal of Clinical Oncology* 1984; **2**: 1115–20.

106 Balker PJM, Danner SA, Lange JMA *et al.* Etoposide for epidemic Kaposi's sarcoma: a phase II study. *European Journal of Cancer and Clinical Oncology* 1988; **24**: 1047–8.

107 Gill PS, Rarick M, McCutchan JA *et al.* Systemic treatment of AIDS-related Kaposi's sarcoma: results of a randomized trial. *American Journal of Medicine* 1991; **90**: 427–34.

108 Present CA, Scolaro M, Kennedy P, Blayney DW, Wiseman C. Liposomal daunorubicin as tumour-targeted chemotherapy: initial clinical results in Kaposi's sarcoma. *Proceedings of the American Society of Clinical Oncology* 1992; **11**: 46 (abstract).

109 Epstein JB, Scully C. Intralesional vinblastine for oral Kaposi's sarcoma in HIV infection. *The Lancet* 1989; **ii**: 1100–1.

110 von Gunten CF, von Roenn JH. Clinical aspects of

human immunodeficiency virus-related lymphoma. *Oncology* 1992; **4**: 894–9.

111 Cottrill CP, Young TE, Bottomley D *et al*. *HIV associated non Hodgkin's lymphoma; the experience of the United Kingdom AIDS Oncology Group*, Third European Conference on Clinical Aspects and Treatment of HIV Infection, Paris, 1992.

112 Gill PS, Levine AM, Krailo M *et al*. AIDS-related malignant lymphoma: results of prospective treatment trials. *Journal of Clinical Oncology* 1987; **5**: 1322–8.

113 Lowenthal DA, Straus DJ, Campbell SW *et al*. AIDS-related lymphoid neoplasia. The Memorial Hospital experience. *Cancer* 1989; **61**: 2325–37.

114 Pluda JM, Yarchoam R, Smith PD *et al*. Subcutaneous recombinant granulocyte-macrophage colony-stimulating factor used as a single agent and in an alternating regimen with azidothymidine in leukopenic patients with severe human immunodeficiency virus infection. *Blood* 1990; **76**: 463–72.

19 Malignant tumours and implant rehabilitation

RM Watson and GH Forman

Intra-oral rehabilitation

Introduction

Successful treatment of malignant tumours of the head and neck by irradiation, surgical ablation and repair frequently compromises the oral and facial tissues. Consequently rehabilitation of the patient is often incomplete because of partial or total loss of teeth and jaw, plus possible resection of the palate, tongue, floor of mouth, lip and cheek.

Removable prostheses such as dentures and obturators, however carefully designed and constructed, fail to restore a completely satisfactory appearance and fully functioning dentition capable of producing efficient comfortable mastication and clearly articulated speech.[1,2] Some improvement in the outcome is produced by additional maxillofacial surgical manoeuvres. These can provide sufficient suitable tissue contours for support and stability of the prosthesis and unimpeded movement of the lips, tongue and mandible. Of particular significance is the acquired skill and determination of the patient needed to control such a dental prosthesis.[3]

The use of bone integrated implants to provide effective support and retention of otherwise unmanageable prostheses has dramatically altered the outcome for carefully selected and appropriately treated patients. Such procedures have been developed by and adapted from the work of one man, PI Branemark. He observed in experiments with animals that 'controlled violence' towards soft and hard tissues led to predictable behaviour and healing. This marked a turning point in bone surgery and endosseous implantation of biocompatible materials.[4]

Observing the microvasculature in relation to soft tissue and bony surgery, and using vital light microscopy as a tool, Branemark and co-workers noted that bone which is cut and thus subjected to mechanical and thermal trauma would predictably repair providing that the surgical assault stayed within certain parameters. Bone could be heated up to 47°C for up to 1 min, subsequently devascularise and then revascularise and repair.[5]

These studies also showed that commercially pure titanium was extremely well tolerated by human tissue. Bone and connective tissue cellular components could be in close ultramicroscopic relation to its oxide surface layer with no intervening discernible inflammatory reaction. Subsequently, other ceramics including hydroxylapatite coated implants have been found to behave similarly and in a predictable manner. These experimental observations encouraged Branemark to state that 'the direct structural and functional connection between ordered living bone and the surface of a load carrying implant could be called osseointegration.[4] Osseo-integration would be more likely to occur if the thermal and mechanical trauma of insertion of such an implant were minimised. The implant would be more likely to be accepted if, after placement, it were not subjected to loading for between 3 and 6 months depending on the quality and site of the bone.

Recent work suggests that the ankylosis between fully mineralised bone and the surface of an implant may occupy 60–80 per cent of the contact, the remainder being marrow vessels and fibrous tissue.[6] Transmission electron microscopy, with a higher resolution, indicates the presence of an amorphous layer of 100–400 nm separating bone from the implant surface.[7]

A strict protocol of surgical manoeuvres and an

armamentarium of instrumentation that preserves bone vitality is the basis of success on which this technique is now practised. Whilst the Branemark system of implants is only one of many currently available, the technique embodies the principles already mentioned and is described briefly. The procedure may be completed under local or general anaesthesia using a strict aseptic technique appropriate for dental and maxillofacial surgery.

The surgical site of implant (fixture) placement is chosen usually with an incision where repair does not coincide with the fixture top. Accordingly a labial incision allows for access to the lower ridge in the mouth.

A logical sequential enlargement of bony access hole is accompanied by copious irrigation with cool saline to restrict the rise in temperature of the bone.

A 2 mm diameter twist drill with depth markings on its shaft is inserted and kept along the vertical access of the shaft and lifted occasionally to allow bone dust to be evacuated. A pilot drill enlarges the channel to allow a 3 mm twist drill to descend to the chosen depth while copiously coated with saline.

After the entry site is prepared with a countersink the prepared bone canal is tapped with a titanium screw thread to the full depth. For suitable (less dense) bone, self-tapping fixtures are available.

Both the tapping procedure and the implant insertion are carried out very slowly (12–15 rpm). After hand cranking to ensure a firm fit the fixture is covered with a small cover screw to prevent the hexagonal end of the implant becoming covered with a regrowth of bone. Precautions to avoid contamination of the titanium surfaces during surgery with metal instruments or gloves are essential.

The principle of coverage and non-loading is designed to lessen the incidence of infection and to encourage optimal conditions for the stabilised fixture to become integrated. Integration occurs after 3–4 months in the mandible and 6 months in the maxilla. In a patient previously subjected to radiotherapy antibiotic cover is given to lessen the risk of overwhelming contamination of compromised bone (Fig. 19.1).

A study of fixed prostheses supported by implants located in the anterior aspects of completely edentulous jaws has revealed a successful survival level of around 90 per cent after 15 years.[8]

Integration in irradiated bone is less certain. A reduced success rate has been reported (with six of 35 fixtures failing) without any incidence of osteo-radionecrosis in nine subjects.[9] In another study of 54 implants in irradiated mandibles and 26 in the maxillae, only three fixtures were lost from the irradiated maxillae and none from the mandible.[10]

The effects of damage to osteoprogenitor cells and of reduced vascularity of bone and soft tissues by radiotherapy appear to be only partially reversible. To allow maximum recovery a delay of 1 year is recommended by some authorities before implant placement.[11]

Applications of the Branemark technique

Resection of the mandible

Previous treatment techniques involving the use of alloplastic materials and free bone grafts for mandibular reconstruction often gave rise to considerable problems.[12,13] Many resected mandibles were therefore left without reconstruction following irradiation. Facial deformity, abnormal muscle and joint behaviour affecting jaw movements and unfavourable intra-oral tissue contours restricting the movements of the lips, cheek and tongue were the outcome. Additionally the construction of a functional prosthesis was unlikely because of the lack of bilateral support.[14]

Recent introduction of biocompatible materials and the use of vascularised free tissue transfer grafts have improved reconstruction.[15] Better jaw function and facial contours are expected using several surgical techniques such as radial forearm and iliac crest microvascular anastamosis procedures. However, the capacity to restore the dentition subsequently is restricted. For example, when using the radial forearm flap the placement of osseointegrated implants has had to be limited to the edentulous sites within the broader contralateral unresected jaw in order to provide a stable prosthesis.[16–21]

The placement of implants within consolidated vascularised iliac crest bone is possible when a sufficient volume of cortical and cancellous tissue has been grafted. It is not uncommon for the subsequent placement of implant fixtures to have been overlooked when planning reconstruction so that the cross-sectional form of the graft has adequate height but insufficient width to accommodate the implants.

Individual case reports of preparatory placement and integration of implants in bone of the hip prior

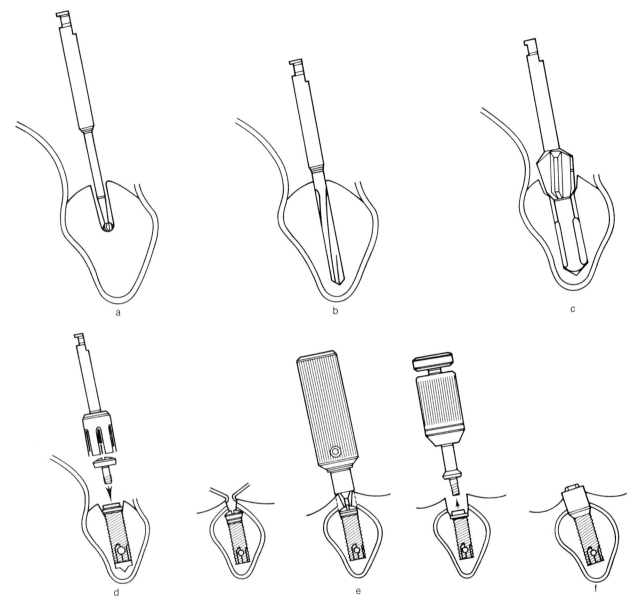

Fig. 19.1 Diagrams illustrating the surgical stages of placing a dental implant in the jaw. (a) and (b) Preparing the canal. (c) Countersink widening the canal orifice. (d) Implant fixture in position and sealed with a cover screen. (e) Removing cover screw seen at second operation. (f) Transmucosal abutment screwed to implant fixture. Reproduced by permission of Nobelpharma and Dental Update.

to grafting are also available. There have been ten studies of long term operative success and implant survival so far.[10]

Following integration of the implanted fixtures, problems may arise with the location of the transmucosal abutments owing to the rise and fall of the sulcus with movement of the tongue or to inad-

equate access because of their close relation with the cheek.[22] The thickness of intervening soft tissue must be considered. It has been recommended, therefore, that the secondary procedure of vestibuloplasty incorporating a skin graft be used to secure fixed cuffs around accessible implant abutments.

Many operative procedures involving only localised rim resection of the mandible are associated with distortion of the neutral zone where teeth would normally sit. (Fig. 19.2). This results in significant loss of prosthetic space following reconstruction techniques for the tongue, floor of mouth and cheeks or lips. When planning the location and direction of the fixtures and the extent of the prosthesis it is therefore essential to evaluate not only the volume of bone available but also the form and function of the investing tissues. Clinical assessment of the gape and access to the jaw surface must be complemented by articulated study casts in order to assess the occlusion and jaw relations in advance of implant placement.

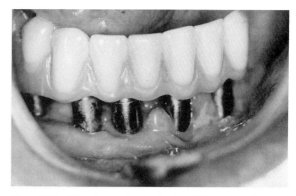

Fig. 19.3 Fixed prosthesis *in situ*. Note the effect of partial glossectomy on the relation of the tongue with the dental arch.

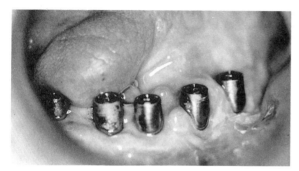

Fig. 19.2 Titanium implants located in the anterior edentulous mandible avoiding the reconstructed left cheek.

Prosthetic outcome

A fixed prosthesis comprising a cast gold alloy beam incorporating a partial dental arch is screwed to the titanium implant abutments. The design for this prosthesis is produced so that the required bulk lies within an acceptable neutral zone between the variable forces exerted by the lips, tongue and cheeks (Fig. 19.3). However, unlike a conventional denture, complete retention, support and stability is achieved from the carefully positioned fixtures in the resected jaw or its associated bone graft. Now the patient is also able to use the often restricted movements of the tongue, lips and cheeks to manipulate the masticated bolus of food and to articulate speech phonemes.

The extent of the cantilever of the dental arch both labially and distally to the supporting implant fixtures is determined by the leverage exerted on the fixtures rather than the requirements of an ideally balanced occlusion. Improvements in the facial profile from enhanced lip support are usually possible, especially when five or more fixtures are

located in the edentulous anterior mandible (Fig. 19.4). Inferiorly the beam is spaced above the oral mucosa to allow access for cleaning the tissues, especially those forming a cuff around the abutments. Ideally 5 mm clearance provides easier cleaning but the design will vary according to the display of the prosthesis during speech, the mobility of the floor of the mouth. and the space between the jaw ridges and the opposing arch (Fig. 19.5).

A number of factors may compromise the prosthetic design and should be carefully considered in the examination of the patient by the surgeon and prosthetist. First, the number of artificial teeth restoring the arch is dependent on the number of fixtures. For example, two fixtures may support three artificial teeth (bridge units) made as an independent free standing fixed prosthesis. For the edentulous jaw the beam may be cantilevered

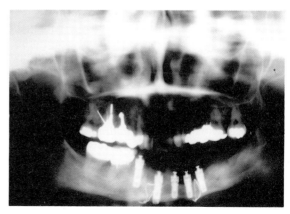

Fig. 19.4 Titanium fixtures with abutments, integrated in the graft restoring a resected mandible.

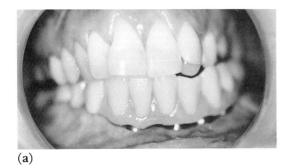

(a)

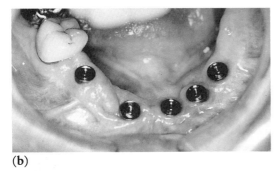

(b)

Fig. 19.5 Abutments penetrating the mucosa, upon which are secured a fixed partial prosthesis.

approximately 13 mm beyond the most distal abutment.[23,24] However, the quality of bone and the length of the fixtures are also important when deciding upon the span of the restored dental arch. Where fewer fixtures can be placed consideration may be given to a removable overdenture.

The limitation of gape on opening the mouth significantly affects not only the capacity of the surgeon to position the implant fixtures and the prosthodontist to record impressions of the teeth and jaws, etc. but also on the ability of the patient to manipulate food between the teeth. A compromise in siting the level of the occlusal plane may only be practical in an edentulous jaw. It is also essential that the relation of the intended restored arch with the location and angulation of the fixtures is fully assessed using a trial prosthesis positioned upon articulated dental casts and again positioned in the mouth. From this trial arrangement a surgical template can be prepared for operation to assist in localising the fixtures. This should then avoid the placement of the abutments too far lingually or labially in conflict with either the elevation of the floor of the mouth or movement of the lip. It may be appropriate to plan to exchange the conventional

straight screw linked abutments for angulated components. These provide the correct access for fixing screws for the prosthesis lingually to the artificial incisor teeth crowns or occlusally in posterior teeth (Fig. 19.6). Finally, it is essential to examine the jaw relations in order to consider effects of occluding a secure implant retained prosthesis with the opposing maxillary arch (Fig. 19.7). Surgical resection and reconstruction may adversely affect the morphology of the opposing edentulous jaw, or alternatively, the skeletal relation may be abnormal so that a conventional upper prosthesis may be destabilised by occlusal forces generated by the fixed prosthesis in the mandible.

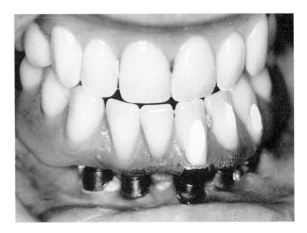

Fig. 19.6 Labial perforations of artificial teeth provide access holes for fixing screws securing a fixed prosthesis restoring a class III malocclusion. (Angulated abutments were not available at this time to position the access holes inside the lower arch.)

Resection of the maxilla

Partial loss of the maxilla affects the support and stability as well as the retention of a dental prosthesis. The situation is frequently made more severe by the total loss of teeth and by deformation of the cavity because of resection of the zygomatic arch. Bilateral support may therefore be severely impeded by a resection which includes the tuberosity or the bony orbital floor on the side from which the tumour is removed.[25]

Conventional approaches to these problems include surgical manoeuvres to eliminate sharp bony contours and to clothe load bearing surfaces with

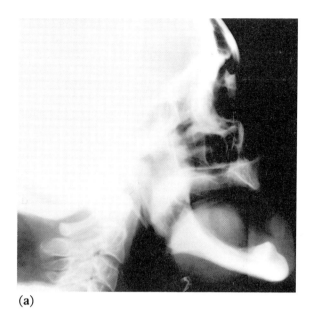

(a)

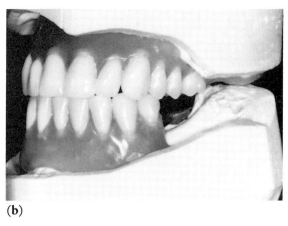

(b)

Fig. 19.7 Abnormal jaw relations may affect the design and stability of the opposing prosthesis.

adequately thick mucosal or skin lined surfaces. Prostheses made in sectional form may gain interdependent support, and by using different paths of insertion so provide mutual retention. Retention may be enhanced where the prosthesis is produced with a silicone hollow box that may be deformed and inserted into the surgical cavity (Fig. 19.8).[25]

Healthy teeth may make a substantial contribution to the support, stability and retention of the prosthesis, provided effective standards of oral hygiene and prevention are practised to preserve the dentition when saliva levels are impaired and the risk of caries is greatly increased. However, the form of individual teeth and their position frequently makes a less than ideal contribution to retention. There are therefore various approaches to gain a favourable result.[26] Some authorities recommend crowning to improve the retentive sites using also a cast metal framework for the prosthesis. Others consider simpler prostheses with wrought gold alloy clasps to be more effective producing long term retention without clasp fracture.

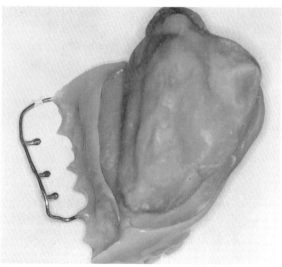

(a)

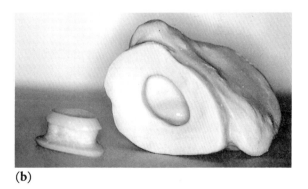

(b)

Fig. 19.8 (a) Use of undercuts by a silicone obturator placed in a well formed cavity. (b) Obturator detached from denture showing acrylic stud to be incorporated in the base of the denture. Reproduced by permission of the *British Dental Journal*.

The placement of endosseous implants achieves two aims. Those positioned in the defect site may produce total stability and retention for the obturator, reducing its size and mobility and thus maximising oral and nasal separation. To do so it is suggested that the malar buttress provides an adequate volume of bone to incorporate up to three fixtures.[27] Access to this site must be secured by a second surgical operation using a skin graft to provide an attached non-mobile tissue surface for accessible abutments. Both a cantilever bar and a bar linked to other implants in the residual maxilla have been described. Retention is then gained by a sleeve incorporated in the fitting surface of the prosthesis.[28]

Use of the residual edentulous maxillary ridge is also appropriate when fixtures can be positioned anterior to or below the unaffected antrum. Hence where there is an absence of natural teeth to provide retention and support, bilaterally placed implants can create an effective substitute.

Prosthetic outcome

Maxillary prostheses retained by implants are constructed as removable units enabling the overdenture to provide obturation to the cavity. Where linked bars are used to provide a frame for retaining the denture, as opposed to individual studs or magnets, it is important to consider the positions of the abutments and gold alloy cylinders. There must be no conflict in locating the bar onto each abutment, nor should there be obstruction to the natural contours of the palate or ridge by the bulkiness of the covering base of the prosthesis. Where convergent opposing anchorage sites are selected then each bar must be constructed in two parts.

Where movement is expected because of a combination of support from implants and mucosa/skin covered bone, undue leverage on the fixtures should be avoided by allowing for a resilient link over the abutments and bar.

Extra-oral rehabilitation

Successful rehabilitation following resection of the nose or external ear or exenteration of the orbit is extremely difficult to achieve since the outcome is only a partial recovery from a disfiguring and psychologically distressing condition. Not uncommonly, loss of an eye or partial loss of the nose is in itself a manifestation of a greater defect arising from a malignancy affecting the jaws and face. While plastic surgery is a useful adjunct in such treatments, to secure a full thickness cover over exposed bone, or to create a continuity of tissue avoiding a facial fistula with the resulting lack of oral seal, a prosthesis may be necessary to compensate for an aesthetic or functional defect. Facial prostheses can be well sculpted and accurately colour matched to the skin using modern silicone, which has adequate colour stability and tear resistance in thin section. They can be made almost indistinguishable even under close scrutiny. A lack of success in their use has been attributable to the need for mechanical retention upon the face. Spectacle frames, head bands, skin adhesives and toupee tape have been employed. By securing the prosthesis to appropriately sited titanium skull implants this major inconvenience has been overcome. Damage to the prosthesis from adhesives or sticky tape is eradicated and irritation of the skin eliminated.

Successful integration of a modified design of bone implant for insertion in the skull was reported in 1983 (Figs 19.9 and 19.10).[29] The abutment penetrated the skin in order to retain an artificial ear prosthesis and a bone conducted hearing aid. Subsequently 82 patients were treated with the insertion of 282 implant fixtures, of which two failed to integrate and eight more were removed.[30] Their use has also been recorded in the zygoma, orbit and maxillae.[31–36] A comparative study between centres in the USA and Sweden details the findings in 95 American and 146 Swedish cases.[37] From this study it would appear that a successful outcome to treatment is influenced both by site of implantation in the skull and the exposure of bone to irradiation.

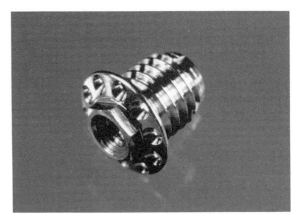

Fig. 19.9 Extra-oral Nobelpharma titanium fixture.

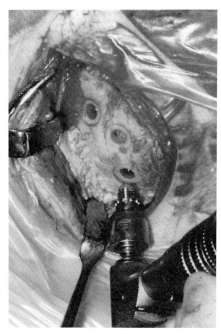

Fig. 19.10 Placement of a fixture into the canal prepared in the skull.

Of 108 implants placed in 27 patients who had been treated with between 40 and 60 Gy of irradiation, 41 failed. Most implants were placed in the orbital region. Success rates in the mastoid region appeared similar in non-irradiated and irradiated cases but numbers were small and irradiation doses tended to be lower. It has also been suggested that survival in the orbital region may be better in the lateral orbital rim and buttress than in the superior rim positions.

By comparison, the success rates for implantation in non-irradiated bone was well in excess of 90 per cent for all sites in cases treated in Sweden. In the USA, however, lower levels of success were recorded for implants placed in the nose and certain 'other' areas of the facial skeleton. Success was however more than 75.9 per cent for the total of 52 implants in this group.

Improvements in the success rates for integration in irradiated bone may be achieved by administration pre- and postoperatively of hyperbaric oxygen on the occasion of inserting the implant fixture. Fixture failure rate in the maxillae and orbit after irradiation and without hyperbaric oxygen was 58 per cent (over an 8 year period). This was reduced to 2.6 per cent with hyperbaric oxygen (in a 2 year study).[38,39]

A patient who has been subjected to irradiation should be treated in the knowledge that there is a higher possibility of implant failure in certain areas of the skull. The age range of patients treated with prostheses supported by implants is extensive and has included children as young as 5 years of age. The response of developing bone and of the body after long term contact with biocompatible materials such as titanium has yet to be fully evaluated.[12]

The behaviour of the skin surrounding the penetrating abutment appears to be dependent upon the production of a tightly bound cuff to the periosteum and an efficient cleansing of the adjacent skin. More than 90 per cent of observations made in the mastoid region over a 5 to 8 year period revealed no soft tissue inflammation.[40–42] However, removal of an implant has been recorded because of persistent staphylococcal infection.[43]

Eye prosthesis

It is important to discover at examination that sufficient depth exists within the orbital cavity. This should accommodate the implant abutments and the retentive elements secured to them, without adversely affecting either the prominence of the prosthesis or the level of the artificial iris.[34]

Location of two or three implants appropriately spaced will depend upon the continuity of the superior orbital rim. However, it should be remembered that the clip to bar retention cannot be employed if the gold alloy cylinders soldered to the retentive bar are not located simultaneously upon convergent abutments (Fig. 19.11). This is likely to occur when the lateral and medial aspects of the orbital rim, as well as the inferior surface of the supra-orbital ridge, retain the skull implant fixtures. If the implants are seen to occupy these positions when the abutments are placed at the second operation, then magnetic retention should be considered. Keepers can be secured into their individual abutment screws and rare earth neodymium boron magnets located in the acrylic resin shell.

The outline form of the facial prosthesis should be determined by an examination of the defective contours, the location of natural skin creases and an assessment of those sites least likely to be distorted by facial movement (Fig. 19.12). To achieve the optimum effect planning is best accomplished using a cast poured from a full face mask impression. The prosthesis is constructed on a localised master cast poured from an impression incorpor-

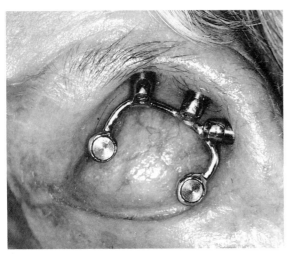

Fig. 19.11 Exenterated orbital cavity showing the retaining bar, and encapsulating magnets for additional retention.

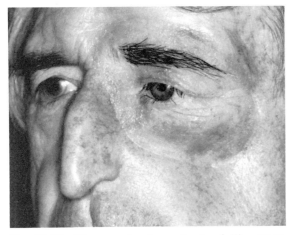

Fig. 19.12 The completed prosthesis of Fig. 19.11 securely retained in position.

ating specially modified transfer copings that position precisely replicas of the implants in this cast.

Since the patient's vision is impaired meticulous cleansing of the skin at implant perforation sites will be the responsibility of a carer.

Nasal prostheses

Replacement of the nose is frequently associated with partial or complete loss of dental palatal structures. Rehabilitation is therefore partly concerned with the construction of a firmly supported, securely

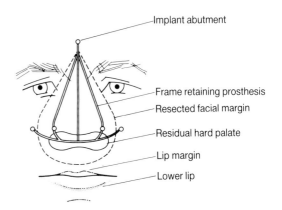

Fig. 19.13 Diagram of a frame secured to titanium abutments in the glabella and malar processes.

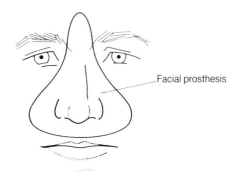

Fig. 19.14 Diagram showing the artificial nose clipped to the frame.

retained maxillary denture and partly with a facial prosthesis. Formerly the maxillary denture might gain support from residual oral and nasal tissues using an obturator. This would in turn offer a means of retention for the nasal facial prosthesis. By linking an individually built framework to the implants positioned in the anterior base of the skull below the glabella, in the root of the zygomas, or in the posterior aspects of the resected palatine bone, fully effective retention can be obtained for both prostheses (Figs 19.13 and 19.14). The framework may simultaneously provide support for the maxillary denture and the facial prosthesis. The denture is designed to provide a palatal roof and a seal for the cavity margin so dispensing with the obturator.[33]

References

1 Jani RM, Schaaf NG. An evaluation of facial prostheses. *Journal of Prosthetic Dentistry* 1978; **39**: 546–50.

2 Chen MS, Udagama A, Drane J. Evaluation of facial prostheses for head and neck cancer patients. *Journal of Prosthetic Dentistry* 1981; **46**: 544–8.

3 Watson RM, Welfare RD, Islami A. The difficulties of prosthetic management of edentulous cases with hemi-mandibulectomy following cancer treatment. *Journal of Oral Rehabilitation* 1984; **11**: 201–14.

4 Branemark PI. Osseointegration and its experimental background. *Journal of Prosthetic Dentistry* 1983; **50**: 399–410.

5 Albrektsson T, Eriksson AR *et al.* Histologic investigations on 33 retrieved Nobelpharma implants. *Clinical Materials* 1993; **12**: 1–9.

6 Eriksson RA, Albrektsson T *et al.* Heat caused by drilling cortical bone. Temperature measured *in vivo* in patients and animals. *Acta Orthopaedica Scandinavica* 1984; **55**: 629–31.

7 Sennerey L, Ericson LE *et al.* Structure of the bone titanium implant interface in retrieved clinical oral implants. *Clinical Oral Implant Research* 1991; **2**: 103–11.

8 Adell R *et al.* A fifteen year study of osseointegrated implants in the treatment of the edentulous jaw. *International Journal of Oral Surgery* 1981; **10**: 387–416.

9 Jacobsson M, Tjellstrom A, Thomsen P *et al.* Integration of titanium implants in irradiated bone. Histologic and clinical study. *Annals of Otolaryngology, Rhinology and Laryngology* 1988; **97**: 337–40.

10 Albrektsson T, Dahl E, Enbom L *et al.* Osseointegrated oral implants. A Swedish multicentre study of 8,139 consecutively inserted Nobelpharma implants. *Journal of Peridontology* 1988; **59**: 287–96.

11 Jacobsson M, Jonsson AK, Albrektsson T *et al.* Short and long term effects of irradiation on bone regeneration. *Plastic and Reconstructive Surgery* 1985; **76**: 841–50.

12 Parel SM, Drane JB, Williams EO. Mandibular replacements: A review of the literature. *Journal of the American Dental Association* 1967; **114**: 605.

13 Adamo AK, Szal RL. Timing, results and complications of mandibular reconstructive surgery. Report of 32 cases. *Journal of Oral Surgery* 1979; **37**: 755.

14 Anderson JD. Implants in the treatment of the maxillofacial patient. *International Journal of Prosthodontics* 1990; **3**: 20–9.

15 Davidson J, Boyd B, Gullane PJ *et al.* A comparison of the results following oromandibular reconstruction using a radial forearm flap with either radial bone or a reconstruction plate. *Plastic and Reconstructive Surgery* 1991; **88**: 201–8.

16 Jewer DD, Boyd JB, Manktelow RT *et al.* Orofacial and mandibular reconstruction with iliac crest free flap. A review of 60 cases and a new method of classification. *Plastic and Reconstructive Surgery* 1989; **84**: 391–403.

17 Urken ML, Buchbinder D, Weinberg H *et al.* Primary placement of osseointegrated implants in microvascular mandibular reconstruction. *Otolaryngology – Head and Neck Surgery* 1989; **101**: 56–73.

18 Sanger JR, Head MD, Matloub HS *et al.* Enhancement of rehabilitation by use of implantable adjuncts with vascularised bone grafts. *American Journal of Surgery* 1988; **156**: 243–7.

19 Parel SM, Branemark PI, Jansson T. Osseointegration in maxillofacial prosthetics – Part 1 intra-oral applications. *Journal of Prosthetic Dentistry* 1986; **55**: 490–4.

20 Keller EE, Desjardins RP, Eckert SE, Tolman D. Complete bone grafts and titanium implants in mandibular discontinuity reconstruction. *International Journal of Oral and Maxillofacial Implants* 1988; **3**: 261–7.

21 Riediger D. Restoration of masticatory function by micro-surgically revascularised iliac crest bone grafts using endosseous implants. *Plastic and Reconstructive Surgery* 1988; **81**: 861–77.

22 Listrom RD, Symington JM. Osseointegrated dental implants in conjunction with bone grafts. *International Journal of Oral and Maxillofacial Surgery* 1988; **17**: 116–18.

23 Rangert B, Jemt T, Jorneus L. Forces and moments on Branemark implants. *International Journal of Oral and Maxillofacial Implants* 1989; **4**: 241–7.

24 Rangert B, Gunne J, Sullivan DY. Mechanical aspects of a Branemark implant connected to a natural tooth – an *in vitro* study. *International Journal of Oral and Maxillofacial Implants* 1991; **6**: 177–86.

25 Watson RM, Welfare RD. Devising retention for maxillary obturator. *British Dental Journal* 1983; **155**: 117–20.

26 Desjardins RP. Obturator prosthesis design for acquired maxillary defects. *Journal of Prosthetic Dentistry* 1978; **39**: 434–5.

27 Block MS, Guerra LR, Kent JN, Finger IM. Hemimaxillectomy prostheses stabilised with hydroxylapatite coated implants. A case report. *International Journal of Oral and Maxillofacial Implants* 1987; **2**: 111–13.

28 Tollman DE, Desjardins RP, Keller EE. Surgical prosthodontic reconstruction of oro-nasal defects utilizing the tissue integrated prosthesis. *International Journal of Oral and Maxillofacial Implants* 1988; **3**: 31–40.

29 Tjellstrom A, Rosenthal U, Lindstrom J *et al.* Five year experience with skin penetrating bone anchored implants in the temporal bone. *Acta Otolaryngologica* 1983; **95**: 568–75.

30 Tjellstrom A, Jacobsson M. The bone anchored maxillofacial prosthesis. In: Albrektsson T, Zarb GA eds. *The Branemark Osseointegrated Implant*. Chicago, IL:

Quintessence Publishing Company Inc, 1989: 235–44.

31 Tollman DE, Desjardins RP. Extra-oral application of osseointegrated implants. *Journal of Oral and Maxillofacial Surgery* 1991; **49**: 33–45.

32 Parel SM, Branemark PI, Tjellstrom A, Gion G. Osseointegration in maxillofacial prosthetics, Part II. Extra-oral applications. *Journal of Prosthetic Dentistry* 1986; **55**: 600–6.

33 Parel SM, Holt GR, Branemark PI, Tjellstrom A. Osseointegration and facial prosthetics. *International Journal of Oral and Maxillofacial Implants* 1986; **1**: 27–9.

34 Seals PR, Cortes AZ, Parel SM. Fabrication of facial prostheses by applying the osseointegration concept for retention. *Journal of Prosthetic Dentistry* 1989; **61**: 712–16.

35 Jackson IT, Tolman DE, Desjardins RP, Branemark PI. A new method for fixation of external prostheses. *Plastic and Reconstructive Surgery* 1986; **77**: 668–72.

36 Nerad JA, Carter KD, Lavelle WE *et al*. The osseointegration technique for the rehabilitation of the exenterated orbit. *Archives of Ophthalmology* 1991; **109**: 1032–8.

37 Parel SM, Tjellstrom A. The United States and Swedish experience of osseointegration and facial prostheses. *International Journal of Oral and Maxillofacial Implants* 1991; **6**: 75–9.

38 Granstrom G, Johnsson K, Harssom Å, Jacobsson M, Albrektsson T, Turesson I. 'Hyperbaric oxygen can increase bone to Titanium implant interface strength after irradiation: In J Schmutz and J Wendline, *Proceedings of the 17th Annual Meeting of EUBS*, Heraclion Greece, 1991; 415–21; and in *Proceedings of the 18th Annual Meeting*, Foundation of Hyperbaric Medicine, Basel, 1992; 151–5.

39 Granstrom G, Jacobsson M. *Titanium implants in the irradiated issue. Benefit from hyperbaric oxygen.* 1st International Seminar on Implants in Craniofacial Rehabilitation and Audiology. Nobelpharma, Sweden 1991: 42–7.

40 Holgers KM, Tjellstrom A, Bjursten LM *et al*. Soft tissue reactions around percutaneous implants used for bone anchored auricular prostheses. *International Journal of Oral and Maxillofacial Implants* 1987; **2**: 35–9.

41 Holgers KM, Tjellstrom A, Bjursten LM *et al*. Soft tissue reactions around percutaneous implants. A clinical study of soft tissue conditions around skin penetrating titanium implants for bone anchored hearing aids. *American Journal of Otolaryngology* 1988; **9**: 56–9.

42 Tjellstrom A. Osseointegrated implants for replacement of absent or defective ears. *Clinics in Plastic Surgery* 1990; **17**: 355–66.

43 Jacobsson M, Tjellstrom A, Thomsen P, Albrektsson T. Soft tissue infection around a skin penetrating implant. A case report. *Scandinavian Journal of Plastic and Reconstructive Surgery* 1987; **21**: 225–8.

Index